Living with Ageing and Dying

Living with Ageing and Dying
Palliative and End of Life Care for Older People

Edited by

Merryn Gott
Professor of Health Sciences
School of Nursing
The University of Auckland, New Zealand

and

Christine Ingleton
Professor of Palliative Care Nursing
School of Nursing and Midwifery
The University of Sheffield, UK

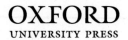
OXFORD
UNIVERSITY PRESS

OXFORD

UNIVERSITY PRESS

Great Clarendon Street, Oxford OX2 6DP

Oxford University Press is a department of the University of Oxford.
It furthers the University's objective of excellence in research, scholarship,
and education by publishing worldwide in

Oxford New York

Auckland Cape Town Dar es Salaam Hong Kong Karachi
Kuala Lumpur Madrid Melbourne Mexico City Nairobi
New Delhi Shanghai Taipei Toronto

With offices in

Argentina Austria Brazil Chile Czech Republic France Greece
Guatemala Hungary Italy Japan Poland Portugal Singapore
South Korea Switzerland Thailand Turkey Ukraine Vietnam

Oxford is a registered trade mark of Oxford University Press
in the UK and in certain other countries

Published in the United States
by Oxford University Press Inc., New York

British Library Cataloguing in Publication Data

Data available

Library of Congress Cataloging in Publication Data

Library of Congress Control Number: 2011921199

Typeset in Minion by Glyph International, Bangalore, India
Printed in Great Britain
on acid-free paper by
Ashford Colour Press Ltd, Gosport, Hampshire

ISBN 978–0–19–956993–9

10 9 8 7 6 5 4 3 2 1

Foreword

This is, literally, a vital book. There can surely be no more compelling call on our solidarity and compassion than the need for comfort, support, and fulfilment in our last few weeks and months.

The story of ageing has changed. We look out on a dramatically different landscape. Commentators range in their opinions about longevity, from those who see no limits to increasing lifespan to those who consider that life expectancy may be about to decrease as a result of the epidemic of obesity. The fact remains that with every recent decade that has passed average life expectancy at birth in the United Kingdom has risen by a staggering two years. This publication is for an international audience but the UK's story is shared across many countries, if not to the same extent.

What is also clear is that the final journey itself is lengthening: more and more of us, we trust, will enjoy a longer retirement with all the opportunities that brings. But with the longer journey is likelier to come a combination of disabilities and illness. As one older person put it, 'It's like living on thin ice,' as one's body gradually experiences, often at the same time, some of the classic ailments of older age.

Meanwhile the story of dying has changed too. So much is for the better, in terms of the quality of clinical support and the capacity of health services to sustain life for much longer. But what has not improved is our ability to talk about it. The latest survey figures from the National Council for Palliative Care show that the proportion of people who have talked about their own wishes regarding their dying has actually fallen in recent years, to a shocking 29%. This reticence seems to be especially strong in the Western World; many other societies seem to do better in their approach to airing the subject and coming to terms with the reality of death.

The vast majority of us, it seems, simply don't want to confront death at all. Such widespread denial prevents us from opening up discussion of how we should respond to dying and how we should support those on those final stages. And so it becomes more likely that people will not have the kind of death they might wish for. The 2008 English government's strategy for end of life care rightly pointed to a climate of increased awareness as the necessary precursor to better support in dying.

Death is universal, but is our approach to dying suitably universal in quality? Far too often, still, experiences of end of life care and support are uneven. These inequalities can be dramatic: witness the relative difficulty of getting pain relief in many developing countries compared to its common availability in richer ones.

There are inequalities within societies too. In the UK research has established that older people are more likely to experience co-morbidities and that extended uncertain trajectory, but less likely than younger people to have social networks and financial resources, or to die in the place of their choosing. It is almost as if there is even ageism at the very end, as well as elsewhere in the experience of older people.

So a concerted approach is needed to the particular situation of older people near the end of their lives, that will tackle their different profiles and difficulties. This book is a rich and commanding resource which leads the way there.

A year or so ago a remarkable and important exhibition of photographs appeared at the Wellcome Collection of Galleries in London. They showed twenty-four people, of different ages but all facing their imminent demise. They had each agreed to be photographed, in their normal clothes, shortly before, and immediately after their death. The shots captured an eloquent mixture of expressions: by turns grave, stoical, fragile, fearful, humorous. But perhaps the most commanding statement of all came with the words of one individual:

> *'I never noticed clouds before. Now I notice every cloud in the sky, every flower in the vase. Suddenly everything matters now.'*

We must hear and act on that passionate embrace of life. The challenge for palliative care is how we, together, can give reality to that impulse to live at full stretch, to drain life to the dregs. So we need to put end of life care in the middle of our lives. It should be the business of schools, workplaces, cinemas, pubs. This is everybody's business.

The start and end is communication. We can never raise the status of end of life care and support, and those who deliver it, unless we make it our mainstream. In the words of the Coalition led by the UK's National Council for Palliative Care, dying matters. So let's talk about it.

Paul Cann
Chief Executive, Age UK Oxfordshire

Acknowledgements

An edited work is always a team effort and we appreciate the help and cooperation of many contributors.

We are indebted to our contributors, from whom we have learned a great deal and who made the process so enjoyable through their commitment, good nature, and patience in responding to our cajoling, pestering, and pleas.

To Paul Cann who has generously contributed to the Foreword.

We also thank our colleagues at the Oxford University Press for their assistance, particularly Georgia Pinteau, Nicola Wilson, Jenny Wright, and Lauren Small.

Simon Halpenny provided valuable administrative support in preparing the final manuscript.

Finally, we would like to extend our gratitude to Kate Chadwick for keeping the project on track. Her quiet patience and usual efficiency was, as always, invaluable.

Contents

Contributors

Sarah Barnes
School of Health and Related Research,
University of Sheffield, UK

Robert H. Binstock
School of Medicine,
Case Western Reserve University, USA

Kevin Brazil
Division of Palliative Care,
Department of Family Medicine,
McMaster University, Hamilton, Canada

Habib Chaudhury
Department of Gerontology, Simon Fraser
University, Canada

Joachim Cohen
End-of-life Care Research Group,
Ghent University & Vrije Universiteit Brussel,
Brussels, Belgium

Luc Deliens
Department of Public and Occupational
Health, VU University Medical Center,
Amsterdam, The Netherlands; and
End-of-Life Care Research Group,
Ghent University & Vrije Universiteit Brussel,
Brussels, Belgium

Murna Downs
School of Health Studies,
University of Bradford, UK

Katherine Froggatt
School of Health and Medicine
Lancaster University, Lancaster, UK

Clare Gardiner
School of Nursing and Midwifery,
University of Sheffield, UK

Barbara Gomes
Cicely Saunders Institute,
Department of Palliative Care,
Policy & Rehabilitation, King's College
London, UK

Merryn Gott
School of Nursing, University of Auckland,
New Zealand

Gunn Grande
School of Nursing, Midwifery and Social
Work, University of Manchester, UK

Barbara Hanratty
Division of Public Health and Policy,
University of Liverpool, UK

Meg Hegarty
Palliative and Supportive Services,
Flinders University, Australia

Irene J. Higginson
Cicely Saunders Institute,
Department of Palliative Care,
Policy & Rehabilitation,
King's College London and Cicely Saunders
International, UK

Jo Hockley
St Christopher's Hospice, UK

Andrew M. Ibrahim
School of Medicine,
Johns Hopkins University, USA

Christine Ingleton
School of Nursing and Midwifery,
University of Sheffield, UK

John Keady
School of Nursing, Midwifery and Social
Work, University of Manchester, UK

Orla Keegan
The Irish Hospice Foundation,
Dublin, Ireland

Allan Kellehear
Department of Social & Policy Sciences,
University of Bath, UK

Jonathan Koffman
Cicely Saunders Institute,
King's College London, UK

Philip Larkin
School of Nursing, Midwifery and Health
Systems, University College Dublin,
Ireland; and
Our Lady's Hospice, Dublin, Ireland

Liz Lloyd
School for Policy Studies,
University of Bristol, UK

Jennifer Lyle
Department of Gerontology,
Simon Fraser University, Canada

Sinead McGilloway
Department of Psychology,
National University of Ireland, Maynooth,
Ireland

Koen Meeussen
End-of-Life Care Research Group,
Ghent University & Vrije Universiteit Brussel,
Brussels, Belgium

Scott A. Murray
Primary Palliative Care Research Group,
Centre for Population Health Sciences:
General Practice, University of Edinburgh, UK

Mike Nolan
Sheffield Institute for Studies on Ageing,
School of Nursing and Midwifery,
University of Sheffield, UK

Margaret O'Connor
Palliative Care Research Team,
Faculty of Medicine, Nursing & Health
Sciences, Monash University, Australia

Deborah Parker
UQ/Blue Care Research and Practice
Development Centre, University of
Queensland, Australia

Sheila Payne
International Observatory on End of Life
Care, Lancaster University, UK

Sabine Pleschberger
Department of Palliative Care and
Organisational Ethics, Faculty of
Interdisciplinary Studies, University of
Klagenfurt, Vienna, Austria

Gloria Puurveen
Department of Gerontology, Simon Fraser
University, Canada

Elisabeth Reitinger
Department of Palliative Care and
Organisational Ethics, Faculty of
Interdisciplinary Studies, Alpen-Adria
University of Klagenfurt, Vienna, Austria

Amanda Roberts
Department of Psychology,
National University of Ireland, Maynooth,
Ireland

Jackie Robinson
Palliative Care Services, Auckland District
Health Board, New Zealand

Bruce Rumbold
Palliative Care Unit, School of Public Health,
La Trobe University, Australia

Tony Ryan
School of Nursing & Midwifery,
University of Sheffield, UK

Anita Sargeant
School of Health Studies,
University of Bradford, UK

Jane Seymour
School of Nursing, Midwifery and
Physiotherapy, Faculty of Medicine and
Health Sciences, University of Nottingham,
UK

Neil Small
School of Health Studies,
University of Bradford, UK

Lieve Van den Block
End-of-Life Care Research Group,
Ghent University & Vrije Universiteit Brussel,
Brussels, Belgium; and
Department of General Practice,
Vrije Universiteit Brussel, Brussels, Belgium

John A. Vincent
Department of Sociology and Philosophy,
University of Exeter, UK

Introduction

Merryn Gott and Christine Ingleton

Older people have been termed the 'disadvantaged dying' (1). Indeed, there is mounting evidence to suggest that, whilst death is increasingly a phenomenon of old age, older people and their families often experience high levels of unmet palliative care need and may be disadvantaged in access to specialist services. Whilst improving palliative care provision for older people has been recognized as an international public health priority by the World Health Organization (2), there is little evidence that the sheer scale of this challenge has been taken on board, either by policy-makers, or by the wider practitioner and academic communities. Indeed, neither gerontology, nor palliative care, have addressed in any detail issues of death and dying specific to older people. This book is an attempt to draw these disciplines together to address this gap in current knowledge and understanding. We have invited a range of leading international experts from different disciplinary backgrounds to contribute to discussions regarding priority areas to consider in relation to ageing and end of life care. Some authors take a theoretical focus, others a very practical approach rooted in their clinical and research experience. This means that the writing styles vary and while some editorial work has been undertaken, we are keen that the chapters reflect the views and insights of our authors, rather than conform to our perspectives. The issues covered are diverse, as are the countries in which discussions are contextualised. However, several common threads have emerged.

Perhaps most prominent of these is the call by authors to consider dying within wider experiences of both living and ageing. Too often, an artificial separation is apparent, both in popular discourses of ageing and dying, and the practices and policies such thinking informs. Indeed, whilst it may seem self-evident that how we age influences how we die, there is often a lack of integration between ageing and dying at an academic level, as well as within practice and policy. Many authors draw attention to the unintended consequences of one example of this—the preoccupation by gerontology with 'successful ageing'. This model of ageing defines 'success' in terms of the ability to stave off disease, functional decline, and, by implication, death. It deflects attention, and research and service development efforts, away from older people's end of life experiences; there is no place for older people who are dying except, perhaps, as cautionary tales of 'failure'.

Whilst this context provides reason enough for the lack of engagement with death and dying by gerontology, the failure of palliative care to acknowledge that, increasingly, people in need of such care will be older and have specific age-(and cohort) related needs is perhaps more puzzling. Historical context provides insight here. As Cicely Saunders reminds us, the original intention was for palliative care to meet those needs of younger and middle-aged cancer patients that she identified were being neglected by contemporary health care (3). It is perhaps a testament to her success, as well as the success (and, arguably, ambition) of the palliative care movement as a whole, that palliative care is now seen as a 'right' for anyone with a life-threatening diagnosis. Many of those who have been brought under the palliative care umbrella by this expansion in remit are older people, dying from the range of chronic conditions referred to as 'non-cancer diagnoses' in the palliative care literature. This terminology is instructive as it highlights that most models of palliative care have been developed with cancer as a reference point. Many of the challenges that affect older people at the end of life arise from their failure to fit neatly into this way of framing, and organizing, dying. They often die too unpredictably, and with too many of the 'messy' trappings of older age. Whilst a mantra of integrated thinking is reiterated in many of the chapters, plenty of examples of 'disintegrated' practice and policy are provided. It is particularly apparent that the desire to distinguish needs related to ageing from those related to dying informs much contemporary health practice. However, for older people and their families, such distinctions are irrelevant and potentially unhelpful. Prioritizing integrated thinking at all levels, from the theoretical to the applied, can be identified as a prerequisite to understanding and mounting appropriate responses to the totality of older people's needs.

Such responses have typically been considered within the framework of health and social care services. Many of our authors highlight the constraints of adopting such a narrow perspective and urge us to think beyond statutory service provision when considering strategies to improve older people's end of life experience. From a public health perspective, the 'solutions' seem very different, and arguably, more achievable. They involve looking to communities for answers. For older people, this way of thinking also offers an alternative to the 'demographic time-bomb' mentality, within which ageing is conceptualized as a problem, if not a potential catastrophe. Indeed, looking to existing and potential community resources entails the recognition that older people make up an increasing proportion of our social capital; the contribution they can, and do, make to the provision of palliative and end of life care within these communities needs acknowledging and supporting. We are urged to think 'bottom-up' rather than 'top-down' and to inform and engage the 'general public' in debates about appropriate care for the dying. It is an issue, after all, in which we all have a vested interest.

One debate that several authors prioritize relates to the role of technology in end of life care. The danger of framing dying as a 'medical' problem for which, given sufficient time, there will be a 'medical' solution is highlighted. Society's ever increasing preoccupation with developing technologies to eradicate the effects of ageing, coupled with the omnipresent hope of mastery over death itself, encourages us all to view ageing, and by extension dying, as a phenomenon we have the potential to control. The clear message that emerges from the book is the need to critically examine this way of thinking of science, and particularly medicine, as promoting straightforward, inevitable progress. When viewed in a historical context, arguably we are not providing better end of life care now than in previous periods.

In considering the nature and extent of our social resources, the work of family carers must be acknowledged. 'Family'—defined in its broadest sense—will provide the bulk of care to most dying people, yet are often inadequately supported in this critical role. As our authors remind us, many family carers are older themselves and the line between 'carer' and 'cared for' can be difficult to draw. Several chapters in the book are devoted to considering issues for the 'family workforce' and the very real need to acknowledge, and support, their role in palliative care provision. Strengthening relationships between family carers and so-called 'professionals' is highlighted as a priority.

Another central argument running through the book is that we know too little about how older people, in all their diversity, understand and define 'good dying'. Evidence is presented that the little we know is not always in line with professional understandings and definitions. For example, the much prized 'home death' may not be desirable, or achievable, for many older people; for example, for those older people who live in poor material circumstances, dying at home may be an unpleasant prospect. That is not to say that they wouldn't prioritize a 'homely' environment, and several chapters consider how this can be achieved within an institutional setting. Nevertheless, we need more evidence from older people themselves to ensure the policies developed are responsive to, and inclusive of, their specific needs, whilst all the time recognizing that commonality by age can never be assumed. Indeed, perhaps the only homogenizing effect of ageing is the experience of ageism in some form or other. Again, this is an issue our authors identify as having been ignored in most palliative and end of life care research.

Within a book of this kind, it is always the case that there will be omissions and we would like to draw attention to the most notable here—our decision to adopt a 'developed country' perspective. Ageing and dying pose different and perhaps even more significant challenges for 'developing' countries. We hope that someone else will explore these challenges and, in so doing, convey the message that those countries we term 'developed' have much to learn from approaches to dying in those countries we term 'developing'. A further and related omission is that, whilst one chapter considers the experiences of minority ethnic older people at the end of life, there is no similar discussion for indigenous older people whose experiences are structured not only through membership of a minority cultural group, but very profoundly by the experiences and legacy of colonialism. Again, we would like to highlight this as a priority area for future discussion.

Having identified countries and peoples that are not included, we would like to caution against assuming too much commonality amongst those that are. 'Developed' countries face similar challenges in improving end of life care for older people and their families, but each population is unique and requires a unique response. Lessons can be shared and learnt, but, in a postmodern age, global solutions cannot be trusted.

We want to end this section by reiterating that this book is aimed at anyone with an interest in issues of ageing and palliative and end of life care. We hope it will provide a springboard to further reflection and debate. It is often said that the mark of a truly civilized society is how it treats its most vulnerable members. For this reason alone, it is to be hoped that these discussions convincingly promote the importance of devoting increased attention to palliative and end of life care for older people, particularly in the minds of those with the potential to effect change.

References

1. Seymour J, Witherspoon R, Gott M, Ross H, Payne S (2005). *End of Life Care: Promoting Comfort, Choice and Well-being for Older People*. Bristol: Policy Press.
2. Macnicol, J (2006). *Age Discrimination: An Historical and Contemporary Analysis*. Cambridge: Cambridge University Press.
3. World Health Organization (2004). *Better Palliative Care for Older People*. Copenhagen: WHO. Available at: www.eapcnet.org/download/forProjects/Elderly/BetterPC.Older%20People.pdf. (Accessed 3 August 2010.)
4. Clark D (2005). *Cicely Saunders: Founder of the Hospice Movement. Selected Letters 1959–1999*. Oxford: Oxford University Press.

Section 1

What is different about dying old?
Introduction

Merryn Gott and Christine Ingleton

The fundamental premise underpinning this book is that, globally, we need to pay increased attention to the specific palliative and end of life care needs of older people and their families. This is for two key reasons. Firstly, there are going to be more older people dying than ever before, and secondly, older people have unique needs for, views about, and experiences of care and support at the end of life. The chapters in this section address these two issues from a number of different perspectives.

In Chapter 1, Barbara Gomes and colleagues map the changing demography of ageing and dying internationally. The numbers speak for themselves: by 2050 there will be two billion people globally aged 60 and over, including 395 million aged over 80 years. Ninety-one million people will die in 2050, compared to 56 million in 2009. By drawing on the best available epidemiological evidence, the authors identify that causes of death, and trajectories of dying, are changing. The challenges for mounting an appropriate societal response are seen to be significant, particularly given that the evidence base to underpin policy and practice is 'embryonic'.

In Chapter 2, Allan Kellehear traces the historical development of end of life care provision for older people. He concludes that, whilst social arrangements to support end of life care for older people have improved over time, this has 'frequently been at the cost of emphasizing quality of life at the expense of recognizing the inevitability of death and dying'. Indeed, what this historical context enables us to recognize is that the failure within contemporary societies to acknowledge the link between ageing and dying negatively impacts upon older people's end of life experiences. Ultimately, Kellehear argues that, when 'seen from the perspective of the history and ethnography of dying… modern care of older people at the end of life falls dramatically short'.

In Chapter 3, John Vincent continues this theme through a critical discussion of 'anti-ageing medicine' which, he argues, is fundamentally changing the relationship between ageing and dying. In common with previous authors, he problematizes the idea that 'progressive' science will necessarily bring benefits to older people. Rather he identifies that the modern quest for immortality prioritizes biomedicine as a means to manage death and brings with it an understanding of both ageing and dying as failure: 'In such a world we struggle to find rituals and to demarcate the sacred or anything meaningful in death.'

Chapter 4 further considers a future where health technology will increasingly shape older people's end of life experiences. Jane Seymour and Merryn Gott consider the complex implications of such technologies for older people, arguing that more debate is needed about their use. In the absence of such debate, and in particular knowing more about how older people define a 'good death', they argue that healthcare practice will increasingly be 'driven by what can be done rather than what, as a humane society, we feel should be done'.

The contemporary tendency to frame ageing negatively is also the focus of Chapter 5, in which Merryn Gott and colleagues consider the potential role of ageism in structuring older people's end of life experiences. Access to specialist palliative care services amongst older people in the UK is explored as one example of the ways in which ageism operates to negatively influence older people's end of life experiences. The discussion makes it clear that, in competition for scarce resources, older people will usually miss out.

The final chapter in this section brings us back to the views and preferences of older people, focusing upon the extent to which they are reflected in current end of life care policy. Liz Lloyd argues that too little is known about what older people prioritize at the end of life and identifies discontinuities between what is known and current policy directives. In common with the previous chapters in this section, she criticizes the artificial divide between ageing and dying, in this instance at a policy level. She concludes that in the absence of joined-up policy-making 'it is difficult to see how older people will obtain the kind of care at the end of life that they wish to have'.

Chapter 1

International trends in circumstances of death and dying amongst older people

Barbara Gomes, Joachim Cohen, Luc Deliens, and Irene J. Higginson

Introduction

A large majority of countries in the world face the same sociodemographic challenge. Their populations are irreversibly ageing, and they should expect rising numbers of deaths and of people dying in older age (1, 2). This phenomenon is happening fast, in some countries earlier and faster than in others, and requires a response.

This chapter explains why end of life care for older people is a pressing global priority. It describes situations in which cross-national comparisons and an international approach have helped to advance knowledge and identify ways forward.

An ageing world

The magnitude and speed of world population ageing is impressive and unprecedented—and will intensify in the future. The issue sparked the United Nations (UN) second World Assembly on Ageing in 2002 (the first was in 1982), and led governments, intergovernmental institutions, and non-governmental organizations to agree a long-term strategy—the Madrid International Plan for Action on Ageing (3). Seminal analyses of international and national trends, indicators of the ageing process, its determinants and consequences, and projections have been produced by the US Census Bureau (2) and the UN Population Division (1). Their estimates differ but both concur that the proportion of people aged 60 and over is steadily increasing in both developed and developing countries (Figure 1.1). According to the latest set of projections (1), the number of people worldwide aged 60 and older is estimated at 737 million as of 2009; by 2050, that number will be two billion. Thus, in 40 years, the proportion of older people will double from 11% to 22% of the total world population. Japan, Italy, Germany, and Sweden are currently the four countries with the oldest populations in the world (1). The greatest rise is expected to be in people aged 80 years and over—their global number was 102 million as of 2009; by 2050, this will be 395 million (1).

The ageing of the population is the result of rapid improvements in survival and a decline in mortality rates on the one hand and past fertility trends on the other. The world population has been growing since the end of the Black Death plague around 1400 through natural increase (more births than deaths) and more recently due to decreasing numbers of deaths. Why has the number of deaths decreased? Initially, this decrease was attributed to rising standards of living, advances in public health knowledge adopted globally by government programmes of mortality control and falling deaths from infectious diseases (especially in childhood) (4). More recent declines have been linked to reductions of deaths caused by cardiovascular disease, in particular ischaemic heart disease (5).

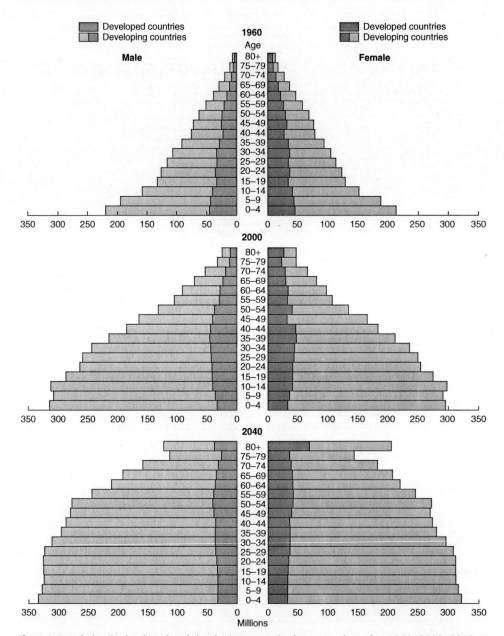

Fig. 1.1 Population in developed and developing countries by age and gender: 1960, 2000, 2040. Reproduced from US Census Bureau 2009 (2), with permission.

In terms of fertility, there are two phenomena that contributed to the ageing of populations. Firstly, many countries experienced baby-booms following the Second World War. These generations are now reaching older age and contribute greatly to raising the numbers and proportions of older people in the population. Secondly, the fertility decline which characterized the second half of the 20th century and the new millennium has decreased the numbers and proportions of people in younger generations. Industrialization, urbanization, and improved survival incited a

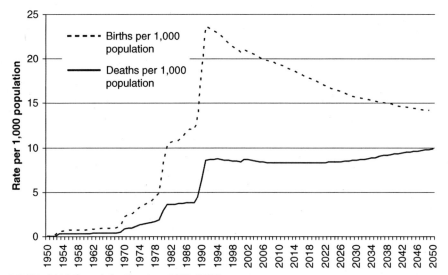

Fig. 1.2 World birth and death rates: 1950–2050.
Source: US Census Bureau 2009 (10).

desire for smaller families and a growing use of family planning and contraception (6, 7). Where smaller younger generations were supplemented by migration, these migrants tend to adopt the fertility patterns of the host population.

In the future, global population ageing is expected to accelerate and in contrast with the past, mortality will assume greater weight than fertility trends in driving population change (2). The world mortality rate is expected to plateau until 2020, and then slowly start to increase (Figure 1.2). However, large cohorts of baby-boomers are entering older age. Given the 'domino effect' of demographic events, the plateau in the mortality rate will not result in a plateau in the number of deaths. The opposite is expected: a dramatic and steady rise in the number of deaths until 2050 (Figure 1.3). According to global predictions, 91 million people will die in 2050 (56 million died in 2009). Compared to this, 122 million babies will be born in 2050 (131 million were born in 2009).

The dynamic process between mortality and fertility described which has contributed throughout time to population ageing is summarized by the demographic transition model (8). This model explains how mortality and fertility decline from higher to lower levels in four stages, and possibly five (Figure 1.4) (9). The majority of developing countries are currently at stage 2 or stage 3, i.e. stages of declining fertility and mortality rates. Most developed countries are beyond stage 3 and there is growing evidence that several countries within Europe have already entered a fifth stage, characterized by higher death rates than birth rates (8). This is the case in Germany, where death rates have been higher than birth rates since 1997 and continue to increase. In this country, the trend in numbers of deaths has been similar to the trend in death rates—deaths first outnumbered births in 1972 and after a period of low fluctuation (1972–1997), the gap has been continuously increasing and is expected to increase further in the future (Figure 1.5) (10). The same transition is expected in the UK in the future. The death rate has been at a plateau since 2001; it is expected to start rising in 2020 and to be higher than the birth rate by 2025. Similar to the world trend (Figure 1.3), the plateau in death rates will not result in a plateau in numbers. This is mainly because large cohorts of baby-boom generations will start to reach the end of their life, raising the numbers of deaths. A sharp and steady rise in the numbers of deaths is expected to take off in the UK in 2012–16 (Figure 1.6) (11, 12).

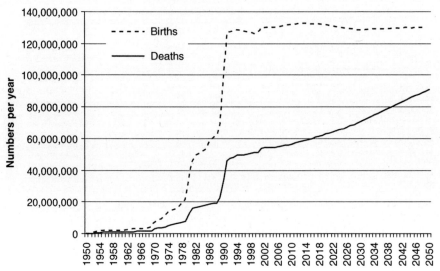

Fig. 1.3 World birth and death numbers: 1950–2050.
Source: US Census Bureau 2009 (10).

The time lag in population ageing and rising numbers of deaths between countries, which for example is about 10 years between Germany and the UK, is important. Countries where the population ageing process is at its peak, e.g. Germany and Italy, have already had to accommodate more older citizens. Others (e.g. UK, the Netherlands, and Norway) still have a few years to learn from these and others countries, to test approaches, and to plan carefully.

Growing need for end of life care

The process of population ageing, its determinants, and consequences have a major impact on the end of life care needs of populations. More people are living longer—in developed countries, after

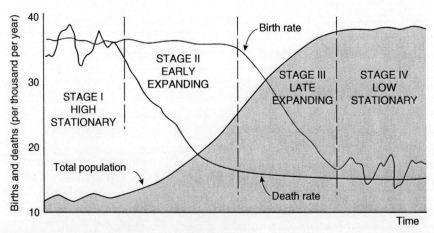

Fig. 1.4 The demographic transition model and its stages.
Reproduced from Haggett, 2001 (9), with permission.

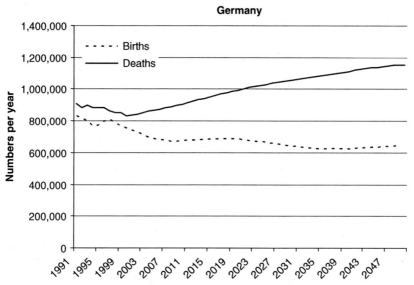

Fig. 1.5 Actual and projected births and death, Germany: 1991–2050.
Source: US Census Bureau 2009 (10).

reaching the age of 60, men now live on average another 20 years and women another 24 years (2). However, these added years of life are not necessarily spent in full health. A recent study commissioned by the European Union (EU) Public Health Programme found that in Europe, an average 50-year-old man could expect to live until his 67th year free of activity limitation, and a woman to her 68th year (13). This means 23–29 years of some illnesses and/or disability before death can be expected. This may vary by socioeconomic status. Studies from the USA, Canada, and European

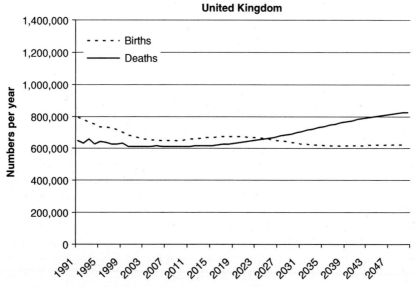

Fig. 1.6 Actual and projected births and death, UK: 1991–2050.
Source: US Census Bureau 2009 (10).

countries have shown that people with lower education, income, and occupational grade tend to experience more disability and to die earlier (2). As rightly pointed out by the authors of the EU Public Health Programme: 'An ageing population in poor health has important implications for future medical and care requirements and pension provision, whereas an ageing population in good health has mainly long-term consequences for pension provision' (13).

Chronic diseases such as heart disease, stroke, cancer, chronic respiratory diseases, and dementia are leading causes of mortality across the world, representing 60% of all deaths and 43% of the global burden of disease (14). By 2020 their contribution is expected to rise to 73% of all deaths and 60% of the global burden of disease. Worldwide, most of the deaths from chronic and degenerative conditions occur in older age (2). These conditions can cause pain and other symptoms, reduced quality of life, and loss of function over many months and sometimes years. For these reasons, although the number of deaths worldwide has been relatively stable, deaths due to chronic disease have increased, resulting in growing numbers of people, particularly of older people, in need of some sort of end of life care. A future in which deaths, chronic illness, and ageing are all increasing will bring even greater needs.

Worryingly, whilst there are more and more people in need of end of life care, there are fewer family and friends around to help them. Families have become smaller and more dispersed, affected by migration, divorce, and other pressures, including work. Increases in the proportion of women working outside the home, for example, limit their ability to provide support and care (15). Fertility rates are currently below replacement levels in practically all industrialized countries, although the latest projections in the UK, for example, predict increasing birth rates again (1, 12). Older dependency ratios are higher than ever before—in Japan, Italy, and Germany, for example, there are fewer than three working-age people (aged 20–64) to support one older person (1). An increasing number of older widowed people choose to live single and independently. Nearly half of older women live alone in European countries such as Germany and Denmark (2). Health and social systems/services are therefore increasingly faced with the needs of those with no family to help take care of them. At the same time, services are also faced with the need to support existing family caregivers, who are themselves ageing. It is increasingly common for middle-aged people to look after their relatives aged 80 years and over.

It is of no surprise that the financial implications of population ageing are being scrutinized, particularly at a time of global economic and financial crisis (1, 2). Health and social care and pension schemes are overstretched and there are concerns with future provision (16). However, it is not yet clear whether population ageing increases health care costs or not (17, 18). As explained in the US Census Bureau report (2), health expenditure by and for older age groups tends to be proportionally higher than their population share, but appears to level off or decline at ages above 80. As more people survive to an increasingly older age, in theory, most age-specific costs may decline. Adding to this, the relationship of country health expenditures and population ageing has been found to be weak, and studies from the USA, the Netherlands, England, and Switzerland suggest there may be cost drivers which are more important than population ageing, such as per capita incomes, health insurance coverage, new medical technology, workforce demographics, and time to death (19, 20). While cost of illness studies and economic evaluations develop to clarify the issue, it is important to note that a large part of health costs for older people is incurred in the year or years just prior to death (20, 21).

There is now worldwide recognition at a policy level of the growing need for end of life care in the context of population ageing. The International Plan for Action on Ageing published by the UN recommends support for the provision of palliative care and its integration into comprehensive health care, for the development of standards for training in palliative care, and for multidisciplinary approaches for all service providers (3). Between 2004 and 2010, the World Health

Organization (WHO) has published two guidance documents on palliative care for older people, most recently with examples of best practice from around the world (22, 23). PRISMA, a project commissioned by the European Commission (2008–2011), is setting up the agenda for future end of life care research in the context of ageing populations, with a component of work dedicated to coordinating best practice and research with older people in nursing homes, where growing numbers in this group die (24).

Where people die across nations

People aged 60 and over account for the overwhelming majority of deaths in developed countries (81%) (25). Where are these people dying? Getting an accurate answer to this question is important because of international recommendations by the WHO for end of life care to be responsive to patient choice for place of care and place of death (26). The information is also instrumental in planning where to allocate resources and develop services to best meet the future end of life care needs of populations.

There is strong international evidence from countries such as the UK, Canada, Italy, and the USA that the majority of people would prefer to die at home (27–30); yet most die in hospitals (23). A European study using death certificate data from six countries on deaths in 2003 revealed that although hospital was the most common place of death, there was considerable cross-national variation (31). Of all deaths, 62.8% in Wales, 62.5% in Sweden, 58.5% in Scotland, 51.6% in Flanders (Belgium), and only 33.9% in the Netherlands, occurred in hospital. Country differences were found to be particularly large for cancer patients and the very old (aged 80 and over). In the Netherlands 30.8% of cancer patients died in hospital as compared to 85.1% in Sweden (31); the proportion of cancer patients who died at home ranged from 12.8% in Norway to 45.4% in the Netherlands (Figure 1.7) (32). Compared to the very old in the Netherlands, those in Sweden were about five times more likely, in England 3.5 times more likely, and in Flanders 1.3 times more likely to die in a hospital, taking into account differences for sex, age at death, cause of death, hospital bed availability, and care-home bed availability (31).

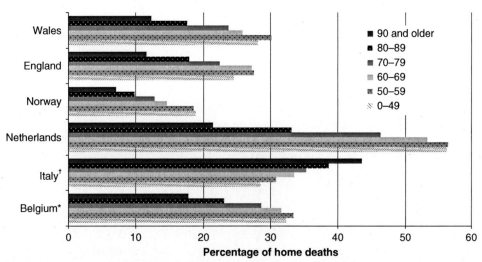

Fig. 1.7 Percentage of home deaths in cancer by age-group in six European countries (2003).
†in Italy the data relates to 2002 and comprises the regions of Tuscany, Emilia Romagna, and the city of Milan; * in Belgium the data comprises Flanders and Brussels.
Source: Cohen et al., 2010 (32).

These striking cross-national differences lead to speculation about their underlying causes. Studies are able to investigate a limited number of possible explanations. The variation between countries is only slightly related to differences in cause of death, sex, and age (31). Availability of hospital beds also appears to play a minor role in explaining European country differences. Availability of alternatives to hospital for older people (i.e. care home beds) seems to explain to a considerable extent why more people die in hospitals in some countries than in others. However, a large part of the cross-national variation in place of death remains unexplained.

A plausible additional explanation—suggested by the fact that cross-national differences are particularly large for older people and for cancer patients—is that countries have different end of life care policies and organizational arrangements, and different hospital admission practices for patients at the end of life; for example, there are country differences with regard to transferring older people from care homes to hospital immediately before their death. The specific nature of Dutch nursing homes as long-term care institutions, with explicit non-transfer policies (aimed at keeping nursing home residents in a familiar environment), is a possible explanation of the considerably lower proportion of hospital deaths in the Netherlands and why 33.5% of all deaths occur in care homes (compared to only 14.1% in Wales, 18.1% in England, and 18.1% in Scotland) (31). There may also be variation between countries regarding what is classified as hospital and nursing home deaths, and this has not been investigated in detail yet.

Additionally, societal expectations and cultural values are likely to contribute to cross-national differences in patterns of place of death. Societies differ in their expectations of how to care for frail older people, for instance. The chances of dying at home for Italian cancer patients increases with age, whilst those of Dutch cancer patients starkly decreases in favour of dying in a care home (32, 33). This can be explained by the fact that Italy has fewer residential homes for older people than the Netherlands and has not developed nursing homes; it also has strong societal expectations of taking care of older and sick people in a home environment (e.g. children taking care of their parents). Another culturally-shaped explanation is the extent of open communication between patient and physician, and the patient–general practitioner relationship that exists within a country. In the UK, the odds of dying in hospital increase with age up to the age of 90, and then the odds of dying in care homes increase (34).

The reality in developing countries is very different. Firstly, people aged 60 and over account for little over half of all deaths. Secondly, given the lack of resources and the distance to hospitals, patients and families may end up staying at home, even if the available care is poor. The provision of end of life care in the community is, for different reasons, equally if not more important in these regions.

In summary, there is some indication that the international variation in place of death has underlying organizational, policy, and cultural differences. Through cross-national comparison and exploration of reasons for such differences, countries can learn from each other and develop appropriate policies and services to enable more people to die in their place of choice, which is generally out of hospital.

The future holds different challenges for different countries though, depending on their past trends in place of death and their projected population ageing stages, magnitude, and speed. Predictions for place of death were made only recently and for the first time in the UK, considering future scenarios in an ageing population (11). In this country, the trend up until 2003 was for decreasing numbers and proportions of deaths at home, especially among older people. A sustained reversal of the trend will be an enormous task considering the rise in total numbers of deaths from 2012 onwards (Figure 1.6). If past trends towards reducing home deaths continue, only one in 10 will die at home in 2030 and there will need to be a large expansion (by over one-fifth) of inpatient facilities. Conversely, if recent trends in numbers of institutional deaths continue, home deaths will need to double and be supported. The health implications of this last scenario should be considered with great care. Although the number of home deaths continues to fall, the last 5 years (2004–2008) have shown a slow but steady increase in home death proportions (11, 35). The English Government's End of Life Care Programme (2004–2006) and National Strategy (2008–2011) may be responsible for this emerging trend, although there may be other reasons related to other factors associated with death at home (36). It is important to ascertain whether the new trend sustains over time and if people who die at home die well and under good care.

Predictions for place of death have been also made for Germany, using similar methodologies to the UK (37). Almost half of all deaths in Germany take place in hospital—the proportion of hospital deaths has been relatively stable since 1995 at around 47%, but slowly decreasing among older people. Considering this past trend and Germany's rising numbers of deaths (Figure 1.5), if hospital death proportions continue as they are, hospital deaths will reach 507,000 in 2050 (as opposed to 397,000 in 2007). In this scenario, there will need to be a major rise in bed availability and provision of end of life care in inpatient settings.

Many countries are committed to increasing choice of place of care and place of death as there is evidence that preferences are not currently translating into reality on this important matter. A hospitalization trend has been clear across nations in the 20th century (38); this still exerts influence as hospital death remains most common. However, trends are now behaving differently between countries, possibly due to organizational, policy, and cultural changes. Whatever the scenario, country or trend, it is still unlikely that death at home will become a reality for the majority of people in the near future. There will still be a large gap between preferences and reality, unless concerted and solid actions are taken to invert the situation.

Age differences in where people die are common and seem to be increasing within countries, but there is no consistent cross-national direction. In some countries, older people are more likely to die at home than their younger counterparts; in others, it is the other way around. It is important to find out how and why older people are dying differently as they increasingly need end of life care.

What is different about dying old?

There are several important differences for older people in end of life care. Not only do more people die in older age groups, but the cause of death is often different to younger people. Compared to younger people, older people more often die from cardiovascular diseases, stroke, some cancers (such as prostate cancer), and following some neurological conditions, such as Parkinson's disease and dementias (Figure 1.8) (23). These conditions often have a very different trajectory of illness than the cancers which traditionally affected younger people. Among older people there is a much more varied trajectory, with a likelihood of improvements and variations, rather than the steady decline found in cancer.

Older people very clearly have special needs because their problems are different, and often more complex, than those of younger people:

- Older people are more commonly affected by multiple medical problems of varying severity
- The cumulative effect of these may be much greater than any individual disease, and typically lead to greater impairment and needs for care
- Older people are at greater risk of adverse drug reactions and of iatrogenic illness
- Minor problems may have a greater cumulative psychological impact in older people
- Problems of acute illness may be superimposed on physical or mental impairment, economic hardship, and social isolation (22, 39).

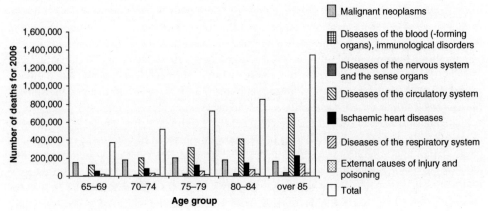

Fig. 1.8 Causes of death by age in 27 European Community countries (absolute numbers) in 2006. Source: Hall et al., 2011 (23).

The complexity of the problems that older people have to suffer is revealed by epidemiological studies in which relatives or key informants are asked about the last year of the patient's life (Figure 1.9)(22, 39, 40). These show, in particular, that mental confusion, problems with bladder and bowel control, sight and hearing difficulties, and dizziness all greatly increase with age.

Challenges for the future: dementia and nursing homes

Dementia is developing into a major public health issue, with 6.4% of Europeans aged 65 and older and 28.5% of those aged 90 and older currently suffering from it (41). It is expected that, through the ageing of the European population, the number of dementia patients will increase

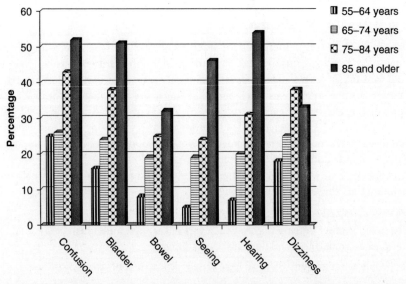

Fig. 1.9 Age at death and percentage of patients where problems were reported for the year before death.
Source: Seale and Cartwright, 1994 (40); Davies and Higginson, 2004 (22, 39).

from about 7 million in 2000 to an estimated 16 million in 2050 (42). Dementia is a complex debilitating disease, and although the trajectory towards death is not as well understood as in cancer, it appears that people live with it over longer periods of time and that the functional decline takes place at a more gradual and slower pace. This trajectory has been described as a period of 'prolonged dwindling' (43). End of life care needs may therefore be present well before a terminal stage, requiring integration of end of life care into a chronic disease management plan (23). The cognitive and functional decline ensuing from the disease, usually going hand-in-hand with gradually-increasing behavioural disturbances, make caring for dementia patients towards the end of life at home, or sometimes even in a nursing home, very challenging. As the illness advances more than 95% of patients need 24-hour care (44).

Though the care needs of patients with dementia are considerable, they often receive poor care towards the end of life, with suboptimal pain control and little access to specialist palliative care services. Although there is very little evidence of the effectiveness of palliative care services for this group of people (45), examples of best practice have been identified by the WHO (23). These include guidelines produced in a long-term unit in a UK psychiatric hospital on managing pain, dyspnoea, constipation, vomiting, agitation, the use of syringe drivers and oral care, a guide for family caregivers which is now being used in Canada, the Netherlands, Italy, and Japan, and a nationwide training programme for care home staff and general practitioners in Germany look-ing at care planning, pain management, interprofessional collaboration, symptom control, and preferences for end of life care.

A European study of dementia-related deaths of people aged 65 and over has found major cross-national differences in the places where these patients die (46). Although the majority died in a care home, there were noteworthy country differences: 50.2% in Wales, 59.7% in England, 60.8% in Scotland, 65.9% in Belgium, and 92.3% in the Netherlands. In the Netherlands, only 2.8% of older dementia patients died in hospital; this was substantially higher in Belgium (22.7%), but particularly high in Scotland (33.9%), England (36.0%), and Wales (46.3%). The proportion dying at home was very low (less than 5%) in most countries except Belgium (11%). The Dutch model of nursing homes with well-equipped long-term care, 24-hour nursing, and physicians skilled in advance care planning, may explain the exceptionally high proportion of nursing home deaths in this country.

With ongoing demographic and societal changes in mind, it is likely that dementia patients (as well as older patients with other diseases) will increasingly be cared for in nursing homes. Countries need to plan the integration of end of life care into care home facilities to ensure people are well looked after and to avoid last minute transfers to hospital and to environments which are unfamiliar to the patient and often undesired. Such transfers discontinue care, can aggravate the disorientation of dementia patients, bring problems of iatrogenesis (e.g. delirium, distress, and pressure ulcers), and become obstacles to ensuring a 'good death'.

There is some indication that interventions to improve end of life care for older people in nurs-ing homes are effective. However, many of the studies are descriptive rather than evaluative. A Cochrane review is currently underway to gather and appraise the evidence on the effectiveness of palliative care interventions such as hospice services, specialist palliative care units, consulta-tion services, and staff educational programmes in care homes (47). The examples of good end of life care practice presented by the WHO may also inspire others to develop, test, and evaluate similar policies and interventions (23).

Challenges for the future: the very old and care at home

Research shows that in countries where older people are less likely to die at home compared with younger people, the difference increases with age. The very old (80 years and over) have consistently reported lower proportions of home deaths and higher proportions of hospital deaths in countries such as the UK and Norway (11, 31). Very old patients have complex health care and social care needs and the lack of support at home may place a greater burden of care on families. Informal caregivers often do not feel equipped to deal with pain management and symptom control, and the needs of patients are likely to be unmet at home as a consequence.

Studies from the UK show that although most of the very old die in hospital (11, 34) between 69% and 86% of people's last months of life is spent at home (48, 49). This suggests that hospital admissions occur close to death, sometimes via emergency departments—these are known to be major gateways into hospital for older people (50). Considerable end of life care needs have been found amongst older people presenting at emergency departments (51,52). For some, an emergency admission may be inevitable and appropriate (e.g. when rapid deterioration from an unknown condition occurs); for others, however, care can be planned ahead and with appropriate home support, admission to hospital may be prevented, enabling death to take place at home.

Home is a preference among older people (30, 53) but it is important that the quality of care at home is high, particularly as there are indications from new policies and emerging trends in countries such as the UK, Canada, and the USA that more might die at home in the future (35, 54, 55). At the moment, there is a lack of evidence to suggest that those who die at home experience better care and a better death, and that their caregivers cope better with bereavement than those who experience institutional deaths. The access to and quality of the home care that older people towards the end of life get varies greatly between and within countries (2, 56, 57). It is still unclear whether home-based models of end of life care which increase the chances of people dying at home, do at the same time improve outcomes for them and their families and are cost-effective.

A Cochrane review is underway to determine the effectiveness and cost-effectiveness of different models of home-based palliative care services for adults with a severe or advanced disease, malignant or non-malignant (58). Recent randomized controlled trials from the USA showed encouraging results derived from a nurse-led educational palliative care intervention and a two-region palliative care programme (59, 60). In addition to health care services, good social care is also needed for the many older people who live alone at home (23).

Conclusions

Population ageing is a real international challenge requiring nations to ensure greater provision of end of life care for their older citizens. This is an increasingly important public health priority. Worldwide recognition by the WHO and other key international and national organizations seems to have taken place already; it is now time to ensure that appropriate and evidence-based actions are taken.

The circumstances of death and dying among older people vary across countries. Examples have been given of differences in where older people are cared for at the end of life and cultural expectations of how to care for older members of families and communities. There are also differences in the solutions found in ways to care for older people at the end of life—diverse interventions and policies developed around the world. This suggests that although the challenge is international, the solutions are likely to be context-specific.

Managing the care of terminally ill people of advanced age is complex both at a population and at an individual level. Older people can die very differently from those who are middle-aged or young. Their illness trajectories are not yet well described but are likely to be more fluctuant and complex, particularly amongst the very old or frail. Problems such as dementia and social isolation are common and pose challenges when dealing with continuity of care, emergencies, decision-making, and planning where people are cared for.

It is unfortunate that in the face of the growing need for end of life care for older people, the evidence which can guide actions is still at an embryonic stage. There is no solid evidence about which models of care best fulfil the complex needs of older people at the end of life although there are examples of good practice from different parts of the world (23, 61). It is tempting to roll out initiatives which seem promising but lack an evidence base. Adoption of untested approaches comes with risk—end of life care services for older people are complex and multifaceted interventions aiming to impact on several outcomes, not just for patients but also for families. Rigorous evaluations are needed to determine the full extent of their effectiveness and cost-effectiveness to ensure sustainability.

Appropriate models of end of life care must be developed and made available in the places where older people currently die, but also in the places where they would prefer to spend their last days. Most older people die in hospitals, and, as age advances, increasingly in care homes. It has been argued that although many older people would ideally prefer to die at home, this is difficult to achieve due to their complex clinical and social circumstances (53). Comparisons of place of death in relation to age between the UK and the USA show this is not necessarily true (62)—in the USA, older people are more likely to die at home which suggests it is possible for older people to die in their place of choice. Whether or not this is because appropriate models of end of life care are in place for older people at home is still a question.

Finally, sharing experiences and examples of good practice across countries needs to be moderated with critical thinking and cultural sensitivity. If done in such ways, much can be learnt from the experience of others so that knowledge advances alongside practice and policies to ensure that more older people receive better care and live the rest of their lives as fully as possible.

Acknowledgements

Barbara Gomes and Irene J. Higginson thank Cicely Saunders International for their continued support which makes work in this topic possible. Irene J. Higginson is supported by the UK National Institute for Health Research as a Senior Investigator. Joachim Cohen and Luc Deliens are supported by the Agency for Innovation by Science and Technology in Flanders, Strategic Basic Research (SBO) programme. All the authors are grateful to the European Commission for funding the PRISMA project under the Seventh Framework Programme, which enabled them to collaborate (Contract number: Health-F2–2008-201655).

References

1. Population Division Department of Economic and Social Affairs, UN (2009). *World Population Ageing 2009*. New York: United Nations.
2. Kinsella K, He W, US Census Bureau (2009). *An Ageing World: 2008. Report No.: P95/09–1*. Washington, DC: U.S. Government Printing Office.
3. United Nations (2002). *Report of the Second World Assembly on Ageing, Madrid 8–12 April 2002*. New York: United Nations.
4. Preston SH(1977). Mortality trends. *Annual Review of Sociology*, **3**: 163–78.
5. Population Division, Department of Economic and Social Affairs, UN (2010). *Health and Mortality — Issues of Global Concern*. New York: United Nations.
6. Caldwell JC (1976). Toward a restatement of demographic transition theory. *Population and Development Review*, **2**(3–4): 321–66.
7. Raleigh VS (1999). Trends in world population: How will the millennium compare with the past? *Human Reproduction Update*, **5**(5): 500–5.
8. Caldwell JC, Caldwell BK, Caldwell P, McDonald PF, Schindlmayr T (2006). *Demographic Transition Theory*. Dordrecht: Springer.

9. Haggett P (2001). *Geography: A global synthesis*, 4th edn. New York: Prentice Hall.

10. Population Division USCB (2009). *International Data base. Population Division*. Washington, DC: US Census Bureau.

11. Gomes B, Higginson IJ (2008). Where people die (1974–2030): past trends, future projections and implications for care. *Palliative Medicine*, **22**(1): 33–41.

12. Office for National Statistics (2009). *National 2008-based national population projections*. Newport: Office for National Statistics.

13. Jagger C, Gillies C, Moscone F, Cambois E, Van Oyen H, Nusselder W, et al. (2008). Inequalities in healthy life years in the 25 countries of the European Union in 2005: a cross-national meta-regression analysis. *Lancet*, **372**(9656): 2124–31.

14. World Health Organization (2005). *Preventing Chronic Disease: A Vital Investment*. Geneva: WHO.

15. International Labour Office (2006). *Changing patterns in the world of work*. Geneva: International Labour Office.

16. Keehan S, Sisko A, Truffer C, Smith S, Cowan C, Poisal J, et al. (2008). Health spending projections through 2017: the baby-boom generation is coming to Medicare. *Health Affairs* **7**(2): 145–55.

17. Zweifel P, Felder S, Meiers M (1999). Ageing of population and health care expenditure: A red herring? *Health Economics*, **8**(6): 485–96.

18. Seshamani M, Gray A (2004). Ageing and health-care expenditure: the red herring argument revisited. *Health Economics*, **13**(4): 303–14.

19. Palangkaraya A, Yong J (2009). Population ageing and its implications on aggregate health care demand: empirical evidence from 22 OECD countries. *International Journal of Health Care Finance and Economics*, **9**(4): 391–402.

20. Seshamani M, Gray A (2004). Time to death and health expenditure: an improved model for the impact of demographic change on health care costs. *Age and Ageing*, **33**(6): 556–61.

21. Shugarman LR, Campbell DE, Bird CE, Gabel J, Louis TA, Lynn J (2004). Differences in Medicare expenditures during the last 3 years of life. *Journal of General Internal Medicine*, **19**(2): 127–35.

22. Davies E, Higginson IJ (2004). *Better palliative care for older people*. Copenhagen: WHO.

23. Hall S, Petkova H, Tsouros A, Costantini M, Higginson IJ (2011). *Palliative care for older people: Best practice*. Copenhagen: WHO.

24. Harding R, Higginson IJ, on behalf of PRISMA (2010). PRISMA: A pan-European Co-ordinating action to advance the science in end of life cancer care. *European Journal of Cancer*, **46**, 1493–501.

25. Population Division, Department of Economic and Social Affairs, UN (2010). *World Population Prospects: The 2008 Revision*. New York: UN.

26. World Health Organization (2004). *Palliative care: The solid facts*. Copenhagen: WHO.

27. Higginson IJ, Sen-Gupta GJA (2003). Place of care in advanced cancer: a qualitative systematic literature review of patient preferences. *Journal of Palliative Medicine*, **3**(3): 287–300.

28. Brazil K, Howell D, Bedard M, Krueger P, Heidebrecht C (2005). Preferences for place of care and place of death among informal caregivers of the terminally ill. *Palliative Medicine*, **19**(6): 492–9.

29. Beccaro M, Costantini M, Giorgi RP, Miccinesi G, Grimaldi M, Bruzzi P, et al. (2006). Actual and preferred place of death of cancer patients. Results from the Italian survey of the dying of cancer (ISDOC). *Journal of Epidemiology & Community Health*, **60**(5): 412–16.

30. McCarthy EP, Pencina MJ, Kelly-Hayes M, Evans JC, Oberacker EJ, D'Agostino RB, Sr., et al. (2008). Advance care planning and health care preferences of community-dwelling elders: the Framingham Heart Study. *Journals of Gerontology Series A-Biological Sciences & Medical Sciences*, **63**(9): 951–9.

31. Cohen J, Bilsen J, Addington-Hall J, Lofmark R, Miccinesi G, Kaasa S, et al. (2008). Population-based study of dying in hospital in six European countries. *Palliative Medicine*, **22**(6): 702–10.

32. Cohen J, Houttekier D, Onwuteaka-Philipsen B, Miccinesi G, Addington-Hall J, Kaasa S, et al. (2010). Which cancer patients die at home? A study of six European countries using death certificate data. *Journal of Clinical Oncology*, **28**: 2267–73.

33. Costantini M, Balzi D, Garronec E, Orlandini C, Parodi S, Vercelli M, et al. (2000). Geographical variations of place of death among Italian communities suggest an inappropriate hospital use in the terminal phase of cancer disease. *Public Health,* **114**(1): 15–20.

34. Lock A, Higginson IJ (2005). Patterns and predictors of place of cancer death for the oldest old. *BMC Palliative Care,* **4**: 6.

35. Office for National Statistics (2010). *Mortality Statistics — Series DR. 2009.* Newport: Office for National Statistics.

36. Gomes B, Higginson IJ (2006). Factors influencing death at home in terminally ill patients with cancer: systematic review. *British Medical Journal,* **332**(7540): 515–518A.

37. Simon S, Gomes B, Higginson IJ, Bausewein C (2009). Future projections of population and mortality in Germany until 2030/2050–and their impact for end-of-life care. *European Journal of Palliative Care,* **165** (abstract).

38. Seale C (1998). *Constructing death: the sociology of dying and bereavement.* Cambridge: Cambridge University Press.

39. Davies E, Higginson IJ (2004). *Palliative care: The solid facts.* Copenhagen: WHO.

40. Seale C., Cartwright A (1994). *The year before death.* London: Avebury Press.

41. Lobo A, Launer LJ, Fratiglioni L, Andersen K, Di Carlo A, Breteler MMB, et al. (2000). Prevalence of dementia and major subtypes in Europe: A collaborative study of population-based cohorts. *Neurology,* **54**(11): S4–S9.

42. Wancata J, Musalek M, Alexandrowicz R, Krautgartner M (2003). Number of dementia sufferers in Europe between the years 2000 and 2050. *European Psychiatry,* **18**(6): 306–13.

43. Lynn J., Adamson D.M (2003). *Living well at the end of life. Adapting health care to serious chronic illness in old age.* Washington, DC: Rand Health.

44. Luchins DJ, Hanrahan P (1993). What is appropriate health-care for end-stage dementia. *Journal of the American Geriatrics Society,* **41**(1): 25–30.

45. Sampson EL, Ritchie CW, Lai R, Raven PW, Blanchard MR (2005). A systematic review of the scientific evidence for the efficacy of a palliative care approach in advanced dementia. *International Psychogeriatrics,* **17**(1): 31–40.

46. Houttekier D, Cohen J, Bilsen J, Addington-Hall J, Onwuteaka-Philipsen B, Deliens L (2010). Place of death of older people with dementia in Belgium, the Netherlands and England. *Journal of the American Geriatrics Society,* **58**(4): 751–6.

47. Hall S., Kolliakou A., Davies E.A., Froggatt K, Higginson I.J. (2008). Interventions for improving palliative care for older people living in nursing care homes (Protocol). *Cochrane Database of Systematic Reviews,* **2**, CD007132.

48. Hinton J (1994). Which patients with terminal cancer are admitted from home care. *Palliative Medicine,* **8**(3): 197–210.

49. Ward AWM (1974). Terminal care in malignant disease. *Social Science & Medicine,* **8**(7): 413–20.

50. Conroy S (2008). Emergency room geriatric assessment-urgent, important or both? *Age and Ageing,* **37**(6): 612–13.

51. Meier DE, Beresford L (2007). Fast response is key to partnering with the emergency department. *Journal of Palliative Medicine,* **10**(3): 641–5.

52. Beynon T, Gomes B, Murtagh F, Glucksman E, Parfitt A, Burman R, et al. (2010). How common are palliative care needs among older people who die in the emergency department? *Emergency Medicine Journal.* (EPub 13 October 2010.)

53. Gott M, Seymour J, Bellamy G, Clark D, Ahmedzai S (2004). Older people's views about home as a place of care at the end of life. *Palliative Medicine,* **18**(5): 460–7.

54. National Centre for Health Statistics (2008). *National vital statistics system, mortality, worktable 309: deaths by place of death, age, race, and sex: United States, 1999–2004.* Hyattsville, MD: National Centre for Health Statistics.

55. Statistics Canada (2009). *Canada vital statistics, death database, table 102–0509: deaths in hospital and elsewhere, Canada, 1991–2005*. Ottawa: Statistics Canada.

56. World Health Organization (2008). *Home care in Europe: The solid facts*. Geneva: WHO.

57. Teno JM, Clarridge BR, Casey V, Welch LC, Wetle T, Shield R, et al. (2004). Family perspectives on end-of-life care at the last place of care. *Journal of the American Medical Association*, **291**(1): 88–93.

58. Gomes B., Higginson I.J., McCrone P (2009). Effectiveness and cost-effectiveness of home palliative care services for adults with advanced illness and their caregivers (Protocol). *Cochrane Database of Systematic Reviews*, **2**: 1–13.

59. Bakitas M, Lyons KD, Hegel MT, Balan S, Brokaw FC, Seville J, et al. (2009). Effects of a palliative care intervention on clinical outcomes in patients with advanced cancer. The Project ENABLE II Randomized Controlled Trial. *Journal of the American Medical Association*, **302**(7): 741–9.

60. Brumley R, Enguidanos S, Jamison P, Seitz R, Morgenstern N, Saito S, et al. (2007). Increased satisfaction with care and lower costs: results of a randomized trial of in-home palliative care. *Journal of the American Geriatrics Society*, **55**(7): 993–1000.

61. World Health Organization (2004). *Better palliative care for older people*. Copenhagen: WHO.

62. Decker SL, Higginson IJ (2007). A tale of two cities: Factors affecting place of cancer death in London and New York. *European Journal of Public Health*, **17**(3): 285–90.

Chapter 2

The care of older people at the end of life: a historical perspective

Allan Kellehear

One of the most enduring and resistant ideas about care of older people is that, in the past and in other societies less modern than our own, communities have cared for their elderly better than we currently do. Rivalling but complementing this idea of a better world in the past for the elderly is another more recent idea about contemporary care of the elderly. Yes, the 20th century has seen a major rise in institutionalization of the elderly but 'post-modern', 'post-industrial', or 'late modern' forms of social relations and technologies are liberating the old from that century's social ills—isolation, crippling disability, and poverty. Modern pension schemes, medical advances, and developments in information technology now conspire to compress morbidity, raise living standards, and connect older people to virtual communities through the Internet. In the specific context of end of life care for older people these two views are simply untrue.

My aim in this chapter is to disassociate ideas and debates about our *general* care of older people from a closely-related but vastly different concern—that of *care for the elderly when they are at the end of life*. I will demonstrate that historical perspectives on care for older people are new, and in any case, the main terms of the debate in that area often omit related concerns about end of life care. Debates about care for older people consistently fail to come to grips with, or gloss over, the equally historical and cross-cultural problem of what to do with the elderly when they become too ill or demented to integrate into family or community.

In focusing on this particular dimension of care I will argue that care of older people at the end of life has *enjoyed a steady improvement in the social arrangements to support end of life care from (admittedly) a very poor start in human history. However, these improved arrangements have frequently been at the cost of emphasizing quality of life at the expense of recognizing the inevitability of death and dying.* Unlike care of older people in general, a topic subject to all sorts of ideal claims and counter claims, care for older people at the end of life is less prone to romancing the past or rationalizing the present arrangements. The diversity of care for older people at the end of life— from ritual killing and abandonment, to household care at great personal sacrifice, to routine medicalization and state incarceration—presents contemporary people everywhere with clearer and more specific political, cultural, and policy challenges. However, without a sketch of the historical background to our current situation we cannot identify future solutions that astutely avoid the mistakes of our past.

To that end, this chapter is organized in the following way. I will first briefly review some re-occurring historical and cultural themes of care for the elderly at the end of life—especially the care of the elderly by hunter-gatherer economies and classical pastoral societies such as Ancient Egypt, Rome, and Greece. I will then describe the major sociological factors behind a creeping historical process of institutionalization before concluding with an outline of the factors that I believe are consistently omitted in debates about the development of institutional care of older people.

Some historical and cultural background

The different histories of ageing can be difficult to compare and evaluate because definitions of who was considered 'old' varied widely. For some hunter-gatherer societies and Ancient Romans, being 'old' might refer to someone in their 40s. Record-keeping societies use different ages to declare someone 'old'—perhaps 50, 60, 65, or 75 as their criteria. Many histories of ageing are histories of male ageing and or ageing of male elites (1). And, of course, the field is also dogged by a lack of written records, particularly in preliterate societies (2).

The classic work on the care of the elderly in hunter-gatherer economies—the economy and social organization that represents most of human pre-history—was written by Leo Simmons and entitled *The Role of the Aged in Primitive Societies* (3). This was a study of 71 tribes from a diversity of countries, climates, and social customs. Simmons (4) concluded that old people have always been viewed as 'a problem' but the methods to deal with this problem have been very diverse. While health was intact the means available to older people to ensure survival and comfort ranged widely. Marrying younger women (to 'absorb their youth' or to ensure a consistent source of household help) was a popular adaptation to ageing. For similar reasons, this was often encouraged by older wives too because they would benefit from home help in this way. Holding on to political, religious, or economic power was also a successful way to secure care, participation, and comfort from the wider and younger group. But as Simmon's argued in later work (5) successful ageing depended on being as active as possible right up to the end. Dependency and frailty caused vulnerability.

And when it came to dependency, hunter-gatherer peoples tended to 'show respect' for the elderly through what we would now call 'assisted dying'—ritual neglect, abandonment, or killing. As Victor (2) observed, 'There seems little cultural variation in the situation of the *frail* elderly; they are almost universally regarded as a burden' (emphasis mine).

The frail aged were vulnerable to forms of assisted dying or mercy killing often irrespective of their political status (6) from societies as diverse as Hopi Indians in North America, the Arawak in South America, the Kalahari in Africa, the Ainu in Japan, Samoans in Oceania, and various aboriginal nations in Australia (4). Since there was no sense of cumulative calendar for the individual—no sense of 'being' 32, 46, or 65—age was determined by appearance and function. This assessment of age through appearance and function is a long standing cross-cultural way of judging who is old and active and who is old and 'dying' (4, 7–9).

As in the animal world from which we emerged, the older member of a group can often provide leadership, experience, and memory for others (5, 8) and this provided respect, protection, and status—not due to ageing for its own sake but for what age could bring to the economic and political welfare of the group. The memories of older people were substitutes for written records, references, information about irregular events and experiences, general knowledge, political and legal precedents, and so on. Hunter-gatherer societies often privilege the old—being 'living proof' of the success of the group. But should age bring illness, disability, or dependency then the fragile economic balances of a nomadic group could not afford to feed an unproductive member and respect and reciprocal obligations would turn quickly into a ritual launch into the world of the ancestors—to protect the group from *that* vantage point. Fear may breed respect but respect and status can lead to mercy killing (8).

The advent and development of pastoral societies in the 12,000 years since the last ice age has been kinder to the elderly in general, and end of life care for the frail age in this newer context took a more generous turn. Simmons (5) argued that farming and handicraft economies were more suited to economically neutral or unproductive people such as an aristocracy, military and professional classes, and the frail elderly. This is nowhere better seen than in Eastern societies where pastoral families in China, Korea, or Japan combined a philosophy of end of life care, ancestor worship, and elder cohabitation under a broader cultural rubric of filial piety (10).

However, despite the importance of family and medicine on most Western pastoral societies, suicide or assisted dying did not disappear altogether because ideas of being a burden to others—as a continuation of hunter-gather economic ideas—also continued in some ancient societies such as those in Greek and Roman times. Nevertheless, throughout the Middle Ages and even until the late 19th century in Britain and Europe cohabitation with older people became common. Historians such as Thane (11, 12), Laslett (13), and Hareven (14, 15) argued that co-residence with older people was *not* the modal arrangement in England or the USA during the few centuries leading up to the 20th century but Ruggles (16) disputes this, arguing that although most people did not live with their elderly parents most elderly did live with their children or borders and lodgers. Ruggles argued that these contrasting views of the historical data are an artefact of the demographic numbers alone, that is, even if all available elderly lived with their children this would only comprise 20% of all households in the 19th century.

Despite these 'internal' discipline-based debates about the data, everyone seems to agree that, at least in farming communities everywhere, both frail and active elderly people lived *either* with their children, next door to their children, or close by their children (16). They also often lived with others—borders, lodgers, or other elderly friends or family. Part of the reason for such companionship lies in the fact that older people did not re-join children at a later stage of life but that some children stayed at home because most 'homes' were in fact family farms. Young men and their families earned a livelihood or would work with the expectation of inheriting and staying at this farm. On other occasions, a widow and her children would *return* to the family home between marriages. Other women would not leave the family home at all but rather assume the responsibility for care of older parents. The life course and life transitions were more flexible than those of the 20th century where transitions were commonly more formal and underpinned by mass occupational mobility, increased life expectancy, and work-related migration (14, 15).

Such 'home care' of the elderly, although self evidently an improvement on ritual neglect, abandonment, and killing, hide a number of social and demographic costs and variations. For one thing, spouses and children were the main carers, especially daughters, who often sacrificed their own work and marriage prospects to say nothing of their own health and fitness. The compassionate living arrangements for end of life care in farming communities from east to west over the last 12,000 years also ignores not simply the gender imbalances in the provision of that care but also the role of social class in the success and generalization of that care.

From family care to institutional care

In farming communities around the world a small plot of land or a share in the harvest and associated products of the farming produce would sustain the older person with or without family. Social isolation was less of a problem because family lived nearby and were not usually drawn to the cities for work until this kind of exodus increased dramatically around the time of the industrial revolution.

However, over the course of 12,000 years of settlement society not everyone lived on farms. Cities were increasingly a significant part of the human landscape. In these places, a loss of wage labour capacity meant instant poverty.

Most theorists of ageing (17–19) agree that whether aged care has worsened over the course of history ('modernization theory') or whether it has improved from better health care and legislation ('revisionist theory'), the key to understanding the broad pattern of care for older people is in understanding class and status. Among the stable petit bourgeoisie on farms, care was consistent because life support was more reliable and direct (e.g. food, housing, kin, etc.) than simply wage income. For the poor, however, food and housing became items tied to monies and often an urban location meant small or absent networks of kin. For these people, particularly in Europe and the USA, large numbers of these older people ended up in institutions for the 'old and infirm' variously called 'poor houses', 'alms houses', asylums, or workhouses depending on the country (20, 21).

The poor houses from the 16th to the 19th century in France and Italy were particularly widespread and the frail and ill were often 'placed' into these institutions by parish authorities (22). It is often argued that in England this was far less common but two factors complicate and qualify this so-called exception. First, asylums and workhouses in England were very large where they did exist, and secondly, when we move away from 'long-term' figures for the inmates and concentrate on, for example short stays, we find that one in six men or one in 13 women spent at least one night in a workhouse before they died (22). These institutions were clearly central social organizations when it came to end of life care for older people—either as long-term stay facilities or to provide 'respite' care for older individuals attempting to eke out an existence away from them.

Modernity, as many have noted, was created in the image of the city (see, 6), with urbanization and industrialization accelerating the process of moving from family farms to wage labour in the last 200 years. This has also resulted in some parallel cultural and attitudinal changes. The reliance on wage labour has encouraged a transition from viewing ageing as 'natural' to one that sees ageing as decline, weakness, and obsolescence (14). The scientific and medical literature after 1880 began to view ageing as a 'social' and 'medical' problem (23); institutions for the aged in the USA paralleled the explosion of institutions for the blind, deaf, and orphans (23); and so-called 'homes' for the elderly in Europe quickly evolved from poor houses and mental asylums as these, in their turn, had evolved earlier from leprosariums (21, 24).

Despite this shift and relabelling of institutions from places that housed the poor in general and the unfit, frail, and elderly in particular, most long-term older residents were a minority of all the older frail people—about 4% or 5% of all elderly—and this did not change substantially for a hundred years from the late 1800s to the late 1900s (22). However, unlike today, most of the inmates did not have relatives nearby or alive, and before the introduction of the pension, no income either. The modern development of institutions for older people—what Pelling and Smith (22) describe as 'the only demonstrable growth'—was for residents over 75 years of age (see also, 21). In the West, the nursing home and the hospital have become the main places of end of life care for the frail older person. Even in places such as Japan, where co-residence is the tradition, many elderly Japanese at the end of life are seeing out their final weeks in hospitals in so-called 'rehabilitation wards' or 'kinstitutions' (10) or seeking greater community support for care to relieve or complement family supports (25).

The contemporary situation of end of life care for older people

In the above 'potted history' of end of life care for older people I have tried to show how, although the relative status and fortunes of older people have varied widely depending on culture and their status within that culture, end of life care for older people has largely improved. End of life care for older people has come from abandonment and mercy killing in hunter-gatherer societies to family care in pastoral societies. However, though the economics of pastoral societies allow for a certain level of dependency, fortunes are not evenly distributed. In urban areas in particular the poor older person at the end of life witnesses the earliest forms of institutionalization. These begin as 'blended' institutions that do not cater solely for older people who are frail and infirm but are shared accommodations with the poor unemployed, the mad, and the disabled.

As urbanization and industrialization spread across the world in the last 200 years, ageing became much more closely linked with concepts of productivity and labour value and soon ageing and concepts of obsolescence began to overlap in the minds of many. Mandatory retirement was soon introduced (14) but so too were state pensions (22). Introduction of public health measures— better food, clean water, introduction of sewerage systems, meat storage standards, and better housing—complemented rising employment, and life expectancy began to soar for the first time in human history. Fertility began to fall dramatically, survival rates at birth began to rise dramatically, and there were major rises in divorce and living alone in all major industrial countries (26–28). The proportion of people living into their 70s and 80s began to rise sharply (29)—the very group who have been the 'traditional' users of institutions. And although most older people now live in communities, most of them will not die there. About one in five people in the USA will experience their end of life care in nursing homes (21, 30). The majority of dying people, and most of these are over the age of 65, will die in nursing homes or hospitals with less than 20% dying at home (31). Numbers of people in nursing homes have tripled in the 20 years preceding the late 1980s alone (30), and the World Health Organization estimates that about half of these residents live with dementia (32).

Dementia is one epidemiological factor often overlooked by the in-house historical debates about whether quality of care for older people has increased or deteriorated in recent years. Thane (33), for example, in a major study of old age in England where she weighs the relative social merits of care across several different periods of time in England, devotes a mere two pages to dementia in her 536-page monograph on old age. Smith and Bengston (34) in their study celebrating the positive consequences of institutionalization of older people in an atypical middle-class residential facility makes almost no mention of the prevailing epidemiological presence of dementia. Clark's (35) early review of sources of dependency in 'later life' does not even cite dementia or neurological disorders. Post-modern writers on ageing may sing the praises of 'genetic interventions', body replacement, or general medical advances for older people and they may declare an 'end to retirement' (36) but dementia has no cure, its prevalence is rising, and 25% of people over 85 and 35% of people over 90 are affected (37). For older people at the end of life the key reason for institutionalization is deteriorating health—falls, debility and frailty, confusion, fractures, strokes, and incontinence (21).

The fact is, while most older people in pastoral/peasant history spent their final days with family (80%) (16), most now do not. The majority of older people who die today do so in institutions such as hospitals, nursing homes, or hospices and not in their own homes (6). But the social picture of care is not so glibly described.

Although most die in institutional care, that care is not similar to institutional care in work-houses, poor houses, or asylums of the past. For one thing, all current institutions are classified as 'healthcare' institutions. There is no forced labour, no meagre food rations, and no routine punishments. Does this mean that a healthcare ideology has improved the end of life care of older people in the present age?

Has end of life care for older people improved?

During the long 12,000-year period of settlement culture most older people preferred a place of their own, with help in the house and access to children and support (13, 21). This was the ideal. Achieving this ideal was another matter altogether, especially among poor, urban-based, older people. For them, institutional care became a tough but humane option that provided basic rations and support as well as shelter from inclement weather. In the last 150 years of modern industrial and urban development older people have moved from the margins of the healthcare system to the centre (38). This has not been achieved as a result of some conspiracy theory against older people to contain their polluting presence or medicalize their identities, although these influences cannot be legitimately dismissed in a broader sociological examination of contributing influences. Rather, both the sheer numbers of older people and their active participation in not only the labour force of the 20th century but also in political governance and policy-making in this period has meant that older people themselves have been instrumental in making their case for greater health and social care attention.

Poor houses were largely for the poor. But these places did provide life support for those without any alternatives and for whom a death in the streets was a genuine and common outcome of a lack of economic and social means. Poor houses did in fact provide a community of sorts and a basic set of provisions where none existed elsewhere. On the negative side, shame was common (39) as were harsh punishments for transgressions against the house rules. And unlike today, there were no medical treatments for the common problems of ageing—organ failure, confusion, chronic pain, or physical disability.

Today, institutions for older people, such as hospitals and nursing homes, do provide medical treatments and support, quality food and accommodation, and basic income is provided for in most countries by way of a pension scheme. It is also common for residents to have families who visit. However, the problem of dependency and shame—linked to institutionalization or physical disability—remains common. Although medical treatments are routine, there has been serious questioning about its medical effectiveness and timely employment (40) as well as in terms of social care (41, 42). Unlike the institutions of the past, nursing homes now house residents from different social cohorts, cultural backgrounds, and occupational groups making 'community' much more difficult and loneliness much more common (6, 43). Furthermore, provision of different 'standards' of care is frequently based on residents' ability to pay, making institutional care from public or private nursing homes and hospitals class-based.

In global terms there are two final observations to make about the quality of end of life care for older people today. First, ritual neglect and abandonment have crept back into the care agenda for older people—not because of some cultural persistence of hunter-gatherer ideas—but because of the rise of AIDS. In developing areas such as Africa and South-east Asia, people living with AIDS live with stigma and social rejection, largely resulting in the widespread belief that such diseases are 'unnatural' or are a result of wrong-doing or witchcraft. Much fear is associated with dying from AIDS in those of any age. Those dying of AIDS do not receive traditional community supports and frequently are abandoned or neglected by communities and sometimes even their own families (44, 45). Furthermore, in affluent countries, there is a policy ambivalence towards care of older people with dementia, with family members assuming that the public sector takes the major responsibility for the frail aged but the public sector assuming that family is the major provider of care with the state as helper (15). The older person with end of life care needs is often caught between this policy ambiguity.

In these ways, we can see that the question about whether end of life care for older people has improved, is not a question about end of life care for older people *living and dying independently or at home with family*. That care seems to have remained more or less the same and the answer to questions of quality about that care must be viewed in the same historical terms. Family care has commonly provided safety from the threat of premature death, with the comfort of care from one's own blood relations, in familiar environments—whether these be affluent or more modest surroundings. On the negative side, children and spouses continue, as they have in the pastoral past, to bear the social, emotional, financial, and health costs of such care—and in the modern context of chronic diseases of ageing, those costs have become more substantial and prolonged with each passing decade.

As for the question of the quality of institutional care of older people at the end of life—the largest organizational development in the modern world for older people—the ultimate answer cannot be divorced from the question of what societies believe constitutes a 'good death'. The debates over improvements to the quality of life for older people in general do not usually speak to the question of what it means to die well. In this way, much of the historical literature on the sociology of ageing and care for older people is written without an academic conversation with the history and sociology of dying. And without that conversation, arriving at an adequately balanced sociological answer to the question about the efficacy and quality of life for older people at the end of their life cannot be derived.

Healthy ageing versus good dying: a modern policy tension

Although hunter-gatherer economies and societies had what, in modern terms, seem to be harsh 'end of life care policies' for their frail aged, they had one thing that modern industrial economies seem to be losing—a community recognition of dying as a social (as opposed to medical) experience. Dying, for most people in hunter-gatherer and pastoral economies, had a set of mutual expectations and obligations. The recognition of impending death called for a specific type of care and responsibility—presence in the form of companionship; giving and receiving; and the value of ritual (6)—these were all essential parts of the dying experience for both the dying person and his or her community. Inside the recognition of dying as the last period of a person's life, in the final gifts exchanged between the dying and their group, or even as someone to leave behind, to kill, or to nurse in those final days, often lay a learning experience about human limitation, fragility, and transience—lessons that are often difficult to learn at earlier ages in the life course (36).

In this way, and by modern criteria for care, the hunter-gathers' approach to end of life care might seem cruel. But by most historical criteria for caring behaviour at the end of life, our reticence to recognize the almost inescapable link between ageing and dying—a reticence so common in institutional care of older people—seem to many observers a denial of 'traditional' rights and status accorded the dying. This denial of the recognition of a life coming to an end also forecloses on a valuable source of learning from one of the great verities in human experience.

Failing to recognize dying as part of ageing and later life is also to fail to offer the care—medical or spiritual—that is specific to the dying experience. These have not been omissions of people from hunter-gatherer or pastoral communities. Seen from the perspective of the history and ethnography of dying, then, modern care of older people at the end of life falls dramatically short of this type of care. Only as a form of chronic illness do we currently debate the merits or otherwise of our care for the older person at the end of life.

Aside from circumstances of family or community care, institutional care of older persons has a long history too, and perhaps counter-intuitively to some, a largely compassionate history. At first, state and church institutions provided for the care of older people when little or no alternative but death existed. In recent years, such institutions have attempted to cater not only for the poor, but also the unwell, disabled, the socially isolated, and the immanently dying from all backgrounds. The sociological problems of this form of end of life care are easily summarized: a lack of consistent standards and regulation of care; a slowness to recognize that quality care for older people must be inclusive of an end of life care approach—medically, psychologically, socially, and spiritually; and that institutional care must be a seamless part of community care if it is to avoid becoming a 'total' institution that disenfranchises its residents from their former social lives and values.

The rise of dementia and frailty as forms of life-threatening illness at the end of life often mean that institutional support will continue to be important part of the way all modern societies provide support to older people. Social isolation, crippling disability, and poverty have not been swept away by 20th-century or early 21st-century social and technological reforms. New forms of isolation, sharp increases in disability associated with advanced ageing, and the continuation of poverty make arguments about family, community, or institutionalization artificial distinctions. In policy and practice terms our ability to support families, communities, or institutions to care for older people will crucially depend on their interdependencies: how closely will institutions resemble the former prisons and asylums of the past? Are care institutions able to model themselves on more socially permeable, modern examples such as schools, universities, libraries, or resorts? How do we support and integrate the new, small, career-oriented families into even newer forms of geographical and 'virtual' communities to support their older family members?

Many older people wish to be taken care of by their healthcare establishments and authorities and can feel abandoned, even victimized, if they are not (46). But at the same time it must also be acknowledged that many older people at the end of life do not fear death, are prepared for death, and are resigned to dying (47–49). Above all, these older people desire their autonomy and value any attempts, formal or informal, to maintain that independence. Acknowledging the end of life and the supports needed to face that prospect is both a state policy and community challenge. There are many current debates about the relative merits of community care versus institutional care, of the introduction of health promotion and community development into end of life care services and practices, and of professional reform in institutional care. These tensions and debates are all challenges that seek to build on the humane organizational responses of pastoral communities but with a recognition of the value of acknowledging death passed down to us by our hunter-gatherer ancestry. The recognition of death between people who care for one another at the end of life does not diminish us but rather permits a greater, more intimate connection with one another during a time of our greatest need.

References

1. Kastenbaum R, Ross B (1975). Historical perspectives on care. In JG Howells (ed) *Modern Perspectives in the Psychiatry of the Old*, pp. 421–49. New York: Brunner.

2. Victor CR (1994). *Old age in modern society: A textbook of social gerontology*. London: Chapman and Hall.

3. Simmons LW (1945/1970). *The role of the aged in primitive society*. New Haven, CT: Yale University Press.

4. Simmons LW (1946). Attitudes toward the ageing: Primitive societies. *Journal of Gerontology*, 1(1): 72–95.

5. Simmons LW (1960). Ageing in pre-inductrial societies. In C Tibbits (ed.) *Handbook of Social Gerontology*, pp. 62–91. Chicago, IL: University of Chicago Press.

6. Kellehear A (2007). *A social history of dying*. Cambridge, Cambridge University Press.

7. Roebauck J (1979). When does 'old age' begin? The evolution of the English definition. *Journal of Social History*, 12(3): 416–28.

8. Minios G (1987). *History of old age: From antiquity to the Renaissance*. Chicago, IL: University of Chicago Press.

9. Johnson P (1998). Historical readings of old age and ageing. In P Johnson, P Thane (eds) *Old Age from Antiquity to Postmodernity*, pp. 1–18. London: Routledge.

10. Thang LL (2000). Ageing in the East: Comparative and historical reflections. In TR Cole, R Kastenbaum (eds) *Handbook of the Humanities and Ageing*, pp. 183–213. New York: Springer.

11. Thane P (1998). The family lives of old people. In P Johnson, P Thane (eds) *Old Age from Antiquity to Postmodernity*, pp. 180–210. London: Routledge.

12. Thane P (2000). The history of ageing in the West. In TR Cole, R Kastenbaum (eds) *Handbook of Humanities and Ageing*, pp. 3–24. New York: Springer.

13. Laslett P (1977). *Family life and illicit love in earlier generations*. Cambridge: Cambridge University Press.

14. Hareven T (1982). The life course and ageing in perspective. In TK Hareven, KJ Adams (eds) *Ageing and Life Course Transitions: An Interdisciplinary Perspective*, pp. 1–26. New York: The Guildford Press.

15. Hareven T (1994). Ageing and generational relations: A historical and life course perspective. *Annual Review of Sociology*, **20**: 437–61.

16. Ruggles S (1999). *Living arrangements and well being of older persons in the past*. Available at: http://www.un.org/esa/population/publications/bulletin 42–43/ruggles.pdf. (Accessed 5 September 2009.)

17. Achenbaum WA, Stearns PN (1978). Essay: old age and modernization. *The Gerontologist*, **18**(3): 307–12.

18. Kertzer DI (1995). Towards a historical demography of ageing. In DI Kertzer, P Laslett (eds) *Ageing in the Past: Demography, Society and Old Age*, pp. 363–83. Berkley, CA: University of California Press.

19. Moody HR (1998). *Ageing: Concepts and controversies*. London: Sage.

20. Brody EM, Spark GM (1966). Institutionalization of the aged: A family crisis. *Family Process*, **5**(1): 76–90.

21. Doty P (1986). Family care of the elderly: The role of public policy. *Milibank Quarterly*, **64**(1): 34–75.

22. Pelling M, Smith RM (eds) (1991). *Life, death and the elderly: Historical perspectives*. London: Routledge.

23. Achenbaum WA (1982). Further perspectives on modernization and ageing: A (p)review of the historical literature. *Social Science History*, **6**(3): 347–68.

24. Foucault M (1973). *Madness and civilization: A history of insanity in the Age of reason*. New York: Vintage Books.

25. 100-member committee to create safe and comfortable communities for people with dementia (2006). *Campaign to build a dementia-friendly community*. Available at: http://www.ninchisho100.net/english/campaign.html.

26. Laslett P (1995). Necessary knowledge: Age and ageing in the societies of the Past. In DI Kertzer, P Laslett (eds) *Ageing in the Past: Demography, Society and Ageing*, pp. 3–77. Berkeley, CA: University of California Press.

27. Klinenberg E (2001). Dying alone: the social production of urban isolation. *Ethnography*, **2**(4): 501–31.

28. Tomassini, C, Glaser K, Wolf DA, Broese van Groenau MI, Grundy E (2004). Living arrangements among older people: An overview of trends in Europe and the USA. *Population Trends Spring* **115**: 24–35.

29. Dunnel K (2008). Ageing and mortality in the UK. *Population Trends*, Winter **134**: 6–23.

30. Shield RR (1988). *Uneasy endings: Daily life in an American nursing home*. Ithica, NY: Cornell University Press.

31. Department of Health (2008). *End of Life Care Strategy: Promoting high quality care for all adults at the end of life*. London: National Health Service. Available at: www.dh.gov.uk/publications.

32. World Health Organization (1986). *Dementia in Later Life: Research and action*. Geneva: WHO Technical Report.

33. Thane P (2000). *Old age in English history*. Oxford: Oxford University Press.

34. Smith KF, Bengston VL (1979). Positive consequences of institutionalisation: Solidarity between elderly parents and their middle age children. *The Gerontologist*, **19**(5): 438–47.

35. Clark M (1972). Cultural values and dependency in later life. In DO Cowgill, LD Holmes (eds.) *Ageing and Modernization*, pp. 263–74. New York: Meredith Publishing Corp.

36. Polivka L (2000). Postmodern ageing and loss of meaning. *Journal of Ageing and Identity*, **5**(4): 225–35.

37. Brown J, Hillam J (2004). *Dementia: Your questions answered*. London: Churchill Livingstone.

38. Conrad C (1998). Old age and the health care system in nineteenth and twentieth centuries. In P Johnson, P Thane (eds) *Old Age from Antiquity to Postmodernity*, pp. 132–45. London: Routledge.

39. Strange JM (2005). *Death, grief and poverty in Britain, 1870–1914*. Cambridge: Cambridge University Press.

40. Aminoff BZ, Adunsky A (2004). Dying dementia patients: Too much suffering, too little palliation. *American Journal of Alzheimer's Disease and Other Dementias*, **19**(4): 243–7.

41. Kitwood T (1993). Frames of reference for an understanding of dementia. In J Johnson, R Slater (eds) *Ageing and Later Life*, pp. 100–6. London: Sage.

42. Kayser-Jones J (2002). The experience of dying: An ethnographic nursing home experience. *The Gerontologist*, **42**: 11–19.

43. Elias N (1985). *The loneliness of the dying*. Oxford: Basil Blackwell.

44. Songwathana P, Manderson L (2001). Stigma and rejection: Living with AIDS in Southern Thailand. *Medical Anthropology*, **20**(1): 1–23.

45. Liddell C, Barrett L, Bydawell M (2005). Indigenous representations of illness and AIDS in sub-Sahara Africa. *Social Science & Medicine*, **60**: 691–700.

46. Gott M, Small N, Barnes S, Payne S, Seamark D (2008). Older people's views of a good death in heart failure: Implications for palliative care provision. *Social Science & Medicine*, **67**: 1113–21.

47. Owen T (ed) (2005). *Dying in old age: reflections and experiences from an older person's perspective*. London: Help the Aged.

48. Hallberg IR (2005). Death and dying from older people's point of view: a literature review. *Ageing Clinical and Experimental Research*, **16**(2): 87–102.

49. Kellehear A (2009). Dying old–and *preferably* alone: Agency, resistance and dissent at the end of life. *International Journal of Ageing and Later Life*, **4**(1): 5–21.

Chapter 3

Anti-ageing and scientific avoidance of death

John A. Vincent

Introduction

The biological processes of ageing and death require a societal response. On one level this is a functional necessity: if society is to continue it has to find ways of replacing those who have died. On a more existential level, societies have to provide explanations of the world which motivate people to live meaningful lives and give them access to explanations and courses of action in the face of problems and fears such as death. In modern society the problems of old age and death are typically constructed as medical problems with scientific solutions based on biological knowledge. We can examine the problems this approach creates for establishing a satisfactory conclusion to old age.

This chapter will use methods of cultural deconstruction to examine scientific attempts to avoid ageing and thus postpone or eliminate death. Secularization and individualism provide the cultural context of the problem of giving a satisfactory meaning to death in the West. I will draw on anthropological materials for comparative evidence to see how death is understood in non-Western cultures and then look at the history of Western ideas about ageing and death and how these have developed and changed, and in particular, look at contemporary changes driven by the institution of science and its cultural products in anti-ageing science and medicine.

In other work I have classified anti-ageing phenomena into four types (1). Firstly there is an approach in which ageing is the *appearance* of old age, a phenomena of the body's surface. This anti-ageing is thus cosmetic in intention. The second approach is to consider ageing to be a *disease* to be tackled by medical strategies with the intention of cure. Ageing from this perspective is a phenomenon of the body interior. The third view of ageing is that it is a fundamental biological process particularly located in the intracellular biochemistry. Biological anti-ageing strategies seek to modify these processes by manipulation of cell chemistry. And fourthly, for some ageing is death. These anti-ageing activities aim to achieve immortality, or at least something close to it. Understanding the development of anti-ageing science provides insights into contemporary cultural changes to old age and death.

Classifications and meaning of old age

The meaning of old age as a cultural category is constructed through establishing its boundaries. Old age as a stage in life is demarcated by the end of middle age and its completion at death. Old age is therefore understood not only by how it is distinguished from middle age but also constructed through the anticipation of death and the meaning culture attributes to death (2). A key concept in understanding the transitions between life stages is that of time. However, time is a socially organized and understood phenomenon and plays an important role in how old age and death are understood (3).

In the Australian Aboriginal world there are two kinds of time. There is sacred time: 'dream time.' 'Dream time' was/is the time of myths and heroes, when sacred ancestors and creators acted/act out the key dramas of the universe. The second type of time is the here and now, a kind of continuous present which is merely a reflection of dream time. This other time is the time in which we live. It does not change or progress but merely shadows what happened/happens in dream time (4–6). The Hindu vision of time is circular. The cycles of the universe are the *yuga*, our current Kali yuga being an evil time awaiting destruction and rebirth. The ideas of an *avatar*, the current reincarnation in a cycle of rebirth, suggest death is but an interlude not an end or a final goal. The (male) individual should proceed through the stages of like from student, to household, to aesthetic (*sanyassi*), to hermit (7).

These views of time contrast with 'modern' understanding of time and with each other. Our modern Western society not only sees time as an arrow and (to mix the metaphor) marching forward, but as something that is precious, must be counted, and that must be saved. In other cultures time is understood as comprising various circles which revolve and recreate the same world, time and time again (8). One logical consequence of the progressive view of time is that the significance of events is seen to fade as they pass into history; the longer ago something happened, the more it loses its significance. The future is the time to come and is seen as new, modern, and fundamentally different than the past. Some societies do not see the future as radically different from the past or present. Ideas of time clearly affect the understanding of the sequence of the life course.

The view that we only have one life and this is marked by death at the end contrasts with the view of death and life merely being opposites sides of a cycle, whereby souls, or *avatars* have continuing existence. One might hypothesize that the close approach of oblivion and irrelevance would lower the status of elderly people. By the same token, where death is seen as translation into a more powerful or desirable state, higher status might be anticipated. The specific modern Western view of time is embedded in science and the knowledge that scientific institutions create. I will return to these themes when considering contemporary 'scientific' culture.

Anthropology of ageing and death

There is considerable anthropological literature on death, in particular death rituals. There is much less on old age. Key analyses in this literature describe the role of collective symbolism and ritual in the way societies understand and manage the transition of the world of the living to the world of the dead. One theme is that of social transition and looks at inheritance of property and resources, and the succession of statuses from one generation to the next. Another theme is that of symbol and ritual, including the way different communities give meaning to this transition through recreating collective or individual identities (9–13). (Chapter 2, this volume, by Alan Kellahear refers to this literature.)

Dinka living in the Southern Sudan in the 1940s and 1950s as described by Leinhardt in *Divinity and Experience* manifest explicit de-individualism; the kin group or clan is the effective social unit which has personality and authority—as in control of the land (14), so much so that the institution of 'burial alive' of the old and ailing 'spear master' is reported as a ritual to preserve the vitality of the lands which are his ritual responsibility. In the Australian desert, the Mardu, who were historically hunters and gatherers as described by Tonkinson, see people as a reflection of the dream world, they have few valued material possessions but associations through song and ritual need to be inherited and kept intact (6). There is an interesting direct contrast between the priority given to announcing death and assembling all parties in this society with an account of death of leaders in Madagascar provided by Woolley where in an agrarian society land is ritually and materially important (15). In this case the burial has to take place in secrecy before anyone outside the immediate group finds out. The Madagascan concerns are to do with the body holding the fertility of the land and fear it will be misappropriated; while the Mardu are most concerned to assemble all the correct kin to be able to successfully transform the person to the other world and safeguard this one (6).

It is significant that the activities described orient towards the survival of the collectivity. The ethnographies describe gathering the family, putting relationships to rights, and ensuring smooth succession, even while the person is still alive. The relevant collective might be kin, or a spiritual community orienting to ancestors or gods, or a political community paying attention to title succession, and even an economic community arranging disposal of property. Thus the key feature of the case examples given are how people in the face of death are not confronted with the impossibility of a continuing individual relationships with a dead body, but the possibility of orientating action to a living collective in a meaningful way. In the West there is a lack of such collectivities. Lafontaine argues that there is a contemporary preoccupation with bodily immortality and that this is fundamentally linked to a lack of attachment to community and the chain of generations (16).

Western culture through time has changed the role of old age and death

In her excellent book *La Société Post-Mortelle* Lafontaine presents an account of the historical changes in Western culture which lead to the loss of sacred meaning of death (16). For Lafontaine, the key factors in understanding modern attitudes to death—what she calls the 'port-mortal' society—are individualization (existential meaning is only to be found in individuals not collectives) and 'de-symbolization' (the lack of ritual and symbolic meanings for death). She sees death as having been removed from a cultural position where it is special and set apart from the everyday world and is now considered within the realms of mundane as merely a biochemical process. As a consequence those experts who have the knowledge of ritual and symbol around death are sidelined and the expertise of medicine and biological science takes first place in our cultural understanding of old age and death.

Lafontaine's theme reflects much classic sociology and philosophy. She examines how the history of ideas in the West has accentuated the individual as the location of moral worth. The image of the rational individual capable of exercising choice is a dominant post-enlightenment image of the moral person. Habermas argues that science and technology and liberal values emphasizing individual choice have historically developed together (17):

> It has always been social change, resulting from technological innovations in the fields of production and exchange, communication and transport, the military, and medicine, which took the lead. Even the post-traditional conceptions of law and morality have been described by classical social theories as a product of cultural and societal rationalization acting *in the same direction* as the advances of modern science and technology . . . And since enlarging the scope of individual choice fosters individual autonomy, science and technology have, to date, formed an evident alliance with the fundamental credo of liberalism, holding that all citizens are entitled to equal opportunities for an autonomous direction of the own lives.

Choice in the modern world has come to be expressed in struggle over the state disciplining of bodies and personal identity—to get the law and state out of the bedroom and the realm of inter-personal relationships, i.e. freedom to be yourself. Thus cultural values are achieved in the contemporary West by self-fulfilment, self-realization, and in particular expressed through the body.

The body becomes the site of cultural display and inscription—of autonomy and control, self-realization, and discipline (18–23).

> The multiple transactions between expertise and subjectivity, and the multiple injunctions and managed desires to reform and remake ourselves through calculated intervention in the name of our authenticity, self realization, and freedom, have been central to the 'government of self' in advanced liberal democracies (Rose 1989). What is new, perhaps, is the centrality accorded to the soma, to the flesh, the organs, the tissues, the cells, the gene sequences, and molecular corporeality to our individual and collective ways of understanding and managing ourselves as human beings . . . our bodies have become ourselves, become central to our expectations, hopes, our individual and collective identities, and our biological responsibilities in this emergent form of live. (24)

These cultural developments create significant problems for the end of life. What choices, what methods of personal fulfilment in bodily terms are possible for an individual with an ageing or dying body?

> Déconstruite et désymbolisée, la mort est devenue une affaire strictement individuelle et se décline sous forme de droit, et même de choix. L'individualisme libéral attaint dans le movement prolongéviste sa forme maximale puisque le droit de prolonger sa prend le pas sur la filiation. Selon Christine Overall, il n'existe, en effet, d'une point de vue individualiste, aucune raison valuable de mourir afin de laisser sa place à une nouvelle génération. (16)

It is possible for increased length of life to be thought of as delay in reaching, rather than the extension of, old age. However, the permanent delay of death is immortality.

In the modern world, longevity and the postponement of death are seen as desirable and to be within the realm of medicine and science. Technical advances, for example the possibility of genetic modification and other methods for establishing human control of biological ageing, seem to hold this out as a realistic possibility (25–31).

Biological theories and research on ageing

Thus, in the 20th century old age has become increasingly associated with the body. As a consequence, biological knowledge takes on a particularly powerful position in shaping the way old age is discussed and thought about. Knowledge of the fundamental biology of ageing in all living creatures, and human beings in particular, is making rapid gains. The field of biogerontology concentrates on intracellular processes, genes, complex molecules, and their transformations. Although such research uses standard models of yeast, worms, fruit flies, and mice, it is largely orientated to understanding human ageing (32–36).

In practice there is no unified theory of ageing within biology as a discipline. There are alternative theories with differing emphases; some highlight the importance of evolutionary explanations using evidence from different lifespans of naturally occurring species, other accounts give priority to ideas rooted in metabolic processes and the functioning of cells, and there are those whose starting point is identifying alleles which correlate with extended lifespan in humans and other experimental species (36–38). Emphasis on cellular ageing concentrates on the processes by which cells replace themselves. Discoveries in the 1950s established that normal cells have a definite limit to their capacity for replication. This phenomenon was conceptualized as 'ageing' at the cellular level. If we could understand how cells 'know' they are old, then perhaps this biological clock could be changed or turned off (39–41). Research into cellular ageing is one of the perceived routes to the scientific control of the biology of ageing. The main problem with translating the understanding of cellular ageing to an understanding of the human life course is the absence of a theoretical basis for generalizing from the constituent cellular parts to the whole person (42).

The politics of death itself

We can explore the cultural impact of biological science on ageing and death through a framework provided by Nikolas Rose in *The Politics of Life Itself* (24). The main thesis of this work is that in the contemporary world at the start of the 21st century, the way 'life itself' has come to be understood has changed. It has been biologized and reconstructed to lie at the subcellular and molecular level. The advances in biochemistry and the understanding of genetics and cell science have atomized the biology of life into a string of complex genetically-induced cascades of complex molecules. We can take this idea about the changing understanding of life and apply it to death. If life has been biologized, fragmented, reduced to a biochemical essence, and rendered political by new potentialities for control, then so too has death. This is the realm of anti-ageing science.

Rose's insightful analysis of the 'politics of life itself' reveals the problem of the 'politics of death itself' (24, 43). The policing and control of life, implies the same processes for death. Not only in the sense of avoiding death and prolonging life, but dealing with the inevitable fact of death. For all the culturally enwrapped denial, we all still die, and this fact has to be managed. The extent of the denial makes this a difficult task. As Lafontaine points out, death has been removed from the world of symbol, ritual, and meaning and turned into a mundane biological fact (16). As such, without its sacred quality and apparently subject to technical biological analysis and control it creates new problems of management. Rose suggests five processes through which to understand changes to 'the politics of life itself' (23). We can look at these in turn and examine what they mean for death in the post-mortal world. They are molecularization, optimization, subjectification, somatic expertise, and the economics of vitality.

The molecularization of death

According to Rose, the essential vitality which animates life is now seen as a molecular process. Modern biology focuses on intracellular biochemical processes and life becomes metabolism of complex molecules. Such 'molecular' life is potentially modifiable and replaceable. Molecularization, or at least modern cell science, has profoundly influenced contemporary understanding of death. Death at the cell level is understood through a number of cell processes involving complex macromolecules. These include 'apoptosis' and 'senescence' (44). However, these cell processes are not unproblematic images and contain metaphors for human death in old age (45).

In this fast moving field, both processes and terminology can be contentious (46–48). However, apoptosis—or 'programmed cell death'—dominate the textbook and teaching literature on cell death. Various internal and external triggers can set off a complex biochemical process involving specific enzymes called capases which shrink the cell, divide it into bits which can be digested by macrophages (the immune system) making the cells resources available for recycling, and cut up the chromosomes in ways which prevent them replicating inaccurately. Apoptosis has been a key development in cell science over the last years of the 20th century. Landecker has mapped some of its cultural significance (49).

> Although many commentators call the insistent presence of narratives of human death in cell death science anthropomorphism and comment on its 'danger' to the practice of science (Clark 1996; Debru 1998; Friedman and Brunet 1995), I believe that these narratives and their tensions point to a more complicated and more interesting role for the cell in contemporary biomedical culture than that of an irrational being incorrectly endowed with human qualities. The cell is a site through which all kinds of changing material, semantic, economic, and conceptual relationships are played out: cell to body, cells to one another, scientists to doctors, patients to laboratories. It is a site in which what it is to be cellular, in life, death, and disease, is constantly being produced. (57)

The biology textbooks and popular science media habitually describe apoptosis as cell suicide. Sometimes they call it murder (when the cell responds to external stimuli but I have only found one case where it is referred to as euthanasia) (50). However, apoptosis is clearly good death. It is a vital part of life and the continued health of the organism. It is a model of good death. It is the individual (cell) playing its part in the overall life of the body. Its death at the right time and the right place is a necessary and desirable outcome for the health of the multicellular soma (people's bodies). On the other hand *senescence* is the cell in old age. The metaphor is a powerful one even if the belief that there is a specific direct link to organism ageing is contentious. Historically in biology the meaning of senescence has shifted from a specific form of decline, loss of efficient function in all aspects, including the accumulation of 'junk', to being used specifically in the sense of replicative senescence—the cessation of mitosis (cell division). Even at the cellular level old age is imaged as bad (43).

Optimization

The second of Rose's themes is that of 'optimization'. He argues that life is no longer simply constrained within the parameters of health and illness, but that it can be manipulated in order to optimize such features as intelligence or longevity. He links these developments to a stress on 'functionality'—enhancing the body's ability to perform what the individual desires from it. The work of Katz and Marshall on the rise of Viagra and sexual functionality in old age is an excellent example (51). As all biofunctions are potentially modifiable, they can, from the post-mortal perspective, be custom-built or rebuilt to function more efficiently. Developments in stem cell research have certainly enhanced hopes for regenerative control of organs. Stem cell research holds out the possibility of replacing worn out or failed bits of the body by growing genetically matched replacements to be transplanted as the need arises (52). Cloning technology not only offers the prospect of cloning your favourite pet so it is replaced by a genetically identical substitute, it offers the possibility of reproducing yourself (53, 54). Death is seen as the ultimate loss of functionality. Optimization requires the body to overcome time and function for ever thus avoiding old age and death.

Politics and control of death

Rose's third theme is that of 'subjectification' and the individual's responsibility for body management. He argues that new ideas about 'life itself' influence what it is to be human in ethical terms. Thus 'the politics of life itself' in his title means the development of a biocitizenship with rights and duties for life, body and risk. He suggests this creates 'somatic ethics'—not ethics as moral precepts but as values about the conduct of a life placing the body and its management at the centre.

> The person, educated by disease awareness campaigns, understanding him- or herself at least in part in neurochemical terms, in conscientious alliance with health care professionals, and by means of niche-marketed pharmaceuticals, is to take control of these modulations in the name of maximizing his or her potential, recovering his or her self, shaping the self in fashioning a life. The forms being taken by contemporary neurochemical selfhood, the blurring of the boundaries between treatment, recovery, manipulation, and enhancement, are intimately entwined with the obligations of these new forms of life. They are intrinsic to the continuous task of monitoring, managing, and modulating our capacities that is the life's work of the contemporary biological citizen. (23)

Thus 'subjectification' relates to the individual's responsibility for how their body ages. Similarly, with death, biocitizenship implies responsibilities. Rose's argument about biocitizenship, the individual responsibility of citizens to maintain their bodies in a healthy state, to strive for bodily improvement with its implied image of perfection, leaves no place for death. Death becomes someone's fault, perhaps the individual who did not look after themselves properly, perhaps the expert who failed to prevent death from a specific disease. The *prologeviste* movement, those striving for immortality take this position to the logical conclusion: death is the ultimate failure, the final sin/dereliction of an individual. For example, Herb Bowie the author of *Why Die? A Beginner's Guide to Living Forever* provided the answers to 'Frequently Asked Questions About Living Forever' on his website (55).

> I tend to think that the 'secret' to living forever is to take advantage of many small, gradual advances. Research has already determined that many of the symptoms of so-called ageing are actually the results of a self-fulfilling prophecy: as people get older, they take gradual deterioration for granted, instead of trying to do something about it. Is it any wonder, then, that they do gradually go downhill? . . . I believe that the key is to change our consciousness – to revise our expectations and belief systems. This is the most fundamental change, and the one that will let us take advantage of all the other advances as they become available. (53)

From this perspective ageing becomes the fault of the individual. It is slackers, morally culpable people who do not follow the best practices of healthy living that will lose out on immortality and die.

Somantic expertise

Rose's next theme is that of somatic expertise which refers to the rights and responsibilities of others for biological control over our bodies. He identifies a professionalization of expertise concerning the body. There is a proliferation of sub-branches of biology and biochemistry and specialisms which control the technical expertise of these sciences. There is also professionalization of the pastoral response to life and death, experts who offer counselling and advice on how individuals should manage grief. Rose notes 'bioethics' as a new discipline in which people claim expertise with which to legitimate research and 'medical' activities:

> Critical analysis needs to move beyond the traditional dichotomies — free will versus determinism, society versus biology — for these cannot help us understand the relations of power, knowledge, ethics, and subjectification that are taking shape within these new practices of control. Instead, perhaps, a critical biopolitics of control needs to ask what are the benefits, what are the dangers, what are gains, and to whom, and what are the costs, and to whom, of strategies of control that seek to identify and govern biologically risky individuals in the name of public protection? (23)

Rose's analysis thus directs us to look at death managers and death avoidance experts and the role they play in policing death. We can divide policing death into two kinds, policing the dead and policing the survivors. Historically policing the dead was the apparatus of church and religion, the proper processing of souls to pass from this world to the next. In the modern secular world it becomes a health issue, hygienic disposal of corpses through properly sanctioned crematoria and prohibition of bodily disposal in any but authorized sites. In the UK, recent changes in law permit a variety of types and places of disposal but strictly under a licensing procedure to accommodate a growth in woodland burials, burials at sea, and other non-religious locations. In a world where death is a biological phenomenon stripped of meaning beyond the functioning of organs and the continuation of metabolism, strict rules about the hygienic disposal of soma are required.

The 'post-mortal' society creates new dilemmas and institutions in the policing of the dead (23). There are those who seek immortality through revival of the corpse when science has progressed to perform such miracles, in other words entrusting their body to future life and death experts. The most well developed of these is the cryonics industry with active facilities in both the USA and Russia (56, 57). Despite the absence of current technology for thawing out and resuscitating those that have chosen this method of bodily disposal, faith in the progress in science is felt to justify such procedures. An essential feature of cryonics is the location of the individual, the persona, personality, in the body, indeed in the brain, and that the preservation of the chemical constituents will preserve the essence of the person. Such a radical approach challenges a number of our key institutions, the legal system recognizes the frozen as dead, inheritance laws apply and there is no way of ensuring the revived are not destitute. The freezers are run by commercial firms who are just as liable to economic failure and bankruptcy as any other economic institution, thus potentially leaving immortality in the hands of administrators.

At a death we have institutions for policing the living. For example, we have institutions to manage the laws on succession and inheritance of property and status. We have judicial and law enforcement institutions to hold to account those who commit homicide. In the modern world psychological well-being of survivors—post-traumatic stress, grief counselling—has become an additional realm of professional expertise. However, individuals are expected to engage in personal self policing. In terms of 'somantic ethics' they have a responsibility for coming to terms with bereavement. The living are required to manage 'the mourning process'—the psychological process of consigning the dead to quiescent memory and there are psychological experts to help people through this process. To fail to do so in due time is to open up moral/medical accusations of being morbid, of insufficient self-control (58).

Policing, and self-policing of the living, also leads us to the realm of euthanasia and choice of one's death. Western culture, with its values of individualism and choice, produces a profound ambivalence to suicide. It is the ultimate act of individual control and choice. It is also in terms of somantic ethics the ultimate sin, destroying the material basis of existence. Euthanasia therefore might be seen as the converse of attempts at immortality such as cryonics. It involves both a rejection of the power of science and reason to solve the problem of disease and pain satisfactorily, and involves the abdication of self. Yet it involves the expression of individuality through choice—the ultimate choice to live or die.

The medical technicians at the scene of death have to work within the moral framework which gives them power and responsibility. They have to strive to avoid being blamed (59). Accidental death has no place in world where science is infallible; the mechanics of life and death are known to experts, someone must be culpable. The moral apparatus of the 'post-mortal' society seeks cause, and therefore blame, in the material facts of a material world scientifically understood, a world of cause and effect. Either the individual deceased is responsible for the cause, not engaging in the necessary risk management, or those responsible for not alerting the individual to making the correct 'safe' choices are at fault. In these circumstances a good death is not possible. Even euthanasia becomes a problematic answer to the construction of a moral death. Somatic expertise implies there must be a discernable cause behind the desire to die—whose failure is behind that desire? Candidates for culpability might include weakness in the moral standing of the individual, or weakness in the psychological make-up of the individual due to parental upbringing, or clinical failure on the part of medical technicians to control pain, to control the course of the illness, or failure of public authorities who have not yet devoted the resources which will (inevitably, eventually) find a cure (60).

Economics of vitality

The final theme from Rose is that of the economics of vitality (23). He suggests that the vital elements of life can be:

> decomposed into a series of distinct and discrete objects—that can be isolated, delimited, stored, accumulated, mobilized, and exchanged, accorded a discrete value, traded across time, space, species, context enterprises—in the service of many distinct objectives. (23).

Hence the idea of 'biovalue'. Biological knowledge and its techniques and products, protected by patents, can be used to generate wealth:

> Energized by the search for biovalue, novel links have formed between truth and capitalization, the demands for shareholder value and the human value invested in the hope for cure and optimality. (23)

This trend is clearly identifiable in the world of anti-ageing science and medicine. Biocapital is being sought by a wide range of anti-ageing entrepreneurs. The market serves as both source of capital and as outlet for consumer products. A good case example is that of the history of the search for a method of using teleomere science to create an anti-ageing therapy (61). Biovalue is the realm of the anti-ageing foundations—institutions which forge links between the scientist in the lab and the market (62). At one level the search for biovalue and ways to exploit it are based in the straightforward entrepreneurial profit motive. A patent on a once-a-day pill which enables you to live for ever is the ultimate cash machine. However, there is a more profound and subtle critique of capitalism in which biocapital can be seen as part of the objectification of people, undermining their humanity and dissolving human relationships and collective solidarity through the market. To the market, as with science, death is impersonal, mundane, and essentially trivial. Without a basis in community and ritual, death will always be unsatisfactory.

Anti-ageing science and time

We can now return to the theme of the cultural nature of time and its role in framing ageing and death. Biological ageing requires a sense of biological time—at what rate does the body age, how can we measure it? Biological time has to be independent from chronological time. In order to establish biological time we need biomarkers, points which indicate its forward march. Measuring functionality—'looking good for our age', 'looking 10 years younger', being 'fit for your age' requires appeal to such biomarkers. Culturally we are very familiar with the visible symbols we identify as signs of old age, grey hair, wrinkles, changes in posture, loss of hearing, eyesight, and mental acuity. The problem, over and above the key issue of defining someone's humanity by their visual appearance, is that these phenomena do not standardize into predictable chronological age with a high degree of accuracy. Finding objective indices of ageing which are independent of chronological time have proved difficult for biological science. In the USA, considerable scientific endeavour has gone into finding biomarkers for ageing in mice. However:

> The fact is, we do not have biomarkers that accurately predict life span in any creatures . . . despite 10 years' research and 20 million dollars from the American National Institute on Ageing funding — We haven't been successful. (63, see also 64)

Optimization can mean more than looking good, or being 'functional' for one's age. It contains an implicit view of the perfect body, the fully optimized body is one that never fails but is immortal. The construction is embedded in the concept of time inherent in modern science. In one sense the view of time as inevitably progressive underlies the optimization drive. Science is seen as making inevitable progress—the future is more knowledgeable than the past-history of science, the history of elimination of error. However, in an important sense, science is understood as outside of time. It is about the universal laws of nature, true for all time. The laws of nature are not seen as subject to time, to history, and to change. Once they are known it is assumed they always were and always will be the same. Thus in the Petri dish or under the election microscope, in an important sense there is no time. The specimens are archetypes, the knowledge produced is not limited to them, but conceptualized as true for all identical similar situations for all time. The scientific experiment seeks to hold all other things equal except the selected independent variable, which includes time. Time is not usually considered explicitly as it is viewed as constant and unvarying. Time and failure do not form part of the research record and publication memory. 'Failed' experiments are false, imperfect while the truth will live on forever. Perfection steps outside time. This is the world of the biogerontologists who see immortality as a practical project (53, 65, 66). It is a world without time; a world which exists in the laboratory at the level of the cell and biochemical processes which animate it. It is not a world with human relationships and history. The logic then becomes—when we discover the laws of life we will be able to prevent death forever because those laws never change. Perfect understanding creates immortal functionality and avoids death.

There are of course other scientific images of time. Time in the universe of theoretical physicists is not the view of time most people in the West would consider as 'common sense'. It is a specific view which challenges our culturally acquired understanding—by, for example, linking time, space, and velocity—in which it is possible for time to go faster or slower. Indeed this world of theoretical physics has its own anti-ageing device. The classic explanatory story used is that of two twins, one stays on earth, the other explores the cosmos at close to the speed of light, and when the traveller returns to earth he (stories are inevitably male) is younger than his twin (67).

Conclusion

Old age is the boundary between life and death. If these boundaries change so does the understanding of old age. Modern Western societies organize their response to old age around the concepts of science and medicine. As life becomes something to be biologized, essentialized, manipulated, and the subject of struggle and contest, so too does death. In the modern world, embedded in the belief in progressive science is the implication that it will provide the solution for death. Scientists claim to have the techniques for increasing human lifespan, if not exactly now, at least the potential for the future. Scientific medicine acts as if it should have, and eventually will, find the cure for death. For the medical technician every death represents a failure. The modern world and its dominant scientific modes of accounting and legitimizing knowledge have their share of the fountain of youth myths. Immortality, and the defeat of disease and injury are a common place of science fiction (68, 69). These cultural manifestations come from the same mind set as that which sees the goal of science as the elimination of death. The timeless individual has no age; the functionally perfect body does not die. In such a world we struggle to find rituals and to demarcate the sacred or anything meaningful in death.

References

1. Vincent JA (2006). Ageing contested: Anti-ageing science and the cultural construction of old age. *Sociology*, **40**(4): 681–98.
2. Elias N (1985). *The Loneliness of the Dying*. Oxford: Blackwell.
3. Vincent JA (1995). *Inequality and Old Age*. London: University College Press.
4. Berndt CH, Berndt RM (1983). *The Aboriginal Australians: the First Pioneers*, 2nd edn. Victoria: Pitman.
5. Sharp L (1952). Steel axes for Stone Age Australians. In E Spicer (ed) *Human Problems in Technological Change*, pp. 69–90. New York: Russell Sage Foundation.
6. Tonkinson R (2002). *The Mardu Aborigines: Living the Dream in Australia's Desert*. London: Thomson.
7. De Bary TAL, Bashar RN, Dandekar N (1958). *Sources of Indian Tradition*. New York: Columbia University Press.
8. Bailey FG (1971). The peasant view of the bad life. In T Shanin (ed) *Peasants and Peasant Societies* pp. 299–321. Harmondsworth: Penguin.
9. Amoss PT, Harrell S (eds) (1981). *Other Ways of Growing Old: Anthropological Perspectives*, Stanford, CA: Stanford University Press.

10. Holmes ER, Holmes LD (1995). *Other Cultures, Elder Years*, 2nd edn. Thousand Oaks, CA: Sage Publications.

11. Keith J (1994). *The Ageing Experience: Diversity and Commonality across Cultures*. London: Sage Publications.

12. Palgi P (1984). Death; A cross-cultural perspective. *Annual Review of Anthropology*, **13**: 385–417.

13. Barley N (1995). *Dancing on the Grave: Encounters with Death*. London: John Murray.

14. Lienhardt G (1961). *Divinity and Experience: the Religion of the Dinka*. Oxford: Clarendon Press.

15. Woolley O (2002). *The Earth Shakers of Madagascar*. London: Continuum.

16. Lafontaine C (2008). *La Société Post-Mortelle*. Paris: Seuil.

17. Habermas J (2003). *The Future of Human Nature*. Oxford: Polity.

18. Foucault M (1973). *The Birth of the Clinic* (trans. AM Sheridan). London: Routledge.

19. Turner BS (1984). *The Body and Society: Explorations in Social Theory*. Oxford: Blackwell.

20. Shilling C (1993). *The Body and Social Theory*. London: Sage.

21. Hancock P, Hughes W, Jagger E, Paterson K, Russell R, Tulle Winton E, et al (2000). *The Body, Culture and Society*. Buckingham: Open University Press.

22. Faircloth CA (2003). *Ageing Bodies: Images and Everyday Experience*, Walnut Creek, CA: AltaMira.

23. Howson A (2004). *The Body in Society*. Oxford: Polity.

24. Rose N (2007). *The Politics of Life Itself: Biomedicine, Power and Subjectivity in the Twenty-First Century*. Princeton, NJ: Princeton University Press.

25. Benecke M (2002). *The Dream of Eternal Life: Biomedicine, Ageing and Immortality*. New York: Columbia University Press.

26. Fukuyama F (2002). *Our Posthuman Future: Consequences of the Biotechnology Revolution*. New York: Farrar, Straus and Giroux.

27. Harris J (2000). Intimations of immortality. *Science*, **288**(5463): 59.

28. Olshansky SJ, Carnes BA (2001). *The Quest for Immortality: Science at the Frontiers of Ageing*. New York: W.W. Norton & Co.

29. Post SG, Binstock RH (2004). *The Fountain of Youth: Cultural, Scientific, and Ethical Perspectives on a Biomedical Goal*. Oxford: Oxford University Press.

30. Warner H, Anderson J, Austad S, Bergamini E, Bredesen D, Butler R, et al. (2005). Science fact and the SENS agenda: What can we reasonably expect from ageing research? *EMBO reports*, **6**(11): 1006–8.

31. Turner BS (2007). Culture, technologies and bodies: The technological Utopia of living forever. In Shilling C (ed) *Embodying sociology: Retrospect, progress and prospects*, pp.19–36. Oxford: Blackwell.

32. Bramstedt KA (2001). Scientific breakthroughs: Cause or cure of the ageing 'problem'. *Gerontology*, **47**: 52–54.

33. Butler RN, Warner HR, Williams TF, Austad SN, Brody JA, Campisi J, et al. (2004). The ageing factor in health and disease: The promise of basic research on ageing. *Ageing Clinical and Experimental Research*, **16**: 104–11.

34. Holliday R (2000). Ageing research in the next century. *Biogerontology*, **1**: 97–101.

35. Westendorp R, Kirkwood T (2007). The biology of ageing. In J Bond, S Peace, F Dittmann-Kohli, G Westerhof (eds.) *Ageing in Society*, pp. 15–37. London: Sage.

36. Carey JR (2003). *Longevity: The Biology and Demography of Life Span*. Princeton, NJ: Princeton University Press.

37. Arking R (2006). *The Biology of Ageing: Observations and Principles*. New York: Oxford University Press.

38. Holliday R (2007). *Ageing: The Paradox of Life: Why We Age*. Berlin: Springer.

39. Hayflick L (2000). The future of ageing. *Nature*, **408**: 267–9.

40. Finch C (2007). Cellular and molecular causes of ageing. In *The Future of Human Healthspan: Demography, Evolution, Medicine, and Bioengineering*. [Internet] The National Academies, Keck Futures

Initiatives, September 27, 2007. Available at: http://www.keckfutures.org/conferences/healthspan/webcast.html. (Accessed 5 November 2007.)

41. Arkus N (2005). A mathematical model of cellular apoptosis and senescence through the dynamics of telomere loss. *Journal of Theoretical Biology*, **235**(1): 13–32.

42. Faragher RG (2000). Cell senescence and human ageing: where's the link? *Biochemical Society Transactions*, **28**(2), 221–6.

43. Rose N (2001). The politics of life itself. *Theory, culture & society*, **18**(6): 1–30.

44. Lockshin RA, Zakeri Z (1996). The biology of cell death and its relationship to ageing. In NJ Holbrook, GR Martin, RA Lockshin (eds.) *Cellular Ageing and Cell Death, Modern Cell Biology*, pp.167–80. New York: Wiley & Sons.

45. Vincent JA (2008). The cultural construction old age as a biological phenomenon: Science and anti-ageing technologies. *Journal of Ageing Studies*, **22**(4): 331–9.

46. Lockshin RA, Zakeri Z (2001). Programmed cell death and apoptosis: origins of the theory. *Nature Reviews Molecular Cell Biology*, **2**(7): 545–50.

47. Levin S, Bucci TJ, Cohen SM, Fix AS, Hardisty JF, LeGrand EK, et al. (1999). The nomenclature of cell death: Recommendations of an ad hoc Committee of the Society of Toxicologic Pathologists. *Toxicologic Pathology* **27**(4): 484–90.

48. Fietta P (2006). Many ways to die: Passive and active cell death styles. *Rivista di Biologia-Biology Forum*, **99**(1): 69–83.

49. Landecker H (2003). On beginning and ending with apoptosis. In S Franklin, M Lock (eds) *Remaking Life and Death*, pp.23–60. Oxford: James Currey.

50. Raloff J (2001). Coming to terms with death: Accurate descriptions of a cell's demise may offer clues to diseases and treatments. *Science News Online*, **159**(1): 378.

51. Katz S, Marshall BL (2004). Is the functional 'normal'? Ageing, sexuality and the bio-marking of successful living. *History of The Human Sciences*, **17**(1): 53–75.

52. Rando TA (2006). Stem cells, ageing and the quest for immortality. *Nature*, **441**: 1080–6.

53. Harris J (1998). *Clones, Genes and Immortality*, 2nd edn. Oxford: Oxford University Press.

54. Shostak S (2002). *Becoming Immortal: Combining Cloning and Stem-Cell Therapy*. Albany, New York: State University of New York Press.

55. Bowie H (1998). 'Frequently Asked Questions (and Answers!) About Living Forever', publicity poster by Herb Bowie on 12 November 1998 for Bowie H (1997). *Why Die?: A Beginner's Guide to Living Forever*. PowerSurge Publishing.

56. *The Guardian Weekend*, 7 November 2009, 51–9.

57. Cryonics Institute (2009). http://www.cryonics.org. (Accessed 25 June 2009.)

58. Johnson CJ, McGee M (2004). Psychosocial aspects of death and dying. *Gerontologist* **44**: 719–22.

59. Seymour JE (2000). Negotiating natural death in intensive care. *Social Science & Medicine*, **21**(8): 1241–52.

60. Vincent JA (2003). *Old Age*. London: Routledge.

61. Hall SS (2003). *Merchants of Immortality: Chasing the Dream of Human Life Extension*. Boston, MA: Houghton Mifflin.

62. Rabinow P, Dan-Cohen T (2005). *A Machine to Make a Future: Biotech Chronicles*. Princeton, NJ: Princeton University Press.

63. Krondracke M (2003). #09—Biomarkers of Aging: Do they hold the key in the search for the fountain of youth? Original Webcast Date: October 28, 2003, 10 a.m. Available at: http://www.sagecrossroads.net/node/74.

64. Krondracke M (2008). #48—Biomarkers of Aging—How are we going to find biomarkers of aging? Original Webcast Date: July 30, 2008. Available at:http://www.sagecrossroads.net/sagecast48.

65. de Grey A (2003). The foreseeability of real anti-ageing medicine: focusing the debate. *Experimental Gerontology*, **38**(9): 927–34.

66. de Grey A (2007). The natural biogerontology portfolio—'Defeating ageing' as a multi-stage ultra-grand challenge. In SIS Rattan, S Akman (eds) *Biogerontology: Mechanisms and Interventions*, **1100**, 409–23. Proceedings of 5th European Congress of Biogerontology, 16–20 September 2006, Istanbul, Turkey.

67. Debs TA, Redhead MLG (1996). The twin 'paradox' and the conventionality of simultaneity. *American Journal of Physics*, **64**: 384–92.

68. Boia L (2004). *Forever Young: A Cultural History of Longevity*. London: Reaktion Books.

69. Slusser G, Westfahl G, Rabkin ES (eds.) (1996). *Immortal Engines: Life Extension and Immortality in Science Fiction and Fantasy*. Athens, GA: University of Georgia Press.

Chapter 4

The challenges of health technology for ageing and dying

Jane Seymour and Merryn Gott

Introduction

The relentless advance of biomedical technology across the course of the last 50 years has fundamentally altered the encounters we have with ageing, dying, and death (1). The use of technology to diagnose, manage, and treat illness, to try to hold back signs of ageing or to defer entry to the dying phase, is so widespread that it has assumed a taken for granted backdrop to all experiences of health and illness. This process of 'medicalization' has resulted in ageing, dying, and death becoming malleable, sometimes even reversible, and subject to human intention and action in ways never imagined possible in previous times (2). Yet medicalization and its impacts are surrounded by paradoxes. For example, on the one hand, we place high value on concepts of 'natural' ageing or 'natural' death, using language such as 'nature taking its course', 'dying naturally', 'ageing gracefully', and other such terms to represent our desire to age or to die unfettered by what might be seen as the 'prison' of medical technology. On the other hand, we rely fundamentally on technologies, even if these are somewhat hidden or unobtrusive, to produce these ideal images: the use of hormone replacement therapy to offset the female ageing process or the use of discrete modes of pain relief during terminal illness are perhaps typical examples. In relation to critical illness, the physician and sociologist Arthur Frank (3) has noted how we, at one and the same time, often welcome and reject technology: 'high tech medicine offers real hopes, [but] resistance to "dying on a machine" is itself resisted by wanting what that machine might offer'.

As a result of these paradoxes and tensions, the predictable relationship between 'dying' and 'death' has become disrupted (4). In the past, serious illness led to death relatively quickly and there were clear expectations of what the journey would be like. Now, with the rise of what has been called the 'indistinct zone' of chronic illness and the concentration of death in older age (5), it is possible to live for a long time with even very serious illness; death may occur relatively unexpectedly. As a result, appropriate plans for end of life care and transitions to palliative care for those who are likely to die may be either delayed or never completed, with the resultant outcome that quality of care and experience during dying falls far short of the ideal (6). The 'protracted and negotiated death' (7) has taken the place of something which used to be short and unproblematic at least from an ethical, if not a personal, point of view.

Aims of this chapter

This chapter examines how these issues intersect to influence the circumstances in which older people die and some key ethical and moral debates that surround some critical issues of decision-making at the end of life. To begin with, we briefly examine the implications of the expansion of new health technologies for death, dying, and ageing.

Technology and death: a paradigm shift

In the developed world, even when it is recognized that death is a likely outcome of disease or injury, widespread access to life-support technologies, defined as those drugs, medical devices, and medical and nursing procedures that keep individuals alive who would otherwise die within a foreseeable, but usually uncertain period of time (8), may radically transform the life expectancy of some potentially dying people from the few days or weeks usually associated with a terminal disease to the several months or years more often associated with a chronic disease (9). Lock, in her study of death and organ transplantation in North America and Japan (10), has referred to this revolution as a 'paradigm shift' in which the old certainties about ageing, dying, and death have been swept away and many clinical, ethical, and social uncertainties about the relative benefits and burdens of new healthcare technologies have taken their place.

Debates about the benefits and burdens of using life-support technologies have been particularly vociferous in the case of older people. For some commentators the use of these may mean a prolongation of dying among those whose life is drawing to a 'natural close' (11) or may mean that there are less resources to spend on other younger people who have not yet had the chance to live out their 'normal' life span (12). Others argue that older people should be afforded equal access to chances of extending and enhancing their lives through the use of life prolonging care, even in situations of terminal illness (13). In a detailed and prophetic assessment made in 1987 of the implications of the ubiquitous use of life sustaining treatments, the US Office of Technology Assessment (8) reported that:

> As the population ages, as once 'extraordinary' measures become commonplace, and as ever more powerful technologies emerge it becomes increasingly important to understand the problems as well as the potential associated with the use of these technologies and to devise policies that reflect this understanding. (8)

Life-sustaining technologies and their impact on ageing

It is noted in the report from the US Office of Technology Assessment (8) that while many of the consequences of the widespread use of life-sustaining technologies are similar across all age groups, there are important factors which make people in older age groups subject to special consideration, including:

- Older people are more likely to be at risk of life-threatening illness than younger people.
- Older people who experience life-threatening illness are more likely to have coexisting comorbidities that affect their quality of life and functioning.
- Older people are more likely to have cognitive impairment due to dementia, depression, or drug toxicity.
- Many health and social care professionals are poorly prepared to look after seriously ill older people, whose needs may be very different to those of younger people.
- Older people are likely to be the largest group of consumers of healthcare costs.
- Older people are more likely than others to have contemplated the meaning and value of life and its end (8).

Seventeen years after this report was published, similar conclusions were reached by the World Health Organization (WHO) regarding the palliative care needs of older people (6). The WHO also highlighted that older people frequently experience serious and life-threatening illness against a backdrop of social isolation, physical or mental impairment, and economic hardship, producing cumulative disadvantage. The current cohort of people in late old age (over 85 years) is particularly affected by the socially structured character of illness.

People who are now in late old age are much more likely than the upcoming generation to be disabled by physical or mental illness due partly to the disadvantages and poor life chances they have faced during the upheavals of the 20th century (14). The three key factors that will affect how all older people experience the last stage of life, regardless of their prior biography, are: 1) health and disability-related impairment (both physical and cognitive); 2) housing circumstances, and 3) family and (informal) carer circumstances (15).

As we see elsewhere in other chapters in this volume, increasing age is not always and necessarily associated with physical illness, disability, or frailty. Compared to their parents, many older people can look forward to many more years of active old age and increased life expectancy (16). However, predications of future demands for support by key disease groups (dementia, stroke, coronary heart disease, and arthritis) indicate a picture of rapid growth. For example, the UK has been shown to be likely to have a 67% increase in the numbers of people with disability due to these causes by 2025 (17). This means that making plans for care and support during older age and at the end of life are imperative, both at an individual level and at the level of health and social care systems. This is a recurring theme in many chapters of this book. In this chapter, we focus particularly on matters of end of life decision-making since these most clearly reveal issues of relevance to new technologies of healthcare. In the next section, we examine some key ethical debates in this field before turning to explore the views and experiences of older people about these issues.

End of life decision-making and older people

In the same way that clinical, social, and economic circumstances encountered by older people vary, so too do their preferences for styles of end of life care. As Jennett notes:

> Some elderly patients face the prospect of death with equanimity, and may say that have had a good innings and don't wish for aggressive treatment. On the other hand, others are willing to accept higher risks of mortality associated with intervention than younger patients might. Yet others confronted with the possibility of survival after treatment with a considerably reduced quality of life are pleased to extend their lives on terms that might be unacceptable to a younger patient. It is therefore unwise to predict which way individual patients will react to the benefits and risks associated with interventions. (8)

One of the central problems in all clinical decision-making relating to end of life care is the fluctuation and variability not only in personal wishes and preferences, but in individuals' abilities to express these. People may have fluctuating capacity and competence to make informed decisions about options for care and treatment, or they may have never discussed or made known their values and preferences of relevance to their care and treatment at the end of life; this makes determination of their best interests extremely complex.

Prognostication

Pervasive prognostic uncertainty—what the outcome will be of any particular decision—overarches individual issues of decision-making and the stances that people may take towards their role within the decision-making process. The conjunction of this with the structural bias towards continuation of high technology medical treatments and a general cultural reluctance to anticipate and discuss issues of end of life care (18) compound decision-making dilemmas. The sociologist and physician Christakis (19) has noted how what he calls a 'key' task of medicine has been eclipsed since the end of the 19th century by the dual emphasis on diagnosis and therapy.

Christakis argues that a re-emphasis on prognostication—which he defines as the process of 'foretelling' i.e. forming an expert judgment about the likely course of an illness and then using excellent communication skills to discuss this with the individual concerned and their family—is vital if care and treatment options and goals are to be assessed, planned, and evaluated and better end of life care achieved (19). Yet research evidence suggests that doctors are poorly prepared to 'foretell', find it stressful to engage in prognostic conversations with their patients and perceive that they have not received appropriate training to do so (20). On the other hand, patients tend to wait for doctors to initiate a discussion about their future care and treatment and are sometimes confused and baffled when this does not occur, believing erroneously that their condition is perhaps less serious than they had first thought (21, 22). The reconstruction of progressive illness and death as 'failures' is largely behind this problem of missed opportunities for communication and discussion in advance of the dying phase. The outcome is often that crisis driven decision-making pervades both the care of individuals at the end of life and wider service delivery.

These issues in prognostication reflect the fact that communication in the whole area of death, dying, and bereavement has always been a problem for the health care professions; 'getting it right' in these sensitive areas remains a considerable challenge, perhaps especially where care of older people is concerned. It is clear that nurses, in similar ways to doctors, tend to feel unprepared for situations which require them to respond to questions and discussions about death and dying (23). Dealing with questions from patients and relatives is a source of stress and discomfort, and many nurses will talk about needing emotional detachment, particularly after having upsetting experiences. In one study (24) based on interviews with nurses about how they dealt with topics related to death, dying, and meaning raised by dementia patients, nurses reported that they tended to ignore the topic, distract the person, refer to God's control in relation to dying, or respond by showing and giving affection to the older person.

Other chapters in this book examine how these issues play out in advance care planning: the process by which individuals are helped to discuss their values, wishes, and preferences for care and to record, in advance of any loss of capacity or communication ability, a statement to inform care and treatment decision-making. In this chapter, we look at three key issues (25) surrounding contemporaneous decision-making at the end of life: 1) the debates regarding the legalization of assisted dying, 2) the distinction between 'killing' and 'letting die', and lastly, 3) the issue of autonomy, paying attention in each case to their particular significance in end of life decision-making in the case of older people. We refer where relevant especially to the situation of those with dementia who can no longer voice their own best interest decisions.

Assisted dying

Assisted dying encompasses voluntary euthanasia and assisted suicide, whether physician or non-physician assisted suicide. In the last 10 to 15 years, debates about the legalization of assisted dying have featured in most of the countries of the developed world, with legalization of assisted dying of one form or another in some states of the USA, Switzerland, Belgium, and the Netherlands. In a widely accepted consensus statement, euthanasia and physician assisted suicide (probably the most common type of assisted suicide) have been defined thus:

> Euthanasia is killing on request and is defined as: a doctor intentionally killing a person by the administration of drugs at that person's voluntary and competent request.
>
> Physician assisted suicide is defined as: a doctor intentionally helping a person to commit suicide by providing drugs for self administration, at that person's voluntary and competent request. (26)

In a sociological analysis of the trends towards legalization of assisted dying, Howarth and Jefferys observed some years ago that 'the current debate . . . is at least partly about agency, about who does and who should control the decisions to hasten or procure death' (27). Those who take a strongly pro-assisted stance see it as protecting patients' rights against the decision-making power of the medical profession. However, many commentators take the opposite position, arguing that legalization of assisted dying is likely to undermine the patients' rights and lead to some people requesting death because of fears of being a burden or worries that their lives have less value than those of others. This 'slippery slope' argument has been observed to be especially relevant to people with disabilities or chronic illnesses, who will often be older people. The fact that there persists a lack of equality of access to the resources that might ensure quality of life even in the face of great impairment, means that fears of discrimination and exclusion from good care are present in the minds of many who oppose legalization. In his discussion of how the disability rights movement has engaged with this issue, Shakespeare draws attention to how these themes coalesce in the concerns of people with disabilities, quoting the reflections of Ed Roberts, a US disability activist, on his situation:

> I've been on a respirator for twenty-six years, and I watch these people's cases. They're just as dependent on a respirator as I am. The major difference is that they know they are going to be forced to live in a nursing home—or they're already there—and I'm leading a quality of life. That's the only difference. It's not the respirator. It's the money. (28)

Shakespeare points out that, for many people with disabilities, the assisted dying debate gives out implicit messages that their lives may be inferior to those of others, while the oft used strap line of the right to die movement—'death with dignity'—sends out messages that those who are dependent on others for assistance or care can perhaps only achieve dignity in death (28). In a memorandum submitted as evidence to the House of Lords Select Committee on Assisted Dying for the Terminally Ill, a disabled peer and leader of the disability rights movement in the UK, Dr Jane Campbell, eloquently details a number of problems with equality of access to health and social care, which mean that 'choices' about assisted dying are unlikely to be fully informed and 'free' in the cases of people with disabilities and impairment:

> Assisted Dying might be a viable alternative if good quality palliative and social care becomes available across the country. At present this kind of support is patchy at best. If someone chooses death in the absence of such support, their decision is likely to be influenced by this fact. . . . While the Assisted Dying Bill aims to address the needs of patients in the last stage of their lives, I am concerned about the underlying message of the Bill that death is the preferable solution for people severely incapacitated or in pain. Much the same message is communicated to older people who fear being a burden to others, and to terminally ill and disabled people with inadequate care packages. These views will be legitimized if the law is changed to concede that they might be better off dead (29).

However, evidence from the Netherlands where euthanasia has been permissible since 2002 suggests that there has not been a rapid increase in the numbers of disabled or older people either receiving or requesting death. In fact, there is some evidence of a slight downward trend in the incidence of registered euthanasia deaths. Some commentators suggest that this is because, once the fight to legalize euthanasia was won, a space was created for the development of palliative care techniques (30). It is likely that vociferous debates will continue, albeit with similar concerns about quality of life, the best way to relieve suffering, and the nature of the 'good death', on both sides of the fence. Different countries are likely to find different solutions to the shared problems wrought by the conjunction of biomedical advance and the increase in ageing, disability, and chronic illness.

Killing or letting die?

As Pabst-Battin (19) indicates, there is a huge literature devoted to the analysis of the distinction, or lack of distinction, between the concepts of 'killing' and 'letting die'. Supporters of the conceptual distinction point to the widely employed differentiation between the withholding or withdrawal of life-supporting treatments to allow a pre-existing terminal condition to cause death (letting die), and assisted dying which involves (as we have described above) an act, for example, the administration of a drug, which results directly in the death of the person to whom the drug is given (killing). In the UK, one of the most pivotal cases that led to a fundamental review of end of life decision-making was that of Tony Bland[1] who was fatally injured in the Hillsborough football ground disaster of 1989. Bland was 19 years old when he was crushed at Hillsborough; he remained in a persistent vegetative state until 1994 when, at the request of his parents and following a prolonged legal battle, his feeding tube was withdrawn and he died.

The case of Anthony Bland pushed forward the establishment of a House of Lords Select Committee on Medical Ethics, which reported in 1994. The committee ruled that Bland's death was a case of 'double-effect' in which death was an unintended, although not unforeseen, consequence of the removal of futile life-prolonging medical therapy (31). This judgement on the Bland case led to a clarification of the distinction between 'killing' and 'letting die', with the recommendation made that where death is inevitable, then life-prolonging treatments such as resuscitation, artificial ventilation, dialysis, artificial nutrition and hydration can be withdrawn or withheld, and the goal of medicine redirected to the palliation of symptoms and the provision of 'basic care' and comfort, which are mandatory (32).

As we noted in the introduction to this chapter, among many older people—especially those who survive to late old age—there may be no definable moment at which 'dying' commences and the complex factors which lead to death can only be understood retrospectively (33). As a result, increasingly it is older people who constitute the majority of those who exist betwixt and between life and death in critical care units and other acute hospital care environments, where making decisions to 'let die' are of particular relevance. However, it should be noted that the general difficulty in establishing the wishes of people who are approaching death means that they are vulnerable to both over- *and* undertreatment, especially where opportunities have not been taken to discuss prognostic and diagnostic information with the individual and his/her family at an earlier stage. In this situation, 'letting die' is less relevant than whether appropriate standards of best clinical practice have been followed to ensure the best chances of survival or the most comfortable death possible. A report published in 2009 in the UK about of the care of patients

---

[1] 'Since April 15, 1989, Anthony Bland has been in persistent vegetative state. He lies in Airedale General Hospital in Keighley, fed liquid food by a pump through a tube passing through his nose and down the back of his throat into the stomach. His bladder is emptied through a catheter inserted through his penis, which from time to time has caused infections requiring dressing and antibiotic treatment. His stiffened joints have caused his limbs to be rigidly contracted so that his arms are tightly flexed across his chest and his legs unnaturally contorted. Reflex movements in the throat cause him to vomit and dribble. Of all this, and the presence of members of his family who take turns to visit him, Anthony Bland has no consciousness at all. The parts of his brain which provided him with consciousness have turned to fluid. The darkness and oblivion which descended at Hillsborough will never depart. His body is alive, but he has no life in the sense that even the most pitifully handicapped but conscious human being has a life. But the advances of modern medicine permit him to be kept in this state for years, even perhaps for decades.' Extract from *Airedale NHS Trust v. Bland (C.A.)*, 19 February 1993, 2 Weekly Law Reports, p. 350, of Hoffman's description of Bland.

who died in hospital within 4 days of admission (34) reveals very clearly that poor communication and poor clinical judgments often surround the care of acutely, seriously, and critically ill older people: on the one hand it seems that ageist attitudes mean that they are sometimes treated with less urgency that younger people might be and are not appropriately referred to senior or specialist staff, while on the other hand, they are sometimes given unnecessarily invasive and futile treatments immediately prior to death.

Where older people are not acutely or critically ill, but rather in a situation of progressive 'dwindling' towards death, then an especially pertinent decision surrounding their care and treatment (as in the case of Anthony Bland) is the provision, withholding, or withdrawal of artificial feeding and hydration, because of the ease with which this treatment can be provided across hospital, home, hospice, or nursing home environments. An examination of the issues here also highlights those that are likely to apply in the context of other types of health technology. A recent systematic review of research among patients with dementia shows that there is inconclusive evidence that artificial feeding by enteral tube provides any benefit in dementia patients in terms of survival time, mortality risk, quality of life, nutritional parameters, physical functioning, and improvement or reduced incidence of pressure ulcers (35). Furthermore, commentators have observed that the need for restraint in older people with dementia who are being artificially fed is a significant contributor to their suffering during the final period of their lives and may lead to increased use of the 'chemical cosh' (36). On the other hand, others have argued strongly that artificial nutrition should be provided on ethical, social, and biographical grounds. Concerns voiced by the family of dying people may be particularly powerful. For example, Kedziera (37) provides an example of an older man dying from cancer who, with his wife, had been a victim of the holocaust. His wife found the idea of discontinuing food and fluids inconceivable and therefore he was supported with artificial feeding until he died. In England and Wales, the code of conduct underpinning the Mental Capacity Act provides helpful guidance about how to balance these competing clinical, social, and existential issues in care decision-making for people who have lost capacity of all ages and at all stages of illness (38), with the essential point being to follow a process of consultation and consensus building about the best course of action in any individual case, rather than making 'blanket decisions' for particular groups of patients.

Autonomy

Where older people retain capacity, it is usually assumed that they will wish to be autonomous in relation to decisions about their care and treatment. However, many older people may not necessarily either be able or will wish to join in the widespread exhortation to 'be assertive' or 'take control' of decisions relating to their care and treatment, which policy and practice discourse tends to demand. Empirical research has found that older people tend to take heterogeneous stances towards decision-making and that their abilities (and indeed wishes) to be 'autonomous' often depend on the context in which they find themselves. For example, a valuable study conducted in the Netherlands (39) followed the cases of 22 hospitalized older people and examined their perspectives on the choices they were faced with at this time. Although the study did not explicitly address end of life care, it has much to tell us of relevance:

◆ Hospital routines meant that the views and values of older people were often not accommodated into decision-making, in spite of the well meaning efforts of individual staff. This diminished patients' influence on what happened to them and made it difficult for doctors to think about what was in a patient's best interests.

◆ There was little attention to a model of collaborative decision-making, in which information is exchanged between doctors and patients during the various phases of decision-making.

This should be understood as having four phases: establishing a relationship, reaching agreement on what the problem and the goals of treatment are; selecting an approach to treatment; deciding which interventions to use; and evaluation and following-up.

◆ Some patients preferred to play a passive role in decision-making. They preferred to 'entrust' their care to doctors. It is argued that that we should respect this type of choice and ensure that the trust is enhanced. Ways of achieving this may include training clinicians to listen to patients and express concern and compassion and paying attention to the organization of care to ensure relationship continuity.

As Lloyd has observed in an essay on ageing and the ethics of care (33), we lack both the language and a set of policies that might adequately address the nature of social justice or inform the sensitive delivery of care for those who are dependent upon others or who do not wish to assert their own interests (33).

Conclusion

One the of the most significant challenges facing modern medicine is how to ensure advances in available technological expertise are translated into improved patient experience. For older people, this balance is particularly difficult to achieve. Medicine, and the technology that supports medical practice, is driven by an ethic of cure, often with scant regard as to what 'cure' may mean for patients and their families. In a similar way, ageing is increasingly framed as a problem with a potential technological solution, rather than a natural process, the only inevitable outcome of which is death. Technologies of end of life care have largely been developed in the absence of critical sociological debate and reflection, with the inevitable result being that current practice is driven by what can be done, rather than what, as a humane society, we feel should be done. The responsibility for end of life decision-making is typically placed upon individual (older) patients and their families who are asked to weigh up the pros and cons of technologies they do not understand, in situations of crisis. A cure culture also limits the ability of health professionals to respond to the needs of patients in these situations; modern medicine lacks a language that enables health professionals to engage in end of life discussions with any degree of confidence or comfort. Within this context, the apparent rise in popular support for legalized assisted dying internationally is unsurprising. For many people, assisted dying appears to offer the only option to deploy technology in such a way that ensures end of life choices can be guaranteed. However, as we have argued, within an 'unequal' society we cannot ensure that such decisions are context free; the ageism inherent in contemporary societies means that older people in particular may feel under pressure to end their lives prematurely. This danger needs to be made visible and not masked by a rhetoric of agency and choice. Indeed, there is an urgent need to bring all these issues into the public consciousness and for each country to develop a coherent socio-legal and ethical framework to guide end of life decision-making rooted in the values of their unique population. However, of universal concern must be ensuring a prominent voice for older people, whose experience is of most relevance and to whom such concerns are most pertinent.

Acknowledgement

This chapter draws in part on a plenary lecture delivered in 2006 to the British Sociological Association (Medical Sociology Group) and published in 2007 as: Seymour, JE (2007). Windows on suffering: sociological perspectives on end of life care. *Medical Sociology Online,* November, (2): 2. Available at: http://www.medicalsociologyonline.org/.

References

1. Webster A (2006). New technologies in health care: opening the black bag. In A Webster (ed) *New technologies in health care. Challenge, change and innovation*, pp. 1–8. Basingstoke: Palgrave Macmillan.

2. Seymour J (1999). Revisiting medicalisation and 'natural' death. *Social Science and Medicine*, **49**: 691–704.

3. Frank A (1995). *The wounded storyteller. Body, illness and ethics*. London and Chicago: University of Chicago Press.

4. Field D (1996). Awareness and modern dying. *Mortality*, **1**: 255–65.

5. Lynn J (2005). Living long in fragile health: The new demographics shape end of life care. *Hastings Center Report*, **35**: S14–S18.

6. Davies E, Higginson I (2004). *Better Palliative Care for Older People*. Copenhagen: World Health Organization Europe.

7. Meier DM, Morrison S (1999). Old age and care near the end of life. *Generations*, Spring, 6–11.

8. Office of Technology Assessment (1987). *Life sustaining technologies and the elderly*, Washington, DC: US Government Printing Office.

9. Jennett B (1995). High technology therapies and older people. *Ageing and Society*, **15**: 185–98.

10. Lock M (1996). Displacing suffering: the reconstruction of death in North America and Japan. Daedalus. *Journal of the American Academy of Arts and Sciences*, **125**: 206–44.

11. Justice C (1995). The 'natural' death while not eating: a type of palliative care in Banaras, India. *Journal of Palliative Care*, **11**: 38–42.

12. Callahan D (1987). *Setting limits: Medical goals in an ageing society*. New York: Simon and Schuster.

13. Department of Health (2001). *The national service framework for older people*. London: HMSO.

14. Seymour JE, Witherspoon R, Gott M, Ross H, Payne S (2005). *End of life care: promoting comfort, choice and well being among older people facing death*. Bristol: Policy Press.

15. Doran T, Drever F, Whitehead M (2003). Health of young and elderly informal carers: Analysis of UK census data. *British Medical Journal*, **327**: 1388.

16. Age Concern (2007). *Perspectives and priorities among older people in rural areas: The research base*. London: Age Concern.

17. Jagger C, Matthews R, Spiers N, Brayne C, Comas-Herrera A, Robinson T, et al. (2006). *Compression or expansion of disability? Forecasting future disability levels under changing patterns of diseases. Wanless Social Care Review Research Report*. Leicester: Leicester Nuffield Research Unit, University of Leicester.

18. Seymour JE, French J, Richardson E (2010). Dying matters: let's talk about it. *British Medical Journal*, **341**: c4860.

19. Christakis N (1999). *Death Foretold: prophecy and prognosis in medical care*. Chicago, IL: University of Chicago Press.

20. Christakis N, Iwashyna T (1998). Attitude of self reported practice regarding prognostication in a national sample of internists. *Archives of Internal Medicine*, **158**: 2389–95.

21. Steinhauser KE, Christakis NA, Clipp EC, McNeilly M, Grambow S, Parker J, et al. (2001). Preparing for the end of life: preferences of patients, families, physicians, and other care providers. *Journal of Pain and Symptom Management*, **22**(3): 727–37

22. Horne G, Payne S (2004). Removing the boundaries: palliative care for patients with heart failure. *Palliative Medicine*, **18**(4): 291–6.

23. Albinsson L, Strang P (2002). A palliative approach to existential issues and death in end-stage dementia care. *Journal of Palliative Care*, **18**(3): 168–74.

24. Hopkinson JA, Hallet C (2002). Good death? An exploration of newly qualified nurses' understanding of good death. *International Journal of Palliative Nursing*, **8**(11): 532–39.

25. Pabst-Battin M (1994). *The least worst death: essays in bioethics on the end of life*. New York: Oxford University Press.

26. Materstvedt LJ, Clark D, Ellershaw J, Førde R, Gravgaard AM, Müller-Busch HC, et al. (2003). Euthanasia and physician assisted suicide: a view from an EAPC Ethics Task Force. *Palliative Medicine*, **17**(2): 97–101.

27. Howarth G and Jeffreys M (1996). Euthanasia: sociological perspectives. *British Medical Bulletin*, **52**: 376–85.

28. Shakespeare T (2007). *Disability Rights and Wrongs*. Abingdon: Routledge.

29. United Kingdom Parliament (2005). Select Committee on Assisted Dying for the Terminally Ill Bill—Written Evidence. Memorandum by Dr Jane Campbell, Chair of Social Care Institute for Excellence (SCIE) and Commissioner, Disability Rights Commission (DRC). Available at: http://www.publications.parliament.uk/pa/ld200405/ldselect/ldasdy/86/86we05.htm.

30. ten Have H (2005). End of life decision making in the Netherlands. In R Blank, JC Merrick (eds) *End of Life Decision Making: A Cross National Study*. Cambridge, MA: MIT Press.

31. House of Lords (1993/4). *Report of the Select Committee on Medical Ethics* (HL Paper 21-I). London: HMSO.

32. British Medical Association (2007). *Withholding and Withdrawing Life-Prolonging Medical Treatment*. London: BMA.

33. Lloyd L (2004). Morality and mortality: ageing and the ethics of care. *Ageing and Society*, **24**: 235–56.

34. National Confidential Enquiry into Patient Outcome and Death (2009). *Caring to the end? A review of the care of patients who died within four days of admission to hospital*. London: NCEPOD.

35. Sampson EL, Candy B, Jones L (2009). Enteral tube feeding for older people with advanced dementia. *Cochrane Database of Systematic Reviews*, **2**: CD007209.

36. Gillick MR (2000). Rethinking the role of tube feeding in patients with advanced dementia. *New England Journal of Medicine*, **342**: 206–9.

37. Kedziera P (2001). Hydration, thirst, and nutrition. In BR Ferrell, N Coyle (eds) *Textbook of Palliative Nursing*, pp. 156–63. Oxford: Oxford University Press.

38. Department of Constitutional Affairs (2007). *Mental Capacity Act 2005: Code of Practice*. London: The Stationery Office.

39. Schermer MN (2003). *The different faces of autonomy. Patient autonomy in ethical theory and hospital practice*. New York: Springer.

Chapter 5

The disadvantaged dying: ageing, ageism, and palliative care provision for older people in the UK

Merryn Gott, Andrew M. Ibrahim, and
Robert H. Binstock

Introduction

Whilst there is a growing body of evidence to suggest that older people are the 'disadvantaged dying', little attention has been paid to the role of ageism in shaping older people's end of life experiences (1). This largely reflects a lack of integration between gerontology and palliative care in the academic literature, particularly at a theoretical level. However, the failure to attend to the role of ageism in relation to end of life care must be considered an oversight given a widespread acceptance that most contemporary societies are inherently ageist (2). The tendency to afford greater value to youth over old age and attribute negative characteristics to older people must influence both expectations of, and experiences at, the end of life for older people. Indeed, the consequences of living within an ageist society for how older people die are likely to be numerous.

In this chapter we examine one important facet of this experience for older people, namely, the extent to which older age influences access to specialist palliative care services. We do this within the context of one country—the UK—where universal health funding means that older people compete with younger people for scarce palliative care resources. To set the stage, we begin this analysis with a brief discussion of ageism and the context within which the term was first coined, namely US health care. Ironically, within the USA, ageism in health care has been substantially mitigated in recent years through the establishment of Medicare, a national health insurance programme for persons aged 65 and older. In contrast with the NHS, in the Medicare programme older people do not have to compete with younger age groups for health care resources, including specialist palliative care.

Ageism and US health care

The term 'ageism' was first introduced 40 years ago by Robert N. Butler, a practising psychiatrist and the first director of the US National Institute on Ageing, part of the National Institutes of Health. In an article entitled 'Age-ism: Another Form of Bigotry' he defined ageism as 'prejudice by one age group toward other age groups' and was particularly concerned with prejudice toward *older* persons (3). In a Pulitzer Prize winning book, *Why Survive? Growing Older in America*, Butler went on to observe that ageism in cultural attitudes manifests itself in discrimination against older persons within a variety of societal institutions and arenas such as in the workplace and health care (4).

Butler's observations regarding ageist attitudes toward older patients in US health care settings were vividly portrayed a few years later in a best-selling autobiographical novel about a recent medical school graduate who was interning at a first-tier hospital in Boston, Massachusetts (5). Among other things, the novel highlighted physicians' irritation toward older patients presenting at emergency room, where effort, time, and other resources were scarce. Such a patient was referred to as a 'GOMER,' standing for 'Get Out of My Emergency Room'. As we document below, similar ageist attitudes and practices reflecting them have been manifest in health care services in the UK, in line with the majority of Western developed nations.

The incidence of ageism in US health care was considerably reduced however, following the establishment in 1965 of Medicare, a programme of national health insurance for which most Americans aged 65 and older are eligible. Despite a dominant American political ideology that is highly individualistic and, for the most part, biased against provision of welfare by the state, the creation of public programmes benefiting older persons has been an exception (6). From the enactment of a Social Security programme in 1935 through the late 1970s the US constructed an old-age welfare state, facilitated by a *compassionate ageism*—a cultural stereotyping of 'the aged' as poor, frail, politically powerful, and, above all, deserving (7). Today, more than one-third of the US federal government's budget is spent on old-age benefit programmes (8).

Medicare was one of a variety of programmes created during the 1960s and 1970s, an era in which just about every issue or problem affecting some older persons (that could be identified by advocates for the elderly) became a government responsibility (7). The enactment of Medicare was particularly notable because efforts to establish health insurance for all Americans had pre-viously failed over many decades (9). In 2009, for instance, fifteen per cent of the US population (46 million persons) still had no health insurance, but largely thanks to Medicare less than 2% of persons age 65 and older lacked it (10).

Although ageism still exists in the attitudes and practices of some US health care professionals, the existence of Medicare means that older Americans generally do not have to compete with younger Americans in access to physicians, diagnostic tests, treatments, hospital beds, and other elements of health care. For 87% of Medicare patients, health care is substantially paid for by the government on an open-ended fee-for-service basis (rather than out of a fixed budget); the remaining Medicare patients are funded in the context of specific fixed-budget groups, in which almost all of their fellow patients are older persons (11).

Due to the specific influence of Dame Cicely Saunders, Medicare eventually added coverage for a hospice benefit for its programme's insurees in the 1980s, thereby making access to specialist palliative care relatively good for those older Americans whom physicians certify as needing it (12). Thus older patients in Medicare are not subject to the possibility that ageism, per se, may lower their priority for receiving specialist palliative care. They have a 'safe harbour' rather than being competitively pitted against younger patients in the allocation of palliative care within the context of a fixed budget. As we will discuss next, this compares unfavourably with the palliative care situation in the UK National Health Service (NHS).

Ageism within the NHS

Ageist attitudes and practices reflecting them have long been manifest in the NHS which is funded by a fixed governmental budget (13). As long ago as 1980, cardiologists in the NHS were frustrated by a high demand for a limited number of hospital beds; in a complaint similar to that expressed about GOMERS in US emergency rooms, they referred to patients aged 65 and older as 'bed blockers' (14). In 2006, a joint report of England's Audit Commission, Healthcare Commission, and Commission for Social Care Inspection concluded that standards of health care for older people were 'unacceptably poor', with mental health services in particular deteriorating in quality with increasing patient age (15).

A recent survey of 201 UK geriatricians indicates ageism remains very significant in influencing older people's experiences of NHS health and health care (16). Sixty-six per cent of participants reported that older people are less likely to have their symptoms fully investigated, and 72% that older people are less likely to be referred for essential treatment, such as neural surgery or chemotherapy. More than half (55%) were worried about how they personally would be cared for by the NHS in old age and 47% concluded that the NHS is 'institutionally ageist'.

This claim has also been made elsewhere, perhaps most pertinently by older people themselves (17). A recently published study exploring the impact of the National Service Framework for Older People concluded that, amongst those older people consulted, 'many, but not all. . . . identified themselves as members of a group that was subject to age prejudice that altered the quality and standard of their care' (18).

Indeed, this claim of ageism is difficult to counter given that older age has been identified as a barrier to accessing numerous specialist services, including chemotherapy, mental health services, cancer services, and stroke care (19–22). For all of these conditions there is compelling clinical evidence for the benefits of specialist services for older patients. Moreover, for most of these services, there are potential cost-saving benefits in facilitating access for older people to the health system as a whole. Nonetheless, it is apparent that in competition for scarce health resources older people typically miss out.

Ageism and experiences of specialist palliative care

Having identified the ways in which ageism is generally manifested within the NHS, we now consider the extent to which ageism may specifically influence older people's experiences of specialist palliative care services in the NHS.

The best evidence of the extent and usage of hospice and specialist palliative care services in England, Wales, and Northern Ireland is provided by the National Council for Palliative Care (NCPC) Minimum Data Sets project which collects information annually. Table 5.1 reports the latest findings from this work which indicates that there are currently 198 inpatient services providing 2782 specialist palliative care beds, 213 day care facilities, 278 services providing home-based specialist palliative care, and 281 hospital-based services. It is this last group which has the highest proportion of usage from people over 85 and with a non-cancer diagnosis (these two variables are related). Overall, the findings indicate a small increase year-on-year in the proportion of older people, and people with non-cancer diagnoses, accessing specialist palliative care in England, Wales, and Northern Ireland.

Whilst the provision of specialist palliative care services has grown in the last decade (Table 5.1), it is apparent that these services only care for a fraction of those dying in the UK annually. Indeed, the UK population is currently estimated to be over 61 million. Extrapolating from data published by Higginson (1997), it is possible to estimate that, within this population annually, there are likely to be 179,200 cancer deaths and 441,600 deaths from progressive non-malignant disease 'where palliative care would have been appropriate' per year (23). Of those people, 448,000 will experience pain, 300,800 will have difficulties breathing, and 211,200 will have symptoms of nausea and vomiting in the last year of life. However, only a minority of people who die in the UK will receive any specialist palliative care services; for example, only 4% of people die in a hospice, although more will have access to other services. Specialist palliative care is obviously a scarce resource for which dying people (and their family and professional advocates) have to compete.

Table 5.1 Provision of hospice and specialist palliative care services in England, Wales, and Northern Ireland in 2006/7

	Inpatient care	Day care	Home care	Hospital support
No. of services	189 services /2782 beds	213	278	281
Response rate to survey	84%	87%	73%	61%
No. of new patients	40,000	19,000	101,000	100,000
Mean length of episode of care	12.9 days	5.5 months	3.5 months	1–3 weeks
% non-cancer patients	7.2%	10.1%	7.3%	13.6%
% under 65	32%	35%	30%	30%
% over 84	10%	9%	13%	15%

Source: http://www.ncpc/org.uk

Moreover, even at a very crude level of analysis, older people appear to be under-represented within the figures reported in Table 5.1 given that 84% of deaths in 2008 occurred in people aged older than 65 years yet specialist palliative care services cared for only 68–70% of people over 65 years; people over 85 accounted for 36.1% of deaths, but only 9–15% of specialist palliative care patients (24). Some of this age-related difference in service access can be explained by the fact that, as indicated in Table 5.1, specialist palliative care in the UK 'is largely synonymous with cancer care, in particular terminal cancer care' (25). Older people are proportionally more likely to die from conditions other than cancer and hence be disadvantaged in access to specialist palliative care by diagnosis (1). Indeed, whilst a philosophy of access on the basis of need rather than diagnosis is now enshrined in health policy (26) there remain fundamental barriers to fulfilling the policy rhetoric of (specialist) 'palliative care for all' (26). However, cancer also occurs predominantly in older age with cancer incidence peaking in men aged 70–74 and women aged 75–79 (27). These figures would therefore appear to indicate differential access to specialist palliative care by age even amongst patients with a cancer diagnosis, something first proposed over 15 years ago (28).

Indeed, there is evidence that older age is negatively associated with access to both inpatient and outpatient specialist palliative care services amongst people dying from cancer. The most extensive data are provided by the UK Regional Study of Care for the Dying, a survey of 2074 bereaved carers of people who had died with cancer in the last quarter of 1990. The study reported that, whilst two-thirds of the deceased under age 75 were admitted to a hospice during the last year of their life, the same was true for only half of those older than 75. Indeed, people over 85 years of age were almost three times less likely to have received inpatient hospice care than people younger than 85 years, even when cancer site, dependency levels and reported symptoms were controlled for (29). This finding persisted when people who had been in receipt of care from a nursing home were excluded. Another interesting finding was that where health districts had a lower than average number of hospice beds, these beds were significantly more likely to be used by patients under the age of 65 than those over this age. This finding confirms earlier reports that older age is negatively associated with inpatient hospice referral (30). Grande et al. also suggests that the age of a family carer, as well as the age of a patient, may be key to explaining who accesses hospices in the UK (31).

That inequalities in access persist at the outpatient level has also been reported (29, 32). For example, patients referred to a Hospice at Home (HAH) service in East Anglia, UK, were found to be almost 5 years younger (mean 70.4 years) than a randomly selected sample of cancer patients from the same region not referred to HAH over a 1-year period (33). This finding is consistent with studies reporting that people aged over 75 years with terminal cancer are less likely to die at home than those under 75 years given evidence that access to home care may be the critical factor in enabling older people to die at home if this is their wish (32, 34, 35).

There is little evidence from which to explore older people's access to inpatient hospital palliative care services. However, one census of palliative care management in an acute NHS hospital found that older people were less likely than younger patients to have been considered for specialist palliative care referral, or to have actually been the subject of such a referral (36). In a recent qualitative study exploring palliative care provision in acute hospitals, this finding was confirmed, with professionals reporting that they felt younger people were more in need of the psychosocial support that specialist palliative care services provide (37).

Establishing an association between ageism and older people's relative under-utilization of specialist palliative care services is not straightforward. Firstly, appropriate use of health services must be related to the need for that service and, within the context of palliative care, this is difficult to establish. Definitions of palliative care need are contested. A recently published discourse analysis concluded that there is 'a broad spectrum of concepts—some of them with conflicting ideas—in the definitions of palliative care, and consequently in the goals and tasks these definitions describe' (38). Higginson and colleagues (39) discuss the difficulties this definitional ambiguity poses for conducting needs assessments for palliative care, arguing that, 'until there is agreement on what it is you are trying to assess, it cannot be properly assessed' (39). The situation is further complicated by the separation between 'specialist' and 'generalist' palliative care. In practice, what is 'specialist' about specialist palliative care can be unclear to both those inside and outside the discipline leading to uncertainty as to which patients deserve 'specialist' attention (40). Given this context, it is unsurprising that eligibility criteria for both outpatient and inpatient specialist palliative care services vary regionally across the UK (26). Ambiguity about the remit of a specialist health service also affords greater influence to those professionals who act as the 'gatekeepers' to that service. In particular, it enables their own individual views of who 'deserves' specialist palliative care to come into play (37).

Burt and Raine discuss the implications of such definitional complexities for understanding the relationship between age and access to specialist palliative care services internationally (41). They conclude that: 'there is some evidence that older people are less likely to be referred to, or to use, SPC'. However, they caution that these findings require confirmation using prospectively collected data which control for patient's need for specialist palliative care. Indeed, they make a good point in highlighting the differences between inequity and inequality of provision of health services, arguing that: 'Unequal use of health care between particular population groups is not inequitable if it reflects an unequal need for care. These findings may therefore reflect a reduced need for SPC amongst older people' (41).

Indeed, in the absence of more robust evidence, whilst it appears that older people (with cancer) are disadvantaged in accessing specialist palliative care, a number of other explanations must be considered. Firstly, it may be that older people are having their palliative care needs met elsewhere in the health- and social-care systems, as suggested by the National Institute for Health and Clinical Excellence in their 2004 report on cancer and specialist palliative care (42). However, a recent review of older people's experiences of end of life care in the UK indicates this is unlikely to be the case (1). Indeed, there is now a significant body of research to show that older people experience unmet physical and psychological symptoms at the end of life (43). Yet, there is little evidence that these needs would be best met by specialist palliative care services as currently configured, partly due to the poor evidence base for specialist palliative care as a whole (44).

However, it is important to consider whether the presence of unmet physical and psychological symptoms amongst older people in the last years of life reflects a need for additional specialist palliative care, additional geriatric medicine/nursing, or additional primary care input. The ability of specialist palliative care to manage older people's typically complex nexus of physical and psychosocial problems has not been established. Therefore, it may be that the relative under-utilization of specialist palliative care services reflects the fact that such services do not always best meet their needs. This warrants further attention.

A further explanation that has been offered for older people's differential use of specialist palliative care services is that they are more accepting of death than younger people and hence have less need for specialist services (29, 45). However, evidence for this is very limited and it could be argued that the popularity of this argument in the health literature may very well reflect ageist assumptions about the value and quality of life at different ages. As Jecker and Schneiderman argue, the death of a younger person, and in particular a child, evokes not only 'greater sorrow, anger, despair or bitterness, but also a greater sense of injustice' (46) than the death of an older person who are seen to have lived a 'full life, have done what they could, and thus are not victims of the malevolence of the forces either of divinity or of nature' (47). This rationale continues to garner popular support for age-based rationing (47).

It is certainly possible that this manifestation of ageism covertly influences who accesses specialist palliative care services, as explored below. Moreover, the logical corollary of invoking death in later life as 'natural' is that older people find facing death 'easier' and thus require less external support, either from health services or elsewhere. This has been implicated in older people's limited access to bereavement services when compared with younger people, despite the limited evidence to suggest that older people are better equipped to deal with grief than younger people (48). In a similar way, there is little evidence that older people as a group are more accepting of death, and the danger of assuming commonality by age must never be underestimated.

That the differential use of specialist palliative care services by older people may be a result of their choice warrants consideration. This issue was explored in a study by Catt et al. in 2005 who concluded from a survey of 256 people aged over 55 years living in London that 'the relative under-utilization of hospice and specialist palliative care services by older people with cancer in the UK cannot be explained by their attitudes to end-of-life issues and palliative care', adding that older people may have lower levels of need for palliative care services (49). However, they identified limitations in their study design pertinent to this discussion. The final participation rate was low (32%) and the authors acknowledge that people with high death anxiety and those in poor health were likely to have been underrepresented. A further difficulty in extrapolating from the data is that the relationship between diagnosis and acceptability of palliative care services was not examined. However, there is evidence from older people with advanced heart failure that not thinking about death and dying, issues synonymous with the terms 'palliative care' and 'hospice', can be instrumental to coping with the day-to-day realities of living with a long-term limiting illness such as heart failure (50). The place of cancer in the public imagination may make palliative care services acceptable for those dying from cancer, regardless of age, in a way that is not the case for other conditions.

A final factor that deserves consideration is the role of the professional as 'gatekeeper' to specialist palliative care services. The lack of clarity regarding palliative care 'need' affords significant influence to the individual practitioner in determining service access. This is pertinent given significant evidence that health professionals are ageist in their beliefs and practices and that such ageism can influence referral decisions (51–53). Harries and colleagues, for example, asked GPs, geriatricians and cardiologists to describe and justify the treatment they would give to selected hypothetical patients of different ages (54). Approximately half of doctors in each specialty would have treated patients aged younger than 65 differently from those over this age, independently of clinical indications, comorbidities, and sex. Older patients were less likely to be offered a range of treatments and interventions, including referral to a cardiologist. NHS rationing was explicitly mentioned as a reason why such referral was not instigated. Similar decision-making would be expected within the context of specialist palliative care services given their limited availability. That older people would miss out as a result is indicated by qualitative research undertaken with staff working on care of older people wards in an acute UK hospital. For example, one nurse reported that she had a different reaction to older patients with a life-limiting illness when compared with younger patients: 'If I'm being honest ... I think when you get people who are not old with an end of life or palliative diagnosis you can feel more sympathy towards them, more empathy, with them' (37). The degree of 'sympathy' that a professional has for a patient is likely to influence how deserving they feel that patient is of scarce specialist palliative care resources. Another interviewee from the same study indicated that such attitudes were particularly likely to influence limit older patients access to psychosocial support such as counselling (37).

Nevertheless, how ageism operates at the individual clinician's level in terms of influencing decisions to refer to specialist palliative care services is ultimately difficult to extrapolate. As Dey and Fraser acknowledge: 'Precisely because clinical judgment is meant to invoke holistic assessment of individual needs, it is no easy matter to assess the way age is used at the clinical level. If clinical decisions involve age-based rationing, they are likely to be covert' (55). They go on to argue that such age-based covert rationing is 'a pervasive feature of clinical practice' in the NHS.

Conclusions: ageism and end of life experiences

Commentators are increasingly keen to emphasize that the experience that people and their families have in the last years of life is not solely, or even primarily, influenced by the health care system (see Kellehear, Chapter 2, and Rumbold, Chapter 7, in this volume). Indeed, whilst the focus of this chapter is on articulating the role of ageism in determining access to specialist palliative care, in line with the emphasis of the book as a whole, it is important to foreground our opinion that access to services is not reflective of older people's total end of life experience. Ageism operates in many other spheres of life, often in combination with the effects of cumulative disadvantage over the life course. Older people themselves invoke ageism as a factor determining their difficulties accessing adequate housing, financial resources, and the physical environment (56). All these factors obviously significantly impact upon older people's end of life choices. For example, research has identified that dying at home, a key tenet of the 'revivalist' good death that underpins palliative care philosophy (57) is not considered an option for older people living in poor material conditions where 'home' may not be a comfortable place to live, or die (58). Whilst establishing the role of ageism in resulting in older people living and dying in inadequate housing may be difficult, it must certainly be a concern when considering reports that 20,000 to 50,000 older people in the UK die of cold-related illnesses annually (59).

Moreover, ageism can certainly be implicated in the negative images of 'old age' that looms large in the popular imagination. Indeed, given the social construction of old age as a time of dependency, sickness, and mental and physical decline (60), it is unsurprising that it represents a life-stage with which few people want to engage, whatever their age (61). This certainly has implications for experiences and expectations of, as well as preferences for, palliative and end of life care. For example, research has identified that what many older people fear most is not dying, but the perceived dependency and loss of status associated with 'being old' (50). In this way, 'social death' becomes more feared than physical death and individual understandings of societal ageism, most likely in combination with personal ageism, can determine end of life experiences. Indeed, this context of deeply entrenched prejudice against ageing and, notably, 'being old', is invoked by charities representing older people as a major impediment to the legalization of euthanasia in the UK (62).

It is for reasons such as this that acknowledging the likely role of ageism in determining older people's end of life experiences is so important. Deficiencies in the evidence base, which are perhaps indicative of the problem itself, have limited our ability to fully articulate the role that ageism plays in influencing dying experiences. However, by drawing on the wider literature regarding the negative influence of older age in accessing NHS health services within the UK, a well as juxtaposing the US situation where Medicare provides a 'safe harbour' for older people, it is apparent that the role of ageism is likely to be significant. This discussion therefore provides another example of the need for palliative care to engage with the research literature accumulating within gerontology. Safe, effective, and humane palliative care provision, which is sensitive to differential needs for care on the basis of age but does not use older age as a criterion for covert rationing of services, must be a priority within the context of globally ageing populations.

References

1. Seymour J, Witherspoon R, Gott M, Ross H, Payne S (2005). *End of Life Care: Promoting Comfort, Choice and Well-being for Older People.* Bristol: Policy Press.
2. Macnicol, J (2006). *Age Discrimination: An Historical and Contemporary Analysis.* Cambridge: Cambridge University.
3. Butler RN (1969). Age-ism: Another form of bigotry. *Gerontologist,* **9**: 243–46.
4. Butler RN (1975). *Why Survive: Being Old in America.* New York: Harper and Row.
5. Shem S (1978). *The house of God: The classic novel of life and death in an American Hospital.* New York: Marek.
6. Esping-Andersen G (1999). *Social foundations of postindustrial economies.* New York: Oxford University Press.
7. Binstock, RH (1983). The aged as scapegoat. *The Gerontologist,* **23**, 136–43.
8. Congressional Budget Office (2009). *The Budget and Economic Outlook: Fiscal Years 2010–2020.* Available at: http://www.cbo.gov/ftpdocs/108xx/doc10871/Frontmatter.shtml.
9. Quadagno J (2005). *One nation uninsured: Why the U.S. has no national health insurance.* New York: Oxford University Press.
10. US Census Bureau (2009). *Income, poverty, and health insurance coverage in the United States: 2008.* Washington, DC: US Government Printing Office.
11. Moon, M (2011). Organization and financing of health care. In RH Binstock, LK George (eds) *Handbook of Ageing and the Social Sciences,* 7th edition. San Diego, CA: Academic Press.
12. Moore PC, McCollough RH (2000). Hospice: End-of-life care at home. In RH Binstock, LE Cluff (eds.) *Home care advances: Essential research and policy issues,* pp. 101–16. New York: Springer Publishing Company.
13. Aaron HJ, Schwartz WB (1984). *The Painful Prescription: Rationing Hospital Care.* Washington, DC: The Brookings Institution.
14. Wilson LA (1980). Blocked beds. *Lancet,* **316**: 1013.
15. Eaton L (2006). Care of England's older people still 'unacceptably poor'. *British Medical Journal,* **332**: 746.
16. British Geriatrics Society, on behalf of Help the Aged (2009). *Specialist doctors label the NHS institutionally ageist and demand a law to bring it to an end.* [Press release, 27 January 2009]. Available at: http://press.helptheaged.org.uk/_press/Releases/_items/_Specialist+doctors+label+the+NHS+instit utionally+ageist+and+demand+a+law+to+bring+it+to+an+end.htm. (Accessed January 2010.)

17. Young J (2006) Ageism in services for transient ischaemic attack and stroke. *British Medical Journal*, **333**: 508–9.

18. Manthorpe J, Clough R, Cornes M, Bright L, Moriarty J, Iliffe S, and OPRSI (Older People Researching Social Issues) (2007). Four years on: The impact of the National Service Framework for Older People on the experiences, expectations and views of older people. *Age and Ageing*, **36**(5): 501–7.

19. Dockter L, Keene S (2009). Ageism in chemotherapy. *The Internet Journal of Law, Healthcare and Ethics*, **6**(1).

20. Burns A, Dening T, Baldwin R (2001). Care of older people: mental health problems. *British Medical Journal*, **322**: 789–91.

21. Turner NJ, Haward RA, Mulley GP, Selby PJ (1999). Cancer in older age—is it adequately investigated and treated? *British Medical Journal*, **319**: 309–12.

22. Kee Y-YK, Brook W, Bhalla A (2009). Do older patients receive adequate stroke care? An experience of a neurovascular clinic. *Postgraduate Medical Journal*, **85**: 115–118.

23. Higginson IJ (ed) (1997). *Health Care Needs Assessment: Palliative and Terminal Care. Health Care Needs Assessment*, 2nd Series. Oxford: Radcliffe Medical Press.

24. Office for National Statistics Cancer Statistics: Registrations Series MB1. Available at: http://www.statistics.gov.uk/statbase/Product.asp?vlnk=8843

25. Addington-Hall J (2008). Referral patterns and access to specialist palliative care. In S Payne, J Seymour, and C Ingleton (eds) *Palliative Care Nursing: Principles and Evidence for Practice*, 2nd edn, pp. 90–107. Buckingham: Open University Press.

26. Department of Health (2008). promoting high quality care for all adults at the end of life. London: Department of Health.

27. Cancer Statistics Registrations (2010). Available at: http://www.statistics.gov.uk/downloads/theme_health/MB1-38/MB1_No38_2007.pdf. (Accessed 30 June 2010.)

28. Seale C (1991) Death from cancer and death from other causes: the relevance of the hospice approach *Palliative Medicine*, **5**:12–19.

29. Addington-Hall JM, Altmann D, McCarthy M (1998). Which terminally ill patients receive hospice in-patient care? *Social Science and Medicine*, **46**(8): 1011–16.

30. Hunt R, McCaul K (1996). A population-based study of the coverage of cancer patients by hospice services. *Palliative Medicine*, **10**: 5–12.

31. Grande G, Farquhar MC, Barclay SIG, Todd CJ (2006). The influence of patient and carer age in access to palliative care services, *Age and Ageing*, **35**(3): 267–73.

32. Cartwright A (1993) Dying when you're old. *Age and Ageing*, **22**(6): 425–30.

33. Grande GE, Farquhar MC, Barclay SIG, Todd CJ (2006). The influence of patient and carer age in access to palliative care services. *Age and Ageing* **35**(3): 267–73.

34. Seale C, Cartwright A (1994) *The year before death*. Aldershot: Avebury.

35. Grande GE, Addington-Hall JM, Todd CJ (1998). Place of death and access to home care services: are certain patient groups at a disadvantage? *Social Science and Medicine*, **47**(5): 565–79.

36. Gott CM, Ahmedzhai SH and Wood C (2001). How many inpatients at an acute hospital have palliative care needs? Comparing the perspectives of medical and nursing staff. *Palliative Medicine*, **15**(6): 451–60.

37. Gardiner C, Cobb M, Gott M, Ingleton C (2011). Barriers to providing palliative care for older people in acute hospitals. *Age and Ageing* doi: 10.1093/ageing/afq172.

38. Pastrana T, Jünger S, Ostgathe F, Elsner F, Radbruch L (2008). A matter of definition–key elements identified in a discourse analysis of definitions of palliative care. *Palliative Medicine*, **22**(3): 222–32.

39. Higginson I, Hart S, Koffman J, Selman L, Harding R (2007). Needs assessments in palliative care: an appraisal of definitions and approaches used. *Journal of Pain and Symptom Management*, **33**(5): 500–5.

40. Hibbert D, Hanratty B, May C, Mair F, Litva A, Capewell S (2003). Negotiating palliative care expertise in the medical world. *Social Science & Medicine*, **57**: 277–88.

41. Burt J, Raine R (2006). The effect of age on referral to and use of specialist palliative care services in adult cancer patients: a systematic review. *Age and Ageing*, **35**(5): 469–76.

42. National Institute for Clinical Excellence (NICE) (2004). *Guidance on cancer services: improving supportive and palliative care for adults with cancer–the manual*. London: NICE.

43. Burt J, Shipman S, Richardson A, Ream E, Addington-Hall J (2010) The experiences of older adults in the community dying from cancer and non-cancer causes: a national survey of bereaved relatives. *Age and Ageing*, **39**(1): 86–91.

44. Zimmermann C, Riechelmann R, Krzyzanowska M, Rodin G, Tannock I (2008). Effectiveness of specialized palliative care: a systematic review. *Journal of the American Medical Association*, **299**(14): 1698–709.

45. Wong PTP, Reker GT, Gesser G (1994). Death anxiety profile - revised: a multidimensional measure of attitudes towards death. In RA Neimeyer (ed) *Death anxiety handbook: research, instrumentation and application*, pp 121–46. London: Taylor and Francis.

46. Jecker NS, Schneiderman LJ (1994). Is dying young worse than dying old? *The Gerontologist*, **34**(1): 66–72.

47. Callahan D (1987). *Setting Limits: Medical Goals in an Ageing Society*. New York: Simon and Schuster, Inc.

48. Scrutton S (1996). 'What can you expect, my dear, at my age?': recognising the need for counselling in a residential unit. *Bereavement Care*, **15**(3): 28–9.

49. Catt S, Blanchard M, Addington-Hall J, Zis M, Blizard R, King M (2005). Older adults' attitudes to death, palliative treatment and hospice care. *Palliative Medicine* **19**(5): 402–10.

50. Gott M, Small N, Barnes S, Payne S, Parker C, Seamark D, Gariballa S (2008). Older people's views of a good death in heart failure: implications for palliative care provision. *Social Science and Medicine*, **67**(7): 1113–21.

51. Bowling A (1999). Ageism in cardiology. *British Medical Journal*, **319**(7221): 1353–5.

52. Billings J (2006). Staff perceptions of ageist practice in the clinical setting: practice development project. *Quality in Ageing*, **7**(2): 33–45.

53. Henderson J, Xiao L, Siegloff L, Kelton M, Paterson J (2008). 'Older people have lived their lives': first year nursing students' attitudes towards older people. *Contemporary Nurse*, **30**(1): 32–45.

54. Harries C, Forrest D, Harvey N, McClelland A, Bowling A (2007). Which doctors are influenced by a patient's age? A multi-method study of angina treatment in general practice, cardiology and gerontology. *Quality & Safety in Health Care*, **16**(1): 23–7.

55. Dey I and Fraser N (2000). Age-based rationing in the allocation of health care. *Journal of Ageing and Health*, **12**(4): 511–37.

56. Minichiello V, Browne J, Kendig H (2000). Perceptions and consequences of ageism: views of older people. *Ageing and Society*, **20**: 253–78.

57. Clark D (2002). Beyond hope and acceptance: the medicalisation of dying. *British Medical Journal*, **324**: 905–7.

58. Gott M, Seymour J, Bellamy G, Ahmedzhai S, Clark D (2004). Older people's views about home as a place of care at the end of life. *Palliative Medicine*, **18**(15): 460–67.

59. Office for National Statistics (2001). *Deaths in 2001: excess winter mortality in 2000–1 and 2001–2*. London: ONS.

60. Gott M (2005). *Sexuality, Sexual Health and Ageing*. Buckingham: Open University Press.

61. Gilleard C, Higgs P (2000). *Cultures of Ageing: Self, Citizen and the Body*. Harlow: Prentice Hall.

62. Help the Aged (2002). *Policy Statement*. Available at: http://policy.helptheaged.org.uk/NR/rdonlyres/83101F3F-A03F-4A6A-B55C-19D177D06AA9/0/hs_end_of_life_12_02.pdf. (Accessed 21 January 2010.)

Chapter 6

What do we know about the congruence between what older people prioritize at the end of life and policy and practices?

Liz Lloyd

Introduction

This chapter considers the question of *congruence* between current trends in policies and practices on end of life care and the expressed priorities of older people. Are older people's priorities and preferences properly understood, and are contemporary policies and practices responsive to older people's priorities and preferences concerning care at the end of life? The issues that are raised in this discussion inevitably point to the processes through which policies and practices are developed, and the extent to which older people are able to influence these processes and articulate their priorities.

In recent years, increased interest in the circumstances in which older people in the UK die has been reflected in increased policy activity—most notably in the 2008 End of Life Care Strategy (1). Other areas of policy activity which are relevant to this discussion because they affect the circumstances in which older people are cared for at the end of life include the Mental Capacity Act 2005, the 2008 Strategy for Carers, current proposals on the reform of social care for older people, and the Dignity in Care Campaign (2–5).

A major impetus for this increased policy activity is the ageing of British society. Demographic trends have generated widespread concerns about the capacity of health and social care services to deal with projected demand and consequently have influenced a range of policies on older people's health and well-being, including those relating directly to end of life care. At the same time everyday practices in health and social care with older people are increasingly under the spotlight and inadequacies in services are seen in sharp relief when they are associated with the end of life. For example, at the time of writing, concerns have been expressed in the UK about the practice of tube-feeding older people with dementia living in care homes and questions have been raised not only about the prevalence of the practice and its efficacy but also about its implications for the dignity and human rights of the older people concerned, when they are at the end of their lives.

It should also be noted that the issues and concerns facing British policy-makers are similarly faced by their counterparts in other parts of the world. This chapter focuses on English policies but, where appropriate, UK-wide research as well as that conducted in other countries will be referred to.

Key themes in policies and the policy process

The first task is to identify key themes and trends in current policies on end of life care, which are encapsulated in the 2008 End of Life Care Strategy (1). An underlying theme, one which is congruent with the expressed views of older people's organizations, is the need for fundamental change to contemporary practices in end of life care in mainstream hospitals. Between 2004 and 2006 it was this sphere of health care that gave rise to over half of all complaints received in relation to acute care in hospitals. The term 'dignity' is frequently invoked in relation to end of life care. The End of Life Care Strategy makes the commitment that people will have access to 'services which treat you with dignity and respect both before and after death' (1).

The British government's Dignity in Care Campaign (5) was launched in 2005 to promote good practice amongst practitioners in all settings where older people might receive services. The understanding of dignity in this campaign encompasses respect, the personalization of services, the promotion of independence, choice and control, helping people to express their needs and wants, respecting their right to privacy, helping them to maintain confidence and positive self-esteem, and engaging with family members and carers as care partners.

Another theme in the End of Life Care Strategy is that despite long-standing evidence that the majority of people would prefer not to die in a hospital this is, in fact, where most deaths take place. Enabling people to die at home if that is their wish is now a key policy aim. This also reflects broader strategies to provide health and social care outside institutions and in primary and community settings. There are age-related differences to take into account regarding place of death: children and those aged 75–84 years have the highest rates of hospital deaths whereas those aged over 85 have highest rate of deaths in care homes. In policy terms, care homes are also considered potentially to be 'home' and certainly preferable to a hospital as a place of death (6).

Providing care at home would be an expensive option if it were not for the willingness and capacity of families to provide care. Families have an increasingly important role to play in providing care for older relatives, including at the end of life. Providing older people and their carers with rapid access to specialist advice and support from palliative care outreach services is also an important theme in the End of Life Care Strategy. This reflects a central focus of the 2008 Strategy for Carers on the ways in which family carers can be enabled to fulfil their caring role through improved access to professional help (3). A related theme is to provide support for bereaved carers and other relatives after death, which, if realized in practice would be an important change. In community nursing, for example, a common practice has been to allocate another case to the nurse as soon as a person dies, leaving the family carer to cope without further involvement by professionals (7).

The End of Life Care Strategy calls for a 'care pathway approach' to provide integrated care to individuals. Critical points on this pathway are the identification of those who are dying, initiation of discussions about preferences for care, care planning, care coordination, delivery of services, management of the last days of life, care after death, and support for the bereaved. Enabling individuals to take an active part and maximizing choice and control is crucial to the care pathway approach. The Mental Capacity Act 2005 might be regarded as epitomizing this approach to a carefully planned death, as it has introduced measures to enable people to make advance statements concerning their future care if they lose capacity to make decisions on their own behalf. The care pathway approach is regarded as relevant to all staff whose work brings them into contact with service users who are dying and Strategic Health Authorities are charged with developing the competences of a wide range of staff, not only specialist palliative care providers.

The 2009 Green Paper on Social Care sets out the government's vision of personalized care, which places as much control as possible in the hands of service users and their families, responds to their specific needs, draws on a range of sources of help to meet those needs, and pays for it through a personalized budget (4). Similar plans are in place for the personalization of health care and policy makers see end of life care as a sphere of practice that lends itself to this agenda.

The care pathway approach reflects the whole systems model of palliative care practice, originally developed in hospices and undoubtedly a major influence on the development of end of life care policies. It encompasses the prevention and relief of suffering of people with life-threatening diseases, treatment, and the maximization of the quality of life of patients and their families. In policy terms, hospices are characterized as 'providing a standard of care against which other service will be measured' (1). The palliative care model has been widely adopted as the ideal end of life care practice and the European Region of the World Health Organization has recently called for palliative care to be provided as a 'right' (8).

The End of Life Care Strategy also focuses on the cultural context of services and calls for greater public awareness and discussion of death and dying, offering a number of suggestions about how to achieve this, which include educational activities and open days at funeral parlours and crematoria. Clearly, greater public awareness is necessary to achieve the policy aim of the well-planned death. It is recognized that such a step-change in cultural attitudes will not happen overnight and the first Annual Report of the Strategy notes that there is widespread reluctance on the part of the public to engage in such discussions (6). As a consequence of this, the National Palliative Care Council has established a coalition to raise public awareness and debate about death and dying. There is, therefore, considerable effort being made to promote the cultural change regarded as necessary.

When considered together, a number of relevant themes can be identified in the policy context of end of life care for older people. These include the responsibility of individual citizens for planning for their own present and potential future needs and engaging actively in the organization of their care, the high value placed on home as the location of care, and on care provided by family members, but also the importance of improving care in hospitals and care homes, which should reflect a 'whole systems approach' to personalized care that promotes the dignity of the individual. The question to be considered next is to what extent do these themes reflect the expressed preferences of older people?

What are older people's priorities and preferences for end of life care?

Discussion of the congruence between older people's priorities and those of policy-makers and practitioners must encompass whether priorities in policies and practices are different from older people's, whether older people's priorities are ignored or overlooked and, more fundamentally, whether older people are able to articulate their views effectively so as to exert influence on policy-making and practice. Obtaining older people's views on end of life care is very challenging, not least because of the ethical issues raised when conducting research. Older people's organizations, such as Help the Aged and Age Concern have played an important part in the development of policies and have also developed their own organizational statements on end of life care. Like government policies, these emphasize the need for better care in mainstream hospitals, an equal right to palliative care for older people, greater choice and control for older people over the provision of care, and the need for greater public awareness and openness about death and dying (9). We might conclude from this that policy-makers have listened to older people and that what is now needed is effective policy implementation to improve front line practice with older people at the end of life. However, recent research conducted with older people indicates a more complex picture than this and raises questions about the direction of current developments. This research will be considered by reference to the themes already discussed.

The well-planned death

The first stage of the end of life care pathway entails the identification of people who are dying. This poses a particular set of challenges for older people whose illnesses might not present such a clear-cut point in their dying trajectory or might not be regarded as 'terminal'. Sampson et al. make this point in relation to dementia and Hudson et al. in relation to Parkinson's disease, although there has been a significant change in the practice of recording dementia on death certificates as the primary cause of death over the past 20 years (10–12).

Whether or not there is professional recognition of an older person's condition as terminal, it might still be considered good practice to initiate discussions with older patients who have life-limiting diseases in order to facilitate a planned 'care pathway' approach. Nicholson maintains that 'the majority of older people facing the end of life appear to come to terms naturally with their mortality' and that encouraging and facilitating an open approach to the awareness of dying is desirable. Indeed, she sees this as a part of a person-centred approach to practice that enhances personhood and dignity (13). However, a different perspective is presented by Gott et al. who observed that discussions about death and dying between people with advanced heart disease and health professionals are rare and that this is due in part to the patients' ambivalence towards discussing their prognosis (14). Gott et al. point out that whereas such ambivalence would be considered by some palliative care practitioners as a pathological form of death denial it would be more accurately understood as a coping mechanism or as the 'psychological bracketing' of the impact the illness on participants' lives. This insight challenges the prevailing view that openness is per se an essential attribute of a good death.

Ten Have comments on what he refers to as the 'late-modern *ars moriendi*', in which individual autonomy and control are values to be promoted not simply in order to satisfy the needs and preferences of the individual but also to delegate responsibility to the individual for their own wellbeing (15). The provision in the Mental Capacity Act 2005 for individuals to make advance statements exemplifies how such responsibilities can and should be exercised. However, Seymour et al. identified a different way of thinking amongst older people in their research on older people's views about planning for the end of life and the use of advance statements (16). Participants in focus-group discussions regarded advance statements not as a form of rational planning for their future care but as a means of helping their families to make decisions on their behalf about medical interventions and thus to reduce the burden of such decisions. Seymour et al. make the pertinent point that the majority of older people do not face such decisions in isolation but as part of a family network. They also argue that an advance decision would be better understood as a process rather than as a one-off event, as this would enable older people to come to terms with changes in their health and with the consequent effects on their relationships. From their research in the Netherlands with patients with advanced heart failure Willems et al. (17) identify how the majority of their research participants rarely thought about their deaths or about decisions that might have to be made.

Exercising choice and control

The emphasis on enabling the dying person to exercise choice and control is an important issue, not least because it has been identified by older people's organizations as a crucial element of a good death. Gott et al., however, found participants were less concerned about being able to control the circumstances of their dying than with having their financial affairs in order (14). As Gott et al. express it: 'they had considered their death as carrying with it a social obligation . . . but they did not do this in regard to their dying' (14). Catt et al. found that older people regarded pain control as necessary to a good death, even if it left people confused. Arguably, for these participants pain relief is a higher priority than the clarity of thought needed for the exercise of choice and control (18).

Place of death

As referred to earlier, a death at home is contrasted very favourably with an impersonalized and routinized death in an institution. This has been a key theme in policies and supported by older people's organizations. However, in this theme also, older people's views are not as clear cut as might be thought. Catt et al. explored the question of age in relation to preferred place of death (18). They found that faced with a scenario where there was no hope of recovery, both younger and older research participants expressed a preference to be cared for in a hospice rather than a hospital, although in contrast to the younger group, older participants would prefer to die in hospital than at home. As they point out, this finding runs contrary to current thinking about people's preferences to die at home. It also demonstrates that equality of access to hospices for older people is a well-founded policy aim of older people's organizations.

Agar et al. point out that that there is a difference between people's expressed preferences for place of care and for place of death (19). The type and quality of care received will influence whether or not a person wishes to remain in the same place until death. This is a particularly pertinent point for older people, who might express a desire for inpatient palliative care services primarily because of the inadequacy of community-based services or because they think there is too great a strain on their family carers. People's preferences concerning their preferred place of death should therefore be understood in the context of health and social care services available to older people at earlier stages of illness.

In addition to age-related similarities and differences it is also important to examine those related to ethnicity, as these highlight further complicating factors that challenge current thinking in policies and practices. Seymour et al., for example, found that both white and Chinese older people expressed concern about the practicalities of care and the potential for burdensomeness on their families that a death at home might entail, particularly in relation to the bodily consequences of dying (20). There were differences between the two groups, however, in relation to hospices. Whereas the white participants regarded hospices as synonymous with a 'good death' the Chinese participants took a markedly different view, seeing hospices as 'inauspicious' places because of their association with death and expressing a preference for hospitals as place of death.

The Annual Report of the End of Life Care Strategy highlights a number of improvements in the environment of end of life care in acute hospitals and hospices (6). An important consideration also is that increasing numbers of older people die in care homes and a number of programmes and initiatives to extend the principles of palliative care to care homes are in place (13). This point, however, raises questions about the cost of care at the end of life. A care home might be a more homely place to die but it will cost the older person, whereas a death in hospital is free. It needs to be recognized, therefore, that the options open to people are not evenly balanced.

Families and carers

Whereas a number of studies have identified how older people's concerns for their families have influenced their view of how and where to die, it is also evident that older people's priorities might not coincide with those of their families and carers. In the research by Willems et al., several participants expressed the wish for a speedy end (17). Indeed, the concern that was raised most frequently was the desire not to have a protracted death. However, consistent with the findings in the study by Gott et al., these participants also recognized that their families might suffer more if the death was sudden (14). On the other hand, Hall et al. found that older people in care homes did not express concerns about the aftermath of death or its effect on their families (21). As they observe, this might well be because not having been given a terminal diagnosis, their deaths were not at the forefront of their thinking. These findings highlight the social dimension of death and dying that is easily displaced in individualistic cultures that place high value of the rights of the individual.

Brazil et al. identified marked differences between the expressed wishes of care givers and care receivers concerning the place of death (22). However, their research also identified how a death at home could be facilitated by the availability of continuous professional support and effective symptom management. Reference has already been made to the strategic aim of supporting carers with easily available expert advice and information and if implemented, this could have a positive impact on facilitating a home death. The key factor would be the ability of older people and their families to trust that expert help and support will be available when it is needed and highlights the point that older people's end of life care preferences will be influenced by their experience of health and social care over the longer term.

Policies, practices, and older people's priorities: a complex relationship

The research findings discussed in earlier sections show a number of points of divergence between older people's priorities and those of policy-makers, as well as those of older people's organizations. In order to understand these it is necessary to consider the nature of policies and to see these as a process rather than as documented decisions. The process of policy-making is complex and at all stages power and influence are exercised very unevenly by a range of involved actors. Exploring the process of policies on end of life care raises the question of how older people's priorities and preferences come to the attention of policy-makers. It has, after all, only been in recent years that the end of life in old age has featured on the policy agenda at all. One contributing reason is that older people's organizations have wanted to promote positive views of ageing with the message that old age is not all about decline and death. The interests of those who are going through a period of decline as they die have tended to be overlooked. More recently, however, older people's organizations have played an important part in developing knowledge of older people's priorities and preferences (16).

Through the policy process the development of end of life policies reflects activity in other spheres of policy making. It is noteworthy, for example, that older people's organizations have emphasized older people's rights to palliative care and an end to age-related discrimination in access to hospice care. This reflects their broader campaigns for an end to age discrimination and coincides with a parallel government policy development on ending discrimination in health care (23). It might appear therefore that this particular policy priority is likely to be realized in practice. However, the implementation of policies is never straightforward and evidence suggests that there will be a number of hurdles to overcome, including the view amongst some professionals about the value and potential of palliative care in the context of the diseases that commonly affect older people.

For example, Spence et al. identified how professionals regarded the dying trajectories of patients with chronic obstructive pulmonary disorder (COPD) as different from those with cancer and the practice of palliative care as a separate specialist area of practice rather than an integral part of COPD treatment (24). Hudson et al. comment that their study highlights how Parkinson's disease is regarded as a life-limiting rather than a terminal disease, which has implications for the issue of identifying an individual as dying (25). The long and uncertain dying trajectory commonly associated with Parkinson's disease presents challenges to the aim of extending pallia-tive care to this group of older people. Willard and Luker found a range of barriers in acute care to the implementation of palliative care, including a preoccupation with treatment, the persistence of established routines, and negative perceptions of palliative care, whilst Stevens et al. found a philosophical gulf between stroke treatment and palliative care (26, 27). They argue that palliative care suffers from its 'Cinderella' status, which prevents practitioners from seeing it as equal in status to treatment.

Stevens et al., however, suggest that a way of bridging the gulf between the two spheres of practice would be an assessment tool that identifies unmet palliative care needs, such as symptom control and psychosocial and spiritual issues. Similarly, Hudson et al. identified a number of ways in which a palliative care philosophy could be applied in cases where people had Parkinson's disease, such as the provision of psychological and social support (25). This raises the broader question of which elements of palliative care would be more likely to be acceptable in the health care settings that provide care to older people at the end of life and what would it mean for palliative care to be integrated into (added on to?) other forms of treatment and care. It is noteworthy that where researchers have found points of common interest between palliative care and other practitioners these reflect not so much the policy emphasis on the promotion of individual choice and control as an emphasis on the success of palliative care in pain control and meeting psychological, spiritual, and social needs.

Policies are frequently inconsistent. For example, in the 2009 Green Paper on Social Care which considers the options for developing social care for vulnerable older people, there is no reference to death and dying, despite the high numbers of older people in the social care system living with diseases that they will eventually die from (4). Instead, the Green Paper is replete with references to the promotion of choice and control and re-ablement. The conceptual and organizational separation of long-term care services for older people and services for the dying is reinforced rather than bridged by such policies. It is also a great irony that whilst pushing for greater public awareness of and openness about death and dying the government is apparently shy of tackling the subject of death in its own policies.

For a number of reasons, then, it appears that the implementation of policies on end of life care for older people will not be straightforward but will reflect differences in perceptions about the direction in which practice should develop and about what older people's needs are as they face the end of life at a near but uncertain time. What happens at the level of encounters between health and social care staff and older people is crucially important, since strategies and policies are worthless unless implemented in practice. Indeed, arguably, what happens in practice *is* policy in reality. The evident divergence between the aims of policy and current practice in many areas of medical practice raises complex questions, not least because evidence of older people's expressed priorities and preferences is being constantly developed as more research is done in this area. It is also evident that this is a period of significant change in both policy and practice and this makes it more likely that older people will have opportunities to exert greater influence.

Conclusion

A number of conclusions can be drawn from the examination of the evidence presented in this chapter. These have implications for the development of policies and practices not only in Britain but in other countries also, since the values of awareness, choice, and control in end of life care are evident at a global level (8). First, it is clear that a better understanding of older people's priorities and preferences is needed and a greater appreciation of the differences between these. Without this there is a danger that the particular model of end of life care envisaged in current policy will be applied blanket-fashion and prove to be counterproductive in terms of older people's well-being. The emphasis on choice and control in the dying process is echoed by older people's organizations, whose focus is on combating the disadvantages associated with paternalistic and overbearing health services. However, whilst the case for change is unarguable, the way in which change is envisaged in policy is open to question.

It is also necessary to consider the deeply ageist culture that is the context in which policies and practices in care at the end of life are being developed. The fear of burdensomeness expressed by the older participants in the research discussed earlier in this chapter and the concerns they have about the impact of their dying on their families is not allayed by policies that emphasize the high cost of an ageing society. Arguably, it is at this point in the life-course that the oppressive impact of cultural discourses about older people's burdensomeness will be felt most keenly (28).

The evidence considered in this chapter shows that older people's relationships with their families in relation to care at the end of life is highly complex and calls into question the individualistic approach currently being pursued in policies. Thus, the exercise of choice and control by older people is better understood in the context of their relationships. As Glendinning points out, choice is better understood as an ongoing process rather than as an isolated one-off action by an individual (29). This echoes the point made by Seymour et al. concerning the need to see advance decisions over end of life care as a process (16). A process view allows for the possibilities of changes in preferences and decisions in the light of experiences.

Taking a process view of choice and decision-making also focuses attention on the importance of taking a longer-term view of older people's needs, including when they are living with a disease as well as when they are dying. There is a great deal of congruence between the holistic model of palliative care and models of person-centred care and there is no reason why the shift from one sphere to another should not be experienced by older people as seamless. Without a clear policy framework that entitles people to holistic care when they become chronically ill it is difficult to see how older people will obtain the kind of care at the end of life that they wish to have.

References

1. Department of Health (2008). *The End of Life Care Strategy: Promoting High Quality Care for all Adults at the End of Life*. London: Department of Health.

2. HM Government (2005). *Mental Capacity Act*. London: The Stationery Office.

3. HM Government (2008). *Carers at the Heart of 21st Century Families and Communities: A Caring System on Your Side, a Life of your Own*. London: The Stationery Office.

4. HM Government (2009). *Shaping the Future of Care Together*. Cm6763. London: The Stationery Office.

5. Cass E, Robbins D, Richardson A (2006). *Dignity in Care*. Adult Services SCIE Guide 15. London: Social Care Institute for Excellence.

6. Department of Health (2009). *End of Life Care Strategy: First Annual Report*. London: Department of Health.

7. Lloyd L (2000). Dying in old age: promoting well-being at the end of life. *Mortality*, 5(2): 171–88.

8. Davies E, Higginson IJ (eds) (2004). *Palliative Care: The Solid Facts*. Copenhagen: World Health Organization.

9. Age Concern England (2008). *Dying and Death*. Age Concern Policy Position Paper. London: Age Concern England.

10. Sampson E, Gould V, Lee D, Blanchard, MR (2006). Differences in care received by patients with and without dementia who died during acute hospital admission: a retrospective case note study. *Age and Ageing*, 35:187–9.

11. Hudson PL, Toye C, Kristjanson LJ (2006). Would people with Parkinson's disease benefit from palliative care? *Palliative Medicine*, 20: 87–94.

12. Griffiths C, Rooney C (2006). Trends in deaths from Alzheimer's disease, Parkinson's disease and dementia, England and Wales, 1979–2004. *Health Statistics Quarterly*, **30**(Summer): 6–14.

13. Nicholson C (2007). End of Life Care. In Report prepared for Help the Aged by the National Care Home Research and Development Forum *My Home Life: Quality of Care in Care Homes. A Review of the Literature*, pp. 118–28. London: Help the Aged.

14. Gott M, Small N, Barnes S, Payne S, Seamark D (2008). Older people's views of a good death in heart failure: implications for palliative care provision. *Social Science and Medicine*, **67**: 1113–21.

15. ten Have H (2001). Suffering and death: introductory comments. In H ten Have, B Gordijn (eds) *Bioethics in a European perspective*, pp. 407–9. Dordrecht: Kluwer Academic Publishers.

16. Seymour J, Witherspoon R, Gott M, Ross H, Payne S, with Owen T (2004). *End-of-Life Care: Promoting comfort, choice and well-being for older people*. Bristol: The Policy Press.

17. Willems DL, Hak A, Visser F, van der Wal G (2004). Thoughts of patients with advanced heart failure on dying. *Palliative Medicine*, **18**: 564–72.

18. Catt S, Blanchard M, Addington-Hall J, Zis M, Blizard R, King M (2005). Older adults attitudes to death, palliative treatment and hospice care. *Palliative Medicine*, **19**: 402–10.

19. Agar M, Currow DC, Shelby-Jones TM, Plummer J, Sanderson C, Abernethey AP (2008). Preference for place of care and place of death in palliative care: are these different? *Palliative Medicine*, **22**:787–95.

20. Seymour JE, Payne S, Chapman A, Holloway M (2008). Hospice or Home? Expectations about end of life care among older white and Chinese people living in the UK. *Sociology of Health and Illness*, **29**(6): 872–90.

21. Hall S, Longhurst S, Higginson I (2009). Living and dying with dignity: a qualitative study of the views of older people in nursing homes. *Age and Ageing*, **38**:411–16.

22. Brazil K, Howell D, Bedard M, Krueger P, Heidebrecht C (2005). Preferences for place of care and place of death among informal caregivers of the terminally ill. *Palliative Medicine*, **19**: 492–9.

23. Department of Health (2009). *Age Equality in Health and Social Care: a consultation on preparing the NHS and social care in England for the age requirements in the Equality Bill that affect the provision of services and exercise of public functions*. London: Department of Health.

24. Spence A, Hasson F, Wladron M, Kernohan WG, McLaughlin D, Watson B, et al. (2009). Professionals delivering palliative care to people with COPD: a qualitative study. *Palliative Medicine*, **23**: 126–31.

25. Hudson PL, Toye C, Kristjanson LJ (2006). Would people with Parkinson's disease benefit from palliative care? *Palliative Medicine*, **20**: 87–93.

26. Willard C, Luker K (2006). Challenges to end of life care in the acute hospital setting. *Palliative Medicine*, **20**: 611–15.

27. Stevens T, Payne SA, Addington-Hall J, Jones A (2007). Palliative care in stroke: a critical review of the literature. *Palliative Medicine*, **21**: 323–31.

28. Pleschberger S (2007). Dignity and the challenge of dying. *Age and Ageing*, **36**: 197–202.

29. Glendinning C (2008). Increasing choice and control for older and disabled people: a critical review of new developments in England. *Social Policy and Administration*, **42**(5): 451–69.

Section 2

What does a public health perspective bring to understandings of ageing and end of life?
Introduction

Merryn Gott and Christine Ingleton

The relatively recent framing of palliative care as a public health issue seems to offer significant opportunities to address the urgent need to improve older people's experiences at the end of life. Indeed, the scant regard given to defining 'health' in the context of palliative care is identified as an oversight in the opening chapter of this section. Bruce Rumbold argues that a 'health promoting palliative care' approach 'can both improve existing services for aged dying people and identify wider social reforms needed to develop age-friendly communities'. He argues that there is a need for health services to hand back ownership of dying to communities so that they become responsive to, rather than directive of, end of life experiences. Whilst public health approaches to palliative care have been developed internationally, Rumbold outlines specific developments in Australia where, by 2003, Palliative Care Australia asked that all palliative care services involve themselves in at least one of the following: community development, community education, prevention strategies aimed at reducing social morbidity, and social policy practice and advice.

The need to seek consumer perspectives and mobilize community participation is recognized and it is this theme that Neil Small and Anita Sargeant take up and expand in Chapter 8. They identify the potential of increased user and community participation at the end of life, as well as the risks, namely that it becomes 'something paternalistic, imposed to colonize a further area of our lives'. The nuances of community and user involvement are drawn out. Barriers to any level of 'involvement' are identified for certain groups, in particular, the 'older old' where practical, generational, and attitudinal factors all seek to mitigate against inclusive involvement. The authors conclude by identifying a need to view user and community participation as processes which must be 'nurtured and grown not switched on and off'.

Chapters 7 and 8 both mention advance care planning (ACP) as a mechanism to further engage individuals in thinking about, and making plans for, their own dying. In Chapter 9, Koen Meeuseen and colleagues from Belgium and the Netherlands outline why they believe ACP is such an important component of palliative care provision globally. They trace the development of the complex legislation concerning ACP from the United States to Europe, and outline some of the key models proposed to implement ACP into practice. The complexities of implementation are also highlighted; to date, the prevalence of ACP remains low internationally. However, the authors argue that overcoming barriers to effective ACP is critical to ensuring greater congruence between the expressed wishes of patients and their families, and the provision of palliative and end of life care.

The diversity of these wishes, and end of life experiences in general, is explored by Jonathan Koffman in Chapter 10 in a critical review of issues affecting experiences of palliative and end of life care amongst older people from minority ethnic groups. The semantic difficulties of categorizing individual identity by 'ethnic' and 'cultural' factors are discussed, as are the complex and multiple ways such 'difference' can impact upon physical and psychological well-being amongst older people at the end of life. A need for culturally appropriate care across increasingly diverse societies internationally is identified, but it is acknowledged that no easy solutions exist. In concluding, Koffman proposes a 'double lens: one that applies a framework of equity to understand and serve population needs of specific communities; and another that never loses sight of the individuals and families before us—those with clinical, psychosocial, and spiritual needs and concerns that may not conform to preconceived or stereotyped patterns'.

If public health approaches to palliative care are to be fully responsive to individual and community needs, the effect of bereavement on health and well-being must be considered. In Chapter 11, Amanda Roberts and Sinead McGilloway discuss community-based initiatives in the area of bereavement care. The tendency to overlook bereavement as an issue affecting the health and well-being of older people is identified and the case made for the importance of addressing the diverse bereavement-related needs of older people. Roberts and McGilloway outline salient issues to be considered when developing or enhancing bereavement support services for older people at a community level, drawing on examples of specific services established internationally. In this discussion, the potential to reframe an ageing population as a resource, rather than a 'demographic time-bomb', is evident. Voluntary bereavement support is typically provided for older people, by older people, a development that brings us full circle to our opening chapter and the argument that communities need to be empowered to support each other.

Chapter 7

Health promoting palliative care and dying in old age

Bruce Rumbold

Introduction

This chapter contends that a public health approach, as exemplified by health promoting palliative care (HPPC), can both improve existing services for aged dying people and identify wider social reforms needed to develop age-friendly communities. Developing such an argument, however, involves a conversation between health care disciplines that have until recently had little to say to each other.

The fact is that the late modern disciplines of health promotion, palliative care, and gerontology, which emerged during the 1970s, took shape with virtually no interaction between them for the remainder of the 20th century. They have only recently moved into conversation and some tentative forms of cooperation. Many conceptual differences and practice difficulties continue to separate those trained in one or other of the disciplines—for very few, if any, are trained in all three. A proposal of new possibilities for collaboration that does not take into account the decades-long estrangement of these disciplines is likely to meet the fate of new wine placed in old wineskins.

It is not particularly surprising that health promotion and palliative care have not been dialogue partners. After all, health promotion has focused upon strategies to avoid morbidity and postpone mortality: death and dying are subjects absent from the health promotion literature, except as outcomes of behaviours that contribute to increased morbidity and early mortality. It is rather more surprising that palliative care and aged care have not engaged with each other from the start, given that death brings an end to all careers as an aged person. Yet health promotion's reluctance to engage with palliative care is matched by that of gerontology. This can be verified quite simply. Take any text on gerontology, particularly texts in the 'successful ageing' genre, and look for 'death' and 'dying' in the index. Often neither term will be found. When 'death' is indexed, it nearly always refers to epidemiological findings (causes of death) rather than an event approached through the universal human experience of dying. Dying as the process and experience that ends people's identity as aged citizens is notably absent from these texts.

Health promotion in aged care has typically focused upon maintaining physical function and overall well-being for as long as possible (1–3). Mental health similarly has been addressed in terms of preventing or reducing the impact of physiological changes to cerebral function, with less focus upon strategies for adjusting to age-related changes (4). There is a remarkable absence in this literature of consideration of whether the relative proximity of death might affect older people's mental state or decision-making, and a corresponding lack of consideration of how well-being might be understood in the face of diminishing capacity and increasing infirmity. Successful ageing, with its focus on continuing active participation, clearly is important. However, a narrow focus upon success in terms of resisting incapacity sets up the situation where inevitably most people's ageing is no longer successful. (To their credit, this omission of 'dealing with death' is noted by Wykle et al. in their epilogue (2)).

Palliative care joins the mainstream

It seems that a necessary condition for developing a conversation between the disciplines was for palliative care to join gerontology and health promotion as part of mainstream health services. During the 1970s and for much of the 1980s palliative care, more often at that stage called hospice care, operated at the fringes of the health system, with funding from local communities and philanthropic organizations supplemented by varied amounts of income from government sources (5, 6). During the 1990s, however, most Western health services moved to incorporate palliative care as one of the services delivered by their public health systems.

One consequence of this mainstreaming of palliative care was that it became clearer that palliative care was not, and was not necessarily equipped to become, the only provider of end of life care. While palliative care philosophy paid attention to the changed forms of dying in modern societies, palliative care practice was largely a response to 'out of time' deaths from cancer (7). As a method of care it was at its best when illness had interrupted expectations of continuing normal work and family life, when the dying person was supported by family and friends, when good communication was at a premium in helping all involved adjust to this radically-changed situation, and when the dying trajectory was relatively predictable so that service provision could be paced with the dying person's decline. As George and Sykes (8) point out, few of these criteria apply to most deaths in old age. Here dying can eventuate from multiple causes and is often not detected until shortly before death, communication can be difficult, and practical social support is limited in comparison with the palliative care 'ideal'. Others have suggested that, unlike people experiencing the disruption of dying 'out of time', old people are somehow accepting of death and thus do not require the supportive care that is integral to palliative care—a suggestion that is singularly lacking in evidential support. In any case, the transfer of palliative care knowledge and skills from cancer care to aged care is not straightforward, and has only been addressed systematically in the last few years.

Another consequence of mainstreaming hospice and palliative care services was to create a new specialism. Specialist palliative care focused on what had become the core business of hospice, cancer care, and generated the associated trappings of specialist associations and career paths for its practitioners. This led to a new set of issues. Questions about the relationship of hospice care with the health system in general now became questions about the relationship of the new speciality with other specialist disciplines within the system (9, 10). Placing palliative care into a health services or population health context also made it obvious that, while it was addressing a particular form of modern dying, the 'out-of-time' death, the majority form of dying in Western societies was death in old age. This in turn raised questions about specialist palliative care's contribution to society's end of life care. From a health systems perspective, policymakers and managers began, and it might be said continue, to ask about the relationship between specialized palliative care delivery and other services offering end of life care (aged care, emergency care, intensive care, primary care), and to explore the possible wider application of palliative care insights and strategies. These discussions were largely confined within health services, although at least some recognized the way health service provision is embedded in, and relies upon, communities that provide informal care and promote a variety of forms of self-care (11–13).

Palliative care and aged care

Individual practitioners and researchers had in the 1990s considered the relationship between aged care and palliative care, but only in the last decade has that relationship been systematically developed. The application of palliative care philosophy and strategies to aged care contexts has followed somewhat different routes in different countries. Australia published Guidelines for a

Palliative Approach in Residential Aged Care in 2004, following a 2-year consultation process (14) (as discussed by Deborah Parker in Chapter 19). Corresponding guidelines for aged care in the community are nearing completion. Increasingly the term 'palliative approach', developed in the project (15), is now being applied generally to care in which primary care providers draw upon their own supplementary training and experience in palliative care and/or consult with a regional specialist palliative care service in order to provide end of life care informed by palliative principles.

Canada and the UK have chosen not to focus overtly on aged care but rather to pursue a general transfer of palliative care principles and practice into the primary care system, using a palliative care and end of life approach. In the UK, general practices have been enlisted in the Gold Standards Framework (GSF) (16), which provides 'strategies, tasks and enabling tools to deliver the best possible care for people nearing the end of their lives'. The programme, which was developed in primary care contexts, is now being implemented in Care Homes. Canada too has focused upon developing palliative care and end of life care within primary care, with some recent specific applications to end of life care for seniors (17). Again, advance care planning is a major part of strategy, directed not only to aged or ill people, but all adults, although admittedly here policy is running ahead of evidence: there has been little rigorous evaluation of these tools to date.

Despite their differences, all these approaches have been largely constrained by the boundaries of the health systems: that is, aged care and end of life care continue to be seen essentially as matters for medical management.

The UK National Health Service (NHS) End of Life Strategy, published in July 2008, has built upon the GSF, and led to a number of important initiatives intended to raise health care practitioner and community awareness of the opportunity and need to be involved in end of life planning (12). Similarly in Canada, implementation of advance care planning has drawn attention to the need for raising awareness and providing information to the community in general, not only to health care practitioners (11). Furthermore, policymakers are becoming increasingly aware that community engagement is needed not only to increase awareness of what health services provide and the decisions they require but also to shape the delivery and character of those services.

This sort of consumer involvement raises boundary issues for clinical models of care that have maintained a clear distinction between professional and lay perspectives and contributions. It is here that a health promoting approach can contribute as it provides a framework that incorporates the insights and concerns of both professional services and communities. Health promotion began by raising, in the face of medical dominance, a question about who owns health. In the same way, health promoting palliative care asks who owns dying? Health promotion answered its question with the assertion that health is created in communities, so that in a sense all policy that shapes community life is health policy. In the same way, health promoting palliative care asserts that dying is a matter for community management, and that health services should respond to, rather than direct, the experience of dying.

What is health promoting palliative care?

Health promoting palliative care stems from a social model of health, and brings into consideration, among other things, the social context of beliefs and practices surrounding death, the tradition of the good death, the role of community, and limits to health services contributions.

The term 'health promoting palliative care' may create cognitive dissonance for at least some readers. As already noted, health promotion for the most part seems interested in death only as something to be avoided or postponed by health promoting practices. The discipline of palliative care, while having the goal of a good death, seldom talks about this as a health outcome.

One of the first systematic attempts to link the health promotion and palliative care literatures was Allan Kellehear's *Health Promoting Palliative Care* (18). Kellehear took a new public health approach, encapsulated in the Ottawa Charter, and considered palliative care through this lens. His intention was to provide a critique of the health service-based understandings of palliative care that had grown out of the community-based hospice movements of the 1970s and 1980s. This critique in turn suggested strategies whereby characteristics of the hospice model of care that were being marginalized in the new mainstreamed palliative care (6) might be reclaimed and incorporated in the revised practice models. Kellehear contended that mainstreaming had skewed palliative care practice, and that as a result aspects that had been integral to the hospice philosophy were now underdeveloped, including:

- Social science and public health perspectives
- Social and spiritual aspects of care
- Early stage care
- Active treatment of disease
- Care for those with life-threatening illness (not just terminal illness) (18).

He saw the dominance of clinical priorities in treating life-threatening illness as encouraging people to be passive recipients of technical care rather than active agents in their own lives. Restoring a holistic perspective, as exemplified in hospice care, required palliative care to be reframed within a participatory model of health. For this Kellehear used the Ottawa Charter (19), the key policy framework of the new public health movement that began with the Declaration of Alma Ata (20). The Charter states that building healthy societies requires governments, agencies, and citizens in general to:

1. Enable, mediate, advocate in pursuit of healthy public policies and practices
2. Create supportive environments
3. Strengthen community action
4. Develop personal skills
5. Reorient health services.

Here health is connected with all aspects of life and is the concern of all citizens. Health promotion should involve a wide range of community and professional groups, while health services should be responsive to the societies they serve. A capacity to be an agent of one's own health, to have access to health education and information, and to work with, rather than submit to, health professionals, are outcomes of policy that recognizes the social character of health.

Bringing together the hospice philosophy of care and the Ottawa Charter, Kellehear developed the HPPC model to redress the effects of mainstreaming. The model reasserted ideals, identified resources that should be provided (such as health education that includes death education), and shared strategies for living with life-threatening illness and for confronting the social conditions that limited or opposed this resourcing and sharing. The goal was to encourage palliative care services to see that their unique insights into the experience of dying today should be offered to their communities so that the attitudes, knowledge, and understandings with which people experience illness in themselves or those close to them might begin to change. People might then encounter life-threatening illness and dying with resources already in place rather than have to assemble or develop them from scratch in the midst of that experience. The key strategies of HPPC aim to provide:

- Health education which includes death education
- Social support

◆ Interpersonal reorientation

◆ Policies that do not separate dying from living (21).

In so doing the model addresses areas neglected by contemporary palliative care models. HPPC:

◆ Complements clinical approaches

◆ Encourages community alliance

◆ Challenges current health policy

◆ Restores social and pastoral interventions

◆ Allows diversity amongst clients

◆ Expands understanding of health

◆ Reclaims an holistic perspective (18).

Reception of the model was mixed. Some practitioners were enthusiastic, seeing the model as tackling problems of which they were aware, but which they felt relatively powerless to address. Others were dismissive, suggesting that their services were already doing health promotion, by which they usually meant marketing their service. Yet others saw the ideas as a good thing, but considered that any such initiatives should be funded from outside the (clinically-focused) palliative care budget: HPPC in their opinion was not 'core business'.

HPPC is not the only public health approach to palliative care, and the recently-formed International Network for Public Health in Palliative Care (http://www.pubhealthpallcare.in/) has promoted sharing amongst these public health programmes and approaches. Here the focus will be upon HPPC in Australia; other countries can draw their own parallels (22).

In Australia, as word spread, local champions emerged to implement HPPC approaches in their own services and regions. The interest generated by the HPPC model, and by projects based upon it, resulted in growing acceptance at the national level of the legitimacy of public health approaches in palliative care, and the need for services to see this as an aspect of practice. By 2003 the national peak body, Palliative Care Australia, in their Service Provision Planning Guide asked that all services involve themselves in at least one of:

◆ Community development

◆ Community education

◆ Prevention strategies aimed at reducing social morbidity

◆ Social policy, practices, and advice (23).

Early health promoting strategies initiated by the La Trobe University Palliative Care Unit, founded by Kellehear, included conducting health promotion groups with people living with life-limiting illness, and providing education for palliative care providers in health promoting approaches (21). Further projects were developed in partnership with palliative care services and community groups (24–27). Responses of practitioners and services to the education programme and project outcomes have provided a basis for implementation and policy development.

The initial focus of HPPC was upon reforming the practice of mainstream palliative care practice services along lines indicated in a set of practice guidelines (28). In this sense the model was subject to the limitations of the hospice and palliative care models of care it wished to reorient. That is, its focus was upon health service responses to modern dying, and to particular aspects of that dying; namely 'out-of-time' deaths from cancer. In addition to providing a ration-ale and strategies by which social and spiritual interventions might be maintained or restored, it also pointed to new horizons in end of life care. Initial work with services made it increasingly clear that any process of reform needed also to involve the communities in which the services operated. This expanded model, published as Compassionate Cities (29) brought palliative care concerns into dialogue with the healthy settings movement (30), in particular the Healthy Cities programme. The Compassionate Cities model provides a broader framework within which end of life issues in general can be addressed, not merely those that fall within the more specialized interests of palliative care. Attention turns to developing communities in which citizens living with dying and loss can continue to participate in meaningful ways.

Health promoting palliative care and aged care

A health promoting approach to the end of life in old age would thus pay attention to the settings in which old people die, their expressed needs in the later years of life, the ways communities in general and health services in particular should seek to meet those needs, and the strategies that should be put in place to prevent distress and minimize harm to those who are dying, their family and friends, and others who care for them. Strategy must take account of all aspects, as public health interventions are systemic, multidimensional, and multidisciplinary. They do not provide lists of possibilities from which a few aspects may be selected as targets for action: individual and structural aspects must be addressed together (19, 31).

Lloyd (32) has in fact outlined such an approach, identifying the key elements as promoting non-institutionalized services, encouraging openness about illness and dying, enabling older people to exercise choice and control over caring interventions, minimizing older people's fear of death, and maintaining family and other social networks. Kellehear's HPPC model applied to dying in old age demonstrates not only a process by which Lloyd's goals might be addressed, but also identifies conceptual and procedural changes that are necessary if these desired outcomes are to be achieved.

Considering the four key strategies of HPPC focuses both possibilities and problems involved in implementing a health promoting response in aged care contexts.

Provide health education that includes death education

It is clear that health promotion in aged care, as expressed both in practitioner texts and government policies, has resolutely separated any discussion of death or dying from health education. This has been noted earlier in the case of aged care texts, but it is equally true of health promotion-influenced 'successful ageing' policies. The WHO *Active Ageing: A Policy Framework* report (33), for example, contains no discussion of death and dying as part of the ageing process (although the discussion paper (34) preceding the report did assert that people are entitled to death with dignity, albeit without commentary on what this goal might imply for aged care policy). The Australian Parliament in a report *Future Ageing* (35) shows some limited awareness of work being undertaken on applying palliative care to death in residential aged care, but otherwise juxtaposes palliative care with physician-assisted suicide as if these two medically-managed processes are the only end of life options available to be considered.

Given the universality of death, and the health care system's determination to develop best-practice interventions throughout the life course, it should be possible to inform citizens about healthy ways to die. The challenge then is to understand health as inclusive of human mortality.

Provide social support

Social support is usually assumed to be diminished or absent for older people, although evidence for this is less clear. Cornwell et al. (36) find for older non-institutionalized adults in the USA that, while network size might decrease with age, the frequency of socializing and social participation increases. They suggest that some late-life transitions, such as retirement and bereavement, may in fact prompt greater connectedness.

A study of loneliness in the UK by Victor et al. (37) complements these findings. For some, loneliness has been a way of life they bring into old age; for others, old age initiates loneliness. Most vulnerable are the 'oldest-old', those living alone and the non-married. Widowhood massively increases vulnerability to loneliness; although loneliness can also decrease as time goes on.

The most important forms of social support appear to be relationships that provide continuity with the past, and this includes relationship with place (38). Occupying particular familiar spaces or places can support a sense of competence, and also help mediate other unavoidable changes. Hockey et al. (39) demonstrate how loss can be engaged through renegotiating familiar spaces, and how, paradoxically, support to do so is provided through continuing bonds with the person whose physical absence is the primary source of loss. The social support provided by continuing bonds has been identified (40–42) but the importance of such support seems not widely recognized. For many old people, relationships with others who have died remain lively sources of encouragement, hope and resilience. Such relationships are further enhanced by contact with people who also have known these others who have died.

Relocation to unfamiliar places and new relational networks will thus affect not only remaining social relationships with the living but also to an extent relationships with important others who have died. The need here is to recognize the changing nature of social relationships that incorporate not only the living but also the dead, and the ways in which all these relationships are mediated by place. The challenge is to develop patterns of social organization, and spatial expressions of those patterns, that protect and maintain social support (43).

Encourage interpersonal reorientation

For health promoting palliative care, interpersonal reorientation involves negotiating a changed identity—that of being a dying person—within current social relationships. Whatever a person's age, this task is not assisted by society's difficulties in seeing dying as a part of living.

The evidence concerning ageing people's capacity to incorporate an identity as a person soon to die is mixed, in part due to the fact that a significant amount of the (relatively sparse) data concerning aged people's experience, concerns, and needs is derived from research questions devised by others rather than old people's own accounts. As an example, consider studies of death anxiety (44) in aged people, undertaken with little attention to how these researcher-selected characteristics might relate to the whole of an old person's experience.

In studies that started with the actual reported experience of older people, a different picture began to emerge (45–47). These studies, along with others by Erikson et al. (48), Howarth (42), and Vaillant (49) eliciting elderly people's reflections on ageing and death, demonstrate a dynamic tension between the limits imposed by dying and death and—in most cases—a continuing affirmation of life. This is further corroborated by Field's study of older respondents' views concerning death (recorded in the Mass Observation Archive of the University of Sussex) (50), showing that to be accepting of death does not mean giving up on living. There is a tension or a balance between maintaining control and losing control (51). Individuals' perception of the balancing point for them is a function of both their personal history and the resources currently available to them. The caregiver's task, argues Hasselkus (52), is to deal realistically with both aspects of experience, and to support an appropriate equilibrium.

Older people thus balance a spectrum of concerns, from staying healthy and being as active as possible, through to maintaining dignity and dying well—concerns which are not necessarily experienced as inconsistent by those who hold them. However, the health system privileges some of these (staying healthy and active) whilst regarding others (reflecting on decline and dying) as detracting from the pursuit of those 'positive' goals. Aged people are thus provided with social roles that privilege some aspects of their concerns and limit or ignore others, allowing their actions to be misinterpreted or misunderstood. Clarke and Warren (53) pick this up very neatly, demonstrating the complexity of experience and (implicitly) cautioning against simplistic interpretations of behaviour alone (for example, a decision to limit activity, which could be seen as 'giving up', may in fact be empowering rather than disempowering). They also show how much of the focus for older people is upon everyday life—ordinary needs, deeds and relationships. This focus needs to be taken seriously when developing strategies for care, particularly at the end of life.

Develop policies that do not separate living from dying

Aged care policies in most Western democracies focus strongly upon maintaining the independence of ageing people, expressed through strategies that reinforce individual responsibility. Increasingly individuals are seen by government, and see themselves, as responsible, through superannuation, for their post-employment life. They are responsible, by following the dictates of health promotion programmes, to age in healthy, successful, active ways (54).

The effect of selecting one dimension of experience, 'successful ageing', and making this the sole focus of public policy is to polarize ageing people's experience. Some elements are publicly acceptable, while others are not. Diminishment, decline, decay are private matters, to be resisted and, when resistance is no longer possible, to be endured with medical support and a consequent loss of independence.

Whether policy makers understand independence in the way older people understand it is debatable (55). The most common conceptualization seems to equate independence with not relying on other people. For older people independence encompasses not only self-reliance but also self-esteem and self-determination. In this understanding, high levels of physical dependence can coexist with high levels of felt independence. Autonomy is probably a better term to use than independence: and indeed Marmot and colleagues (56, 57) have shown the significance of personal autonomy for health status throughout the life course, not merely in old age.

Plath (58) argues that interpretations of independence affect the way policy is translated into strategy. Particularly at the end of life, where reliance on others is usually unavoidable, these interpretations can impinge upon dying people's autonomy as frailty and decline are managed largely in clinical contexts, where patients lose control of the everyday issues that have to this point expressed their independence. Daily schedule, activities, social contacts, and information are now regulated by others. Independence is impossible, and preserving autonomy—control over one or two aspects of life important to the person—becomes a struggle. In contrast with this, the focus of end of life care, as Wilkes expressed it, should be 'not to prolong life but independence [autonomy], for as long and as comfortably as possible' (59).

Aged care policy until quite recently has failed to address the horizon at which the life course is completed. When it has ventured to discuss death and dying, it has usually treated them as medical, rather than social, events. Discussion quickly moves from discussing the problems of life-prolonging treatments to considering life-shortening treatments, as if the antidote to medically-constructed problems of over-treatment might be compensated for by offering an alternative treatment of physician-assisted suicide. In such discussions, death and dying remain medicalized.

Health promotion contributes to palliative care in old age

Applying the four key HPPC strategies to old age has highlighted several important themes. One is the need to understand old people's experience better. It is clear that much health care practice, strategy, and policy contains assumptions about older people's experience and attitudes that are not supported by evidence, or even fly in the face of evidence that is available. At present, however, the evidence available is partial and uneven. We need some focused and concentrated research upon which to build better process.

A second theme is the importance of settings, including both the social networks that shape the experience and attitudes of older people and the health care institutions that become increasingly influential in most people's lives as they age and die. Society's choice to manage old age in terms of perceived health deficits leads to an increasing segregation of older people from the general community as they are placed in retirement communities, sheltered housing, residential aged care facilities, and nursing homes, largely on the rationale that this clustering increases social support and allows the most effective delivery of scarce medical resources.

A third theme is the way that organizing aged care around health service delivery imposes a framework in which dying tends to be seen as the antithesis of living. The medicalization of old age—which is a social strategy administered, rather than determined, by health systems—appears as a major barrier to achieving healthy dying in old age.

Health promotion based on the new public health offers strategies that can move society from the current situation where expert management of death is invested in clinical approaches toward a situation where communities can develop different approaches. Ageing can then be recovered as a social event, with people's citizenship rather than their patient status shaping the discussion. Palliative care might then develop from a health services response to end of life care towards being a community concern and responsibility. Examples of such strategies can be found in work on strengthening palliative care in Victoria through health promotion (60) and in initiatives outlined in the NHS End of Life first annual report (61). Awareness is raised through poster campaigns, café conversations, theatre productions, and school-based projects. Training in 'how to care, what to say' is offered to primary care health practitioners, volunteers, family caregivers, and people such as hairdressers and taxi drivers who are the accidental listeners to end of life conversations. Information is offered at festivals and street markets about patient rights, advance care planning, and palliative care services. These, and many other grass-roots strategies like them, are aimed at raising community awareness of issues in the current governance of death and dying, and encouraging citizens both to exercise the options already available to them and to ensure that their needs and preferences are included in end of life policy development. In a sense these activities are part of a wider movement toward increased community participation in health service design and delivery, ranging from the health social movements (62) that have reformed, for example, breast cancer services through to the patient-centred and person-centred models of care (63). All seek in one way or another to restore autonomy to those who receive health services.

Policies promoting autonomy

The need for autonomy has been recognized in different ways in aged care and palliative care. Both have recognized the structural constraints upon individual responsibility and decision-making. Both have developed policies to address these constraints. Two in particular are worthy of further comment.

Incorporating a consumer voice: advance care planning

Advance care planning (ACP) as a means for individuals to express end of life care preferences has been available for decades in some jurisdictions, although the scope and status of these plans has varied. In practice, even when preferences have been documented (see Chapter 9, this volume), they have often been ignored, overridden by standard clinical practices, or expressed family wishes.

They have not had binding force, and implementation has relied upon the presence at the bedside or in the clinical meeting of an advocate determined to argue the dying person's case. As an individual's preference, an ACP has focused more upon resisting the possible decisions of others than on creatively constructing conditions for a 'good death'. ACP risks remaining a conversation held on professional territory, driven by professionals' desire to clarify their own options and actions.

End of life decisions need to be made in age-friendly communities, but are too frequently initiated in contexts characterized by ageism and avoidance. End of life decisions need to be seen as completing life's narrative, not shaped excessively by loneliness, marginalization/ageism, guilt or despair. Again, this suggests that focusing end of life discussions around clinical treatment preferences, as much ACP tends to do, misses an opportunity to engage with aged people's actual end of life preferences and issues. As Clarke and Warren (53) remind us, everyday living is the focus of concern, and end of life decisions involve everyday relationships, activities, and interests, identifying those things that need to be retained, those that can be negotiated, those that can be relinquished.

Only in the last few years has ACP become an interest of governments. Now ACP strategies have been produced (12, 17) or foreshadowed (64) by health services. A recent Australian report even presents ACP as a consumer tool for shaping end of life services (65). Perhaps the best integrated response is that of the UK, where the NHS End of Life Care Strategy expresses the intention that all citizens be given the opportunity to register an End of Life plan, and that all health care practitioners be trained to participate in end of life conversations (12). The first annual report on implementation of the Strategy (61) outlines a range of infrastructure developments and resources that have been prepared to support implementation of the Strategy. Interestingly, this preparatory work has led to the realization that community involvement is an essential context for effective development of the Strategy. From the initiatives and programmes now emerging, of particular interest from a health promoting point of view are the North East Patients' Charter for a Good Death (66) and *A Guide to Involving Patients, Carers and the Public in Palliative Care and End of Life Services* (67).

Settings: age-friendly communities

The importance of place is recognized in various ways in policies such as Australia's Ageing in Place (68) and Lifetime Neighbourhoods in the UK (69). The function of place has not been investigated as fully as it might be, but one study shows a plausible link between place, occupation, and sense of identity (70). Perhaps the most graphic demonstration is the research reporting differing responses of aged people engaged in the same activity—sitting in a chair—in different contexts. In their own home, sitting in their own chair, people report remembering and imagining, recalling past events and making new journeys in their minds. In a residential facility, sitting in an institution's chair, people typically report: 'I just sit here all day'. It would of course be naïve to assume that maintaining aged people in familiar settings would ensure successful ageing: but it is equally naïve to assume that people can experience radical changes to their setting without major disruption to their activities, occupation, and sense of self.

An age-friendly community is one in which aged people continue to contribute, in which autonomy is respected so that change is negotiated and supported. Liu et al. (71) in a review of international literature identify as core themes an integrated physical and social environment, and a model of participatory, collaborative governance. Thus individual decisions can be made in a context that respects continuity between the past, the present, and the future.

In the WHO Global Age-friendly Cities report (72), however, there is—again—no reference to death or dying as part of aged experience. The same is true of corresponding national reports: lifetime environments in the UK (69), elder-friendly communities in North America (73). Similarly, the Humanitas projects, held up as practical examples of age-friendly planning, make no mention of death or dying in their key documentation (74). End of life decisions remain relegated to the clinically-organized environments in which much end of life care is offered, and these environments do not offer 'an integrated environment' and 'participatory governance'. Until dying is an issue included in the age-friendly discourse, death and dying will remain clinical concerns, accompanied by the surrender of much of what has sustained ageing people for the majority of their lives (75).

Conclusion

The core argument of this chapter is that insights of both health promotion and palliative care are essential for developing appropriate and sustainable end of life care, particularly in old age. But in order to do so, health promotion needs to find a concept of health that incorporates the idea of a good death. Palliative care needs to move beyond its limited horizons as a health care discipline that promotes a particular idea of a good death for people with degenerative illness, mainly cancer. Both need to re-evaluate their relationship with aged care in order to address the fact that most people today die after a long life, many living with chronic illness and disability during their later years.

As we have seen, conversations between aged care, health promotion, and palliative care encounter communication problems. Some of these are conceptual: their understandings of health, and in particular a possible relationship between health and death, differ. But the fundamental barrier is that collaborative discussions of dying in old age in Western societies are fundamentally compromised by the relentless separation of living and dying that permeates policy, health care systems, health and welfare practice, community planning, and much of popular discourse. Even the initiatives bringing health promoting principles to bear upon ageing through successful ageing and age-friendly communities programmes focus on extending wellness rather than engaging constructively with the end of life. These forms of health promotion remain captive to a professionalized health services perspective. They aim to defer the problem for which apparently no solution is seen—the problem of diminishment, disability, dying, and death in human life.

A new public health approach takes us beyond a health services perspective to consider not merely amended or added professionalized strategies near the end of life, but the settings in which life draws to a close, the resources with which people come to the end of life and—closely linked with both of these—the communities that shape these settings and resources. To put it another way, it invites us to reflect upon what health means over the life course: to develop an idea of a good life that can encapsulate the idea of a good death. Life and death may be binary opposites—but living and dying are not, and should be linked seamlessly in our policies and practice.

Health promotion strategies can incorporate consumer perspectives and mobilize community participation, and such strategies are readily available. The issue is not just one of reforming our health services to become more responsive to consumer perspectives, as important as this may be. Health Promoting Palliative Care, as we have seen applies these health promotion and community development strategies to end of life experiences and needs in order to reform health services and engage community participation. These initiatives will not on their own overcome the separation of living and dying in our understanding of health and the practice of care. This separation is not a health services invention to be overcome by the reintroduction of popular opinion; rather, in this respect health services reflect the societies in which they are embedded. A philosophical or cultural shift in social understanding is involved in reforming the attitudes and policies that separate dying from living.

The possibilities for such a shift can be seen in the origins of today's palliative care movement. It was renewed philosophical, psychological, and social interest in human mortality that prepared the soil that grew the practical strategy of hospice. In subsequent decades, however, the openness to existential questions with which hospice and palliative care began was muted through health service alliances seen as necessary to ensure survival of the movement. Palliative care became incorporated in a clinical framework, focused around cancer treatment, and relegated to the margins of health care practice. The wider existential and reflective framework was downplayed or forgotten.

It may be that increasing longevity in Western society has allowed the postponing of existential questions that were more immediate in previous generations. It is unlikely that this can persist as increasing numbers of people born in the post-Second World War baby boom enter old age. The debates that will ensue—that are already beginning to take place in, for example, the revival of spirituality in a post-religious world—are debates that have at their heart questions of value and meaning. They will drive us to re-evaluate the resources of the past, and develop fresh resources for the future.

Traditionally, both religion and philosophy have concerned themselves with finding meaning in the face of human mortality. Health and death have been connected through transcendent frameworks of value and belief. Some people today still understand health and death through these frameworks, whether formally through religious belief or informally through personal conviction that draws upon cultural memory. Those approaching death may still be exhorted with propositions that range from detailed images of a (religiously-accessed) afterlife to a challenge to be courageous in choosing to live constructively in the face of extinction, or at least the radically unknown. However these propositions tend to be fragments of past belief systems, not an integral part of a contemporary understanding of what it is to be human. We need a fresh normative vision of a good life throughout the life course, including the end of life.

Such a vision can only be effective in reforming end of life care if it emerges within broad social consensus. But a disciplined, critical, multidisciplinary conversation between aged care, health promotion and palliative care can contribute to the wider social and cultural conversation that will take us forward.

References

1. Haber D (2003). *Health Promotion and Ageing: Practical Applications for Health Professionals*, 4th edn. New York: Springer.
2. Wykle M, Whitehouse P, Morris D (eds) (2005). *Successful Ageing through the Life Span: Intergenerational Issues in Health*. New York: Springer.
3. Zeng Y, Crimmins E, Carriere Y, Robine J (eds) (2006). *Longer Life and Healthy Ageing*. New York: Springer.
4. Finch J (2004). *Evaluating Mental Health Services for Older People*. Oxford: Radcliffe Publishing.
5. Hockley J (1997). The Evolution of the Hospice Approach. In Clark D, Hockley J, Ahmedzai S (eds) *New Themes in Palliative Care*, pp. 84–100. Buckingham: Open University Press.
6. Rumbold B (1998). Implications of Mainstreaming Hospice into Palliative Care Services. In Parker J, Aranda S (eds) *Palliative Care: Explorations and Challenges*, pp. 24–34. Sydney: MacLennan & Petty.
7. Howarth G (2007). *Death and Dying: A Sociological Introduction*. Cambridge: Polity Press.
8. George R, Sykes J (1997). Beyond Cancer? In Clark D, Hockley J, Ahmedzai S (eds) *New Themes in Palliative Care*, pp. 239–54. Buckingham: Open University Press.

9. Field D (2004). Palliative Medicine and the Medicalization of Death. *European Journal of Cancer Care (England)*, **3** (2): 58–62.

10. Glare PA, Auret KA, Aggarwai G, Clark KJ, Pickstock SE, Lickiss JN (2003). The Interface between Palliative Medicine and Specialists in Acute-Care Hospitals: Boundaries, Bridges and Challenges. *Medical Journal of Australia*, **179**: S29–31.

11. Implementation Guide to Advance Care Planning in Canada: A Case Study of Two Health Authorities [Internet] (2008). Available at: http://www.hc-sc.gc.ca/hcs-sss/pubs/palliat/2008-acp-guide-pps/index-eng.php.

12. Department of Health (2008). *End of Life Care Strategy–Promoting High Quality Care for All Adults at the End of Life*. London: Department of Health.

13. New South Wales Health (2005). *Guidelines for End-of-Life Care and Decision-Making* [Internet]. North Sydney: NSW Health. Available at: http://www.health.nsw.gov.au/policies/gl/2005/GL2005_057.html.

14. Australian Government Department of Health and Ageing (2004). *Guidelines for a Palliative Approach in Residential Aged Care*. Canberra: Rural Health and Palliative Care Branch, Australian Government Department of Health and Ageing.

15. Kristjanson L, Toye C, Dawson S (2003). New Dimensions in Palliative Care: A Palliative Approach to Neurodegenerative Diseases and Final Illness in Older People. *Medical Journal of Australia*, **179**: S42–4.

16. National Health Service. *Gold Standards Framework* [Internet]. (Accessed 21 January 2010.) Available at: http://www.goldstandardsframework.nhs.uk/.

17. Health Canada (2007). *Canadian Strategy on Palliative and End-of-Life Care–Final Report of the Coordinating Committee*. Ottawa: Health Canada.

18. Kellehear A (1999). *Health Promoting Palliative Care*. Melbourne: Oxford University Press.

19. World Health Organization (1986). *The Ottawa Charter for Health Promotion*. Geneva: WHO. Available at: http://www.who.int/healthpromotion/conferences/previous/ottawa/en/.

20. World Health Organization (1978). *Declaration of Alma Ata*. Geneva: WHO. Available at: http://www.who.int/publications/almaata_declaration_en.pdf.

21. Kellehear A (1999). Health Promoting Palliative Care: Developing a Model for Practice. *Mortality*, **4**(1): 75–82.

22. Sallnow L, Kumar S, Kellehear A (eds) (2009). First International Conference on Public Health and Palliative Care–Conference Proceedings [Internet]. Bath UK and Calicut, India: University of Bath and Institute of Palliative Medicine. Available at: http://www.pubhealthpallcare.in/Palliative%20care%20for%20conference.pdf.

23. Palliative Care Australia. (2003). *Palliative Care—Service Provision in Australia: A Planning Guide*, 2nd edn. Canberra: Palliative Care Australia.

24. Kellehear A, Young B (2007). Resilient Communities. In: Monroe B, Oliviere D (eds) *Resilience in Palliative Care: Achievement in Adversity*, pp. 223–38.London: Oxford University Press.

25. Salau S, Rumbold B, Young B (2007). From Concept to Care—Enabling Community Care through a Health Promoting Palliative Care Approach. *Contemporary Nurse*, **27**(1): 132–40.

26. Kellehear A, O'Connor D (2008). Health-Promoting Palliative Care: A Practice Example. *Critical Public Health*, **18**(1): 111–15.

27. Gardner F, Rumbold B, and Salau S (2009). *Strengthening Palliative Care in Victoria through Health Promotion: Final Report to the Department of Health*. Melbourne: La Trobe University Palliative Care Unit. Available at: http://www.pallcarevic.asn.au/resources—links/resources.

28. Kellehear A, Bateman G, Rumbold B (2002). *Practice Guidelines for Health Promoting Palliative Care*. Melbourne: La Trobe University Palliative Care Unit. Available at: http://www.latrobe.edu.au/pcu/guide.htm.

29. Kellehear A (2005). *Compassionate Cities: Public Health and End of Life Care*. London: Routledge.

30. World Health Organization (1980). *Introduction to Healthy Settings*. Geneva: WHO. Available at: http://www.who.int/healthy_settings/about/en/.

31. Commission on Social Determinants of Health (2008). *Closing the Gap in a Generation: Health Equity through Action on the Social Determinants of Health. Final Report of the Commission on Social Determinants of Health*. Geneva: WHO.

32. Lloyd L (2000). Dying in Old Age: Promoting Well-Being at the End of Life. *Mortality*, **5**: 173–88.

33. World Health Organization (2002). *Active Ageing: A Policy Framework*. Geneva: WHO Department of Health Promotion, Non-communicable Disease Prevention and Surveillance.

34. World Health Organization (2001). *Health and Ageing: A Discussion Paper*. Geneva: WHO Department of Health Promotion, Non-communicable Disease Prevention and Surveillance.

35. House of Representatives Standing Committee on Ageing, 40th Parliament of Australia (2004). *Future Ageing: Report on a Draft Report of the 40th Parliament*. Canberra: Commonwealth of Australia.

36. Cornwell B, Laumann E, Schumm L (2008). The Social Connectedness of Older Adults: A National Profile. *American Sociological Review*, **73**: 185–203.

37. Victor C, Scambler S, Marston L, Bond J, Bowling A (2005). Older People's Experiences of Loneliness in the UK: Does Gender Matter? *Social Policy and Society* **5**(1): 27–38.

38. Cook C, Martin P, Yearns M, Damhurst M (2007). Attachment to 'Place' and Coping with Losses in Changed Communities: A Paradox for Ageing Adults. *Family and Consumer Sciences Research Journal*, **35**(3): 201–14.

39. Hockey J, Penhale B, Sibley D (2001). Landscapes of Loss: Spaces of Memory, Times of Bereavement. *Ageing and Society*, **21**: 739–57.

40. Bennett K (1998). Longitudinal Changes in Mental and Physical Health among Elderly, Recently Widowed Men. *Mortality*, **3**: 265–73.

41. Bennett G, Bennett K (2000). The Presence of the Dead: An Empirical Study. *Mortality*, **5**: 139–57.

42. Howarth G (1998). 'Just Live for Today'. Living, Caring, Ageing and Dying. *Ageing and Society*, **18**: 673–89.

43. Dovey K (1999). *Framing Places: Mediating Power in Built Form*. London: Routledge.

44. Tomer A (ed) (2000). *Death Attitudes and the Older Adult: Theories, Concepts and Applications*. Philadelphia, PA: Taylor & Francis.

45. Hockey J (1990). *Experiences of Death: An Anthropological Perspective*. Edinburgh: Edinburgh University Press.

46. Williams R (1990). *A Protestant Legacy: Attitudes to Death and Illness among Older Aberdonians*. Oxford: Clarendon Press.

47. Young M, Cullen L (1996). *A Good Death: Conversations with East Londoners*. London: Routledge.

48. Erikson E, Erikson J, Kivnick H (1986). *Vital Involvement in Old Age*. New York: Norton.

49. Vaillant G (2002). *Ageing Well*. Melbourne: Scribe.

50. Field D (2000). Older People's Attitudes toward Death in England. *Mortality*, **5**(3): 277–97.

51. Walter T (1994). *The Revival of Death*. London: Routledge.

52. Hasselkus B (1993). Death in Very Old Age: A Personal Journey of Caregiving. *American Journal of Occupational Therapy*, **47**(8): 717–23.

53. Clarke A, Warren L (2007). Hopes, Fears and Expectations about the Future: What do Older People's Stories tell us about Active Ageing? *Ageing and Society*, **27**: 465–88.

54. Kemp C, Denton,M (2003). The Allocation of Responsibility for Later Life: Canadian Reflections on the Roles of Individuals, Government, Employers and Families. *Ageing and Society* **23**: 737–60.

55. Secker J, Hill R, Villeneau L, Parkman S (2003). Promoting Independence: But Promoting What and How? *Ageing and Society* **23**: 375–91.

56. Marmot M (2004). *The Status Syndrome: How Social Standing Affects our Health and Longevity*. New York: Henry Holy.

57. Syme L (2004). Social Determinants of Health: The Community as Empowered Partner. *Public Health Research, Practice and Policy*, **1**(1): 1–5.

58. Plath D (2009). International Policy Perspectives on Independence in Old Age. *Journal of Ageing and Society Policy*, **21**: 209–23.

59. Wilkes E (1986). Terminal Care: How can we do it better? *Journal of the Royal College of Physicians*, **20**(3): 216–18.

60. La Trobe University Palliative Care Unit (2010). *Toolkit for Strengthening Palliative Care through Health Promotion* [Internet]. Melbourne: La Trobe University Palliative Care Unit. Available at: http://www.latrobe.edu.au/pcu/toolkit.

61. Department of Health. (2009). *End of Life Care Strategy: First Annual Report*. London: Department of Health.

62. Brown P, Zavestoski S, McCormick S, Mayer B, Morello-Frosch R, Altman R (2004). Embodied Health Movements: New Approaches to Social Movements in Health. *Sociology of Health & Illness*, **26**(1): 50–80.

63. World Health Organization (2007). *People at the Centre of Health Care: Harmonizing Mind and Body, People and Systems*. Geneva: WHO.

64. National Health & Hospitals Reform Commission (2009). *A Healthier Future for All Australians–Interim Report December 2008*. Canberra: Commonwealth of Australia.

65. National Health & Hospitals Reform Commission (2009). *A Healthier Future for All Australians–Final Report May 2009*. Canberra: Commonwealth of Australia.

66. Public Health Intelligence North East (PHINE) (2010). *A Good Death–Regional Advisory Group* [Internet]. (Accessed 10 January 2010.) Available at: http://www.phine.org.uk/group.php?gid=44.

67. National Council for Palliative Care (2010). *A Guide to Involving Patients, Carers and the Public in Palliative Care and End of Life Services* [Internet]. London: NCPC. Available at: http://www.ncpc.org.uk/users/index.html.

68. Australian Government Department of Health and Ageing (2003). *Aged Care in Australia*. Canberra: Australian Government Publishing Service.

69. Department for Communities and Local Government (2008). *Lifetime Homes, Lifetime Neighbourhoods: A National Strategy for Housing in an Ageing Society*. London: Department for Communities and Local Government.

70. Hearle D, Prince J, Rees V (2006). An Exploration of the Relationship between Place of Residence, Balance of Occupation and Self-concept in Older Adults as Reflected in Life Narratives. *Quality in Ageing*, **6**(4): 24–33.

71. Liu C, Everingham J, Warburton J, Curthill M, Bartlett H (2009). What Makes a Community Age-friendly: A Review of International Literature. *Australasian Journal on Ageing*, **28**(3): 116–21.

72. World Health Organization (2007). *Global Age-Friendly Cities: A Guide*. Geneva: WHO.

73. Austin C, Flux D, Ghali L, Hartley D, Holinda D, McClelland R, Sieppert J, Wild T (2001). *A Place to Call Home: Final Report of the Elder Friendly Communities Project* [Internet]. Calgary: Faculty of Social Work, University of Calgary. (Accessed 3 February 2010.) Available at: http://www.gov.calgary.ab.ca/community/publications.

74. Becker H (2003). *The Art of Living in Old Age: Happiness-promoting Care in an Ageing World* [Internet]. Rotterdam: Eburon Delft. (Accessed 21 January 2010.) English version available at: http://www.humanitas.nu/static/index.html.

75. O'Connor M, Pearson A (2004). Ageing in Place–Dying in Place: Competing Discourses for Care of the Dying in Aged Care Policy. *Australian Journal of Advanced Nursing*, **22**(2): 32–38.

Chapter 8

User and community participation at the end of life

Neil Small and Anita Sargeant

Introduction

> . . . in this world nothing can be said to be certain, except death and taxes.

> (Benjamin Franklin: Letter to Jean-Baptiste Leroy, 13 November 1789.)

It may seem contrary to be presenting a chapter about user and community participation at the end of life, after all what does 'user' in such a context mean? We all experience the death of people we know and we all contemplate our own death. Death has always, and everywhere, been a social or a community event as well as a personal one. Perhaps as we think about Franklin's aphorism in relation to end of life care it is taxes that is the important word. Is the intrusion of government in end of life concerns what is new? Or has the idea of what is social, or of what is a community, changed? Or has the way we contemplate things like death and governments changed? In this chapter we will consider the relationship between those things that are considered personal and those things that are seen to be social. We will also look at what falls under the domain of the government and we will present a concept that helps us rethink what government does, the concept of governmentality. We will also think about changes in the way we see ourselves and express our thoughts and feelings, that is we will examine our individual and collective subjectivities.

Our argument will consider the implications of thinking about end of life care as a public health issue. We will link this with a concern, evident in policy and in practice, to explore user and community participation at the end of life. This approach will allow us to think about changes in the way we understand the relationship between self and society. To preview our conclusion, we will make the case that the expansion of public health approaches into end of life care incorporates concerns to improve and control a new area of what was the social and personal. It risks being something paternalistic, imposed to colonize a further area of our lives. But, in the 21st century, it encounters a new sort of subjectivity, one in which self-knowledge interacts with the social and the governmental to further the evolution of a questioning person able to negotiate their own route and make their own choices. User and community involvement offers an example of these new sorts of relationships. These more theoretical considerations will be augmented with examples of innovation in palliative care and in user and community participation at the end of life.

The development of public health

The idea of what public health consists of, what its priorities should be, and how these should be pursued has changed over time and assumes different forms across the world today. Public health priorities and the means for achieving them in countries with high levels of infectious disease are very different from those in countries where chronic illness is seen as more challenging for society and the state. How we see public health is also linked to the perception we have about what disease is and about the nature and extent of the responsibilities of government.

In the UK the modern history of public health begins with innovation and reforms in the nineteenth century; vaccination to treat smallpox after the discoveries of Jenner in 1796, the Poor Law Reforms of 1834, Chadwick's *Report on the Sanitary Condition of the Labouring Population of Great Britain* (1) in 1842, Snow's identification of polluted water as a source of an 1854 cholera outbreak in London, the development of Pasteur's germ theory, and then artificial vaccines from the 1880s. The context of these changes was the rapid urbanization of the UK following the Industrial Revolution. The enforced proximity of the urban population produced the circumstances required for the rapid spread of disease and it provided the necessity for reforms such as the provision of sewers, the need to remove rubbish, and the importance of providing clean water. Urbanization also led to the breakdown of traditional family and village networks of support; Poor Law Reform included the requirement for the provision of support for the destitute and incapable in workhouses. These were reforms instigated in a hierarchical society by reformers who were prompted by fear of disease, cholera in London knew no class boundaries, and fired by a belief in the potential of science. Chadwick's philosophy of pursuing public health was one that sought an increase in reliance on the role of trained experts rather than the good offices of locally elected representatives (1).

Diseases like cholera also changed the way society understood disease. The established idea was that one quarantined those with infectious disease. They were to be controlled by being excluded, via an enforced segregation. But this did not work for cholera; to combat this the focus of interventions had to be society wide. What was emerging was a 'social medicine', a focus on everyone and everything, replacing sequestration of the problem people. It is the work of Foucault (2) that captures changes like this and presents them as illustrative of 'governmentality'. This is, 'the ensemble formed by the institutions, procedures, analysis and reflections, the calculations and tactics, that allow the exercise of this very specific albeit complex form of power, which has at its target population' (2).

A new subjectivity

Governmentality is not just concerned with responding to the bad but also with promoting the good. It is not just concerned with the technical but also involves the development of a particular subjectivity. 'How do we understand ourselves, and how are we understood by those who would administer, manage, organize, improve, police and control us?' (3). Note that this formulation includes 'improve' as well as 'control'. The inclusion of subjectivity in governmentality is not, according to Rose, developing 'the inappropriate technologisation of some ineffable humanity'. Rather it is helping 'fabricate subjects . . . capable of bearing the burdens of liberty' (3).

Thinking about what public health is, how we think about what is a health and/or a social problem, what the responsibilities of the individual and of government are, and how all these things change over time is necessary if we are going to consider dying, death, and loss in the context of public health. Is end of life care everybody's business? Back in the days of sanitary reform there were voices of opposition to the pursuit of public health, the wonderfully named 'Dirty Party' stated, 'they would rather take their chances with cholera than be bullied into health' by the reformers. In that same spirit perhaps we could argue for the importance of the private, the value of reticence, the legitimacy in believing that there are times when we should just be taken care of and not be expected to be heroically pro-active, when we wonder if we are being bullied into being involved. As Reiff (4) put it, 'We are, I fear, getting to know one another. Reticence, secrecy, concealment of self have been transformed into social problems; once they were aspects of civility' (4). But Reiff (4), in the same way as Rose (3), has a guarded optimism about the changing characteristics of human's as subjects. In 1966 in considering the case for, and implications of, *The Triumph of the Therapeutic,* he wonders if we might be replacing a 'believing man' with a 'knowing man' and in so doing finding that, 'Self-knowledge again made social is the principle of control upon which the emergent culture may yet be able to make itself stable'. Not only stable but able to avoid the damage done by 'moral demands claiming the prerogatives of truth, exercised through creedally authoritative institutions' (4). Both Reiff and Rose quote a prescient Goethe from 1787, ' I too believe that humanity will win in the long run; I am only afraid that at the same time the world will have turned into one huge hospital where everyone is everybody else's humane nurse.' (4).

Public health and palliative care

The focus for public health has continued to be an orientation to prevention and a concern with population level health issues. There has also always been a focus on surveillance and on the promotion of healthy behaviours. Sometimes public health includes treatment of those with a disease when this is vital to prevent its spread to others. But from within public health, throughout its history, there have been those who see its remit as being more than the top down guidance of experts. A 20th century US pioneer, Charles-Edward Amory Winslow, defined public health as, 'the science and art of preventing disease, prolonging life and promoting health through the organized efforts and informed choices of society, organizations public and private, communities and individuals' (5). This much more expansive approach, now science and art, recognizes communal effort and the importance of choice.

Amongst his many achievements Winslow founded the Yale University Department of Public Health and was also instrumental in founding the Yale School of Nursing. It was the latter that, under its head Florence Wald and with the help of UK visitor Cicely Saunders, became the point of origin for the first palliative care and hospice services in the USA. It was both the conceptual and the professional space afforded by a department of Public Health that allowed the nurse Florence Wald to develop her programmes. Those programmes included a key tenet in the development of hospice and palliative care, the commitment to caring for the whole person, all their needs, in order to maximize their quality of life (the approach of total care for total pain).

We can see similarities between the history of public health and emerging palliative care. There was the development of expert knowledge, from pain relief to knowledge about the psychological impact of bereavement. There was an area that had been previously excluded, the sequestration of the dying shifting to a recognition that as mortality from infectious diseases reduced (at least in the West) many more of us would experience a lengthy period of dying. This sort of change in the epidemiology of death would impact on all of us—as we cared for the dying or were ourselves approaching death.

Palliative care recognized the need for support for the social pain resulting from life limiting illness. That social pain included the pain felt by family and friends. Thus the family network was seen as a legitimate and necessary part of the palliative care teams' focus. Within this focus there were two main areas of concern. The first was the likely practical impact on the family of one persons' illness. The provision of welfare benefits advice became a role for the social worker within the palliative care team. The second focus was on the impact of death on the family.

Bereavement support, often via a specialist bereavement counsellor, was the response. But palliative care was not just about the development of expertise and its imposition on those in need. It also incorporated the enthusiasm and expertise of volunteers, it instigated changes based on the experience of service users and its pattern of spread and development was greatly influenced by the activities of local communities.

In recent years work by Kellehear and colleagues has led to an expansion of what is perceived as the domain of the social within palliative care. Kellehear (6) has developed the World Health Organization *Healthy Cities* framework to highlight the potential of linking palliative care with other public and private services for communities and to make robust links with communities themselves. Kellehear and O'Connor (7) point to the importance of social support in fostering wellbeing. 'The fostering of hope and support, or the prevention of depression or social rejection in workplaces, schools or recreational sites is crucial to a sense of quality of life' (7). The case is being made here for palliative care that is both remedial, that is it responds to the impact of loss in individuals, and formative in that it is developing social competencies. In this it is a 'health-promoting palliative care' (8). For our purposes in this chapter the crucial dimension of this approach is that while it might be started and supported by professionals it requires them to move away. Communities own ideas about support develop and not only enable that community to better respond to the specific needs of its members around dying and death but also a community building on its capacities to offer such support is fostering its own resilience (7).

Kellehear and O'Connor (7) offer an example of this professional initiated/community sustained process from Australia. Members of the hospital palliative care team initiated 'cafe conversations' with members of their community (see http://www.theworldcafe.com). As the name suggested these were held in a local cafe and saw small groups of people discussing questions set by the team. Questions included; 'Imagine you had twelve months to live. What does this mean for you and for your community?' and, 'Is it OK to die?' Participants reported an increase in comfort and confidence in talking about death and Kellehear and O'Conner conclude this can enhance the possibility of, 'meaningful social support for the person with a life-threatening illness and enhance the quality of all our lives' (7).

Assumptions about user and community involvement

This approach to health promoting palliative care conflates public health and user and community involvement. The idea of community and user involvement links with two powerful assumptions, one about structures and processes and the other about the nature of knowledge. The first assumption is that there should be, 'a deliberative approach to democracy' (9). Here deliberative democracy can augment or replace representative democracy. That is, the conventional model of agenda setting in politics is that our representatives (MPs and Councillors) present themselves for election with manifestos of their intentions once in office. We select them and hold them to account for their actions at the next election. Between elections the citizen has the right of redress under the law. Deliberative democracy, 'aims to develop citizens capacity to engage in critical reflection' (9) so that they can more effectively hold representatives to account. But there is more, they hold representatives and the professionals implementing services to account as those services are being delivered. That is they do not see agendas unfold and then make judgements, rather they scrutinize and intervene to both set agendas and to scrutinize performance continuously.

The second assumption is that experiential knowledge is sanctioned and valued as providing evidence for what is required, what should change and to make judgments both about what is provided and how it should be provided. A personal involvement in the subject under discussion serves as a qualification to express this experiential knowledge.

User and community involvement suggests a new idea of citizenship and a rethinking of rights. Rights that focus on protections and on access to redress are changed into obligations to participate as active members of the community for the common good (10, 11). It is this sort of reconstituting of citizenship that might prompt the sorts of objections that would be reminiscent of those of the Dirty Party, 'I don't want to be bullied into participating'. We have to return to Reiff (4) and Rose (3) who suggest such an objection is out-of-date. We are not being bullied, nor is our privacy being colonized. This is not part of an expansion of a colonizing power seeking control of the population. Rather we are enacting our humanity via being a knowing 'man' shaping our own experiences.

We now turn to an examination of this rather poetic conceptualization of user and community involvement and of citizenship in the context of examining if the people we are thinking about as 'users', that is those nearing the end of their lives, display the characteristics of this new humanity. In particular we want to consider if there are any particular characteristics of the older-old that might call into questions the Reiff/Rose grounds for optimism.

Generations

What we currently understand as the characteristics of older people is changing (12). There are significant differences in the lived experiences, values and beliefs of people aged over 75 years and the younger 65–75-year-olds (13). These differences will impact on public and user involvement over the next decade (12–14). We may consider older UK and European citizens as a generation characterized by having lived through the Second World War. Those over 75 years old now are likely to have delayed careers and families and to have experienced more economic and social deprivation than those born after the war (14). They share a common identity and a sense of community. This is manifest in their showing more community oriented values related to health and social care provision. They are the generation who saw the inception of the NHS and welfare state within the UK. They are likely to remember experiencing the problems in accessing health care that preceded it and the enthusiasm and pride in having access to free care at the point of need that followed its inception in 1948 (9). This group are also predominantly female, poor, and either isolated or living in age related accommodation (12). They are, perhaps paradoxically, a group who grew up with and retain a stoicism and a deference for the professions. In this cohort there is a sense, for example, both that one gets what one deserves and that doctor knows best.

In contrast, the generation born after the Second World War acquired greater prosperity, in part through a greater engagement in the labour market, rising wages, much wider property acquisition, improved pensions, and increased gender equality (14, 15). Women have had greater opportunities to engage within the public arena and develop economic independence compared to the predominantly domestic focus of the oldest old (10). This generation are challenging previously held stereotypes about what it means to be old. They have also lived their adult years in a culture that has seen the rise of a rights discourse, an emphasis on autonomy, and a scepticism about expert knowledge (11, 16). The irony of this idea of two cohorts amongst the old—the fairly old and the old old—for community and user involvement is that the old old are more likely to be communitarian and so inclined to seek to act for others but are too resigned to what is, and too in thrall to professionals, to do anything about things that are bad. They also are likely to face more practical barriers, something explored in more detail below. The fairly old are better equipped to assert their rights and are not so inhibited by hierarchical power. But they are more individualist and while they may want to improve things for themselves they are less motivated to pursue collective needs—they might be inspired to complain about their own care but not be interested in community involvement. They are good candidates for user but not community involvement.

Of course these two positions are caricatures but they are presented here to serve as indicators of the importance of age cohort effects and of the political and social culture initiatives that promote user and community involvement encounter.[1]

As well as generations there will be wide between country differences. The argument in this section has been built around the historical break of the Second World War and its aftermath, specifically the establishment of the UK's National Health Service. There will be similar experiences across Western Europe with the growth of social democratic governments and social insurance schemes. But in the wider world both the evolution of a new governmentality, changes in subjectivity and the defining characteristics of 'generations' will vary (e.g. see Munday (18) on Central and Eastern Europe).

User and community involvement in palliative and end of life care

We will now shift our focus from the more theoretical and historical to consider examples of user and community involvement. As one of us has argued before, 'user involvement has been taken as well as given' (19). That is, there has been a series of initiatives emerging from the government that have provided direction for the development of user and community involvement. There have also been developments consequent on user initiatives and grassroots campaigns. User and community involvement thus provides examples of both governmentality and the 'self-knowledge made social' that is a feature of changed subjectivity.

There have been numerous legislative and guidance documents from the UK Government (20–23). Guidance from NICE (National Institute for Health and Clinical Excellence) the body that rules on what is evidence-led best practice, was forthcoming in 2004. The National Council for Palliative Care developed a guide in 2004 called *Listening to Users* (24) This provides a wide range of approaches, techniques, and tips to engage with service users within palliative and end of life care. We will go on to present examples of involvement but note that reviews of progress made so far (25, 26) have found that most end of life care user involvement remains challenging with many services incorporating a minimal level of participation through satisfaction surveys and occasional consultation.

These caveats about progress remind us of the importance of recognizing different sorts of participation, this is not a zero-sum concept. A long-standing categorization of the level of involvement by service users is Arnstien's 'ladder of citizen participation' (27). This identified eight levels of involvement which could be reduced to three subcategories: non-participation, tokenism, and citizen power (27). The idea of progressive levels, moving from a minimum that could still be identified as user involvement to user initiated and led projects has been widely used; INVOLVE, a UK organization promoting user and carer involvement, used the categories of consultation, collaboration and control (28); one of us (19) has offered learning from the patient, joint working and user at the heart. But if the idea of levels of involvement has been widely used it has also been criticized. Tritter and McCallum (29) argue that linear and hierarchical models fail to account for the dynamic interactions and processes encountered in user engagement and participation. There are times in any history of involvement when the defining relationship with professionals is likely to vary according to the task being undertaken. There is also a sense

---

[1] The 26th British Social Attitudes Report (17), published in January 2010, asked people if they felt it was a civic duty to vote in elections. In 1991 68% said yes, in 2008 it was 56%. In 1997 62% supported increases in taxation to fund higher spending on health and education, the figure is now 40%. 38% of people agree that the government should create a more equal society, in 1994 the figure was 51%.

in some situations that involvement stops on one level and in others that, over time, the user develops, taking on more initiative and responsibilities.

An example of a complex initiative which demonstrates a shifting, evolving, role for users is provided by Seymour and colleagues in their exploration of older people's beliefs and understandings in relation to end of life care, the use of health technologies and advanced care planning. This work, with a cohort of older people, has developed over a series of studies using participatory and action research methodologies. From initially collecting views from older people aged 60 to over 85 years of age, drawn from different ethnic, religious groups and community organizations (30–32), work developed into a participatory action research study involving older people from Sheffield as community advisors and educators in the development of a peer education programme for advanced end of life care planning (33). This programme is extensive and includes one hundred and fourteen older people aged 50–90 years from care homes and extra care housing in the north of England, community groups, an African and Caribbean community association, lesbian, gay and bisexual older people, a seniors forum and representation from two cancer networks (34).

If we take two phrases, a phrase from Tritter and McCallum and a phrase from Seymour and colleagues, 'history of involvement' and 'a shifting evolving role', we can begin to pull together a picture of involvement that is not a tick box exercise designed to give a spurious legitimacy to what professionals and policy makers want to do anyway. Rather it is something that helps develop what Reiff has called 'self-knowledge made social' in a way that democratizes authoritative institutions. That picture is of involvement as a process not an event, something that has a history and evolves.

Projects in which people in later life are enabled to develop their knowledge, understanding and the capacity to think critically to improve their skills and competence at communicating are being championed by the UK charity Age UK, formerly Help the Aged (35). Such approaches recognize that older people need support to develop the skills and knowledge to become active citizens in relation to health and social care issues. What things are possible, how is policy made, what are the structures for service provision? If this service is supported what are the effects on other services? This sort of learning then needs to go through two more stages to maximize its potential to have a significant and lasting impact. Firstly, there has to be a recognition that even if these older people are not 'health literate' in terms of knowledge of the esoteric language and confused structures of professional health providers they are rich in experience and carry a complex lay perspective of health and illness with its own logic developed within their social context (15). That is, as we have said above, a different sort of knowledge has to be accorded the same status as the previously dominant professional knowledge. Secondly, to create a change it is not just lay views that have to be translated into a language that will influence professional discourse but professional discourses that have to change to engage with lay perspectives. User and community involvement needs to lead to the development of shared knowledge, created through active partnership with older people. (This is an approach that echoes Friere's work on pedagogy (36). He argues that a prevalent culture of silence has been created by socializing the majority into acquiescence with the powerful. Education needs to be hazardous, liberating, and enabling so that people can participate in the historical process.) Tritter and McCallum (29) conclude that evidence of the complex interactions and processes which inform user involvement and the outcomes that result may be less associated with power shifts than with gains for all parties, including expanding shared knowledge, skills, and experiences.

While there is evidence that participation in user involvement initiatives can provide positive affirmation of an individual's sense of dignity and self respect (34, 37) and support the development of political awareness and moral responsibility (38) this is only part of the picture. We need to identify a change in political awareness and moral responsibility on the part of the professionals and policy makers. We also need to know if involvement makes a difference. Improving dignity and self-respect in older people, characteristically socially marginalized, may be positive in itself but it is a pyrrhic victory of we keep the same inadequate services.

It is also a pyrrhic victory if user and community involvement creates new groups of the privileged. A new more socially active citizenship should involve a moral obligation to consider the application of beneficence when involving service users in the development of socially just health and social care services. That is, they should not just pursue their own sectional/personal interests. Having a sense of wider responsibilities would counterbalance the new influence of a section of user and community voices while there remains the underrepresented voices of the still silent, those still socially excluded (16, 39). A common issue across all spheres of user involvement is the reliance on people who are articulate, easily available (12, 13, 35) and motivated (40) who can become over engaged, even professionalized, by continually being invited to participate in a range of projects.

Barriers for the older old

With the exceptions of two examples, the Australian 'Cafe Conversations' (7) and Seymour and colleagues evolving cohort in the UK (30, 31, 34), we have concentrated on general trends underpinning the development of user and community involvement. Given the fast changing nature of this area and the wide between-country differences we think this a useful path for us as we add to the literature in this area. But in this section we will be more detailed. We have considered why the older old might be particularly challenged when we examined the generations context, here we will identify some more prosaic barriers to overcome. We will also present brief details of some initiatives that illustrate how user and community involvement are shaped by particular circumstances.

Abbott and colleagues reported a reduction in civic participation as people get older due to increased dependency, the construction of older people as passive by others and themselves and by a preference of the older people interviewed in their study to focus on everyday decision-making (38). Some barriers to older people's participation are practical ones; economic disadvantage making costs for attending meetings a barrier, transport availability, and accessibility of buildings and meeting rooms. Lack of internet access and IT skills also increases the social exclusion of the older population (35). Some barriers link to health problems more prevalent in older people; greater morbidity, reduced mobility, and a combination of hearing, visual, or cognitive impairments (41). Some barriers arise from the difficulties professionals have in sticking to accessible language or from demands they make on older people, for example when there are managerial 'top down' requirements for meeting tight deadlines or when contributions to reports are required in language more familiar in academic or professional discourse. Reduced levels of stamina and tiredness can also affect involvement (42, 43).

Some of these barriers are easily overcome by an adjustment from the professionals. Others are more deep seated, they relate to discrimination which affects older peoples' participation in political activity, generating a sense of powerlessness, disillusion and alienation (43). Promoting community and user involvement occurs in the context of inherent and often unchallenged assumptions about age, gender and ethnicity within society (10, 44, 45). Given the majority of older people are women there can be a compounding of disadvantage. Gendered assumptions about personal agency within the public domain have constructed our understandings of male and female citizenship. Women have not only been excluded from public life due to their domestic and hierarchical family relationships, but also disadvantaged economically, particularly if we take an international perspective (10, 16).

Both attitudes to older people and to women vary. Social, economic, and cultural dynamics in a country will influence these as they will also shape the relationship between individuals, civic society, and government activity. The evolution of governmentality and a new subjectivity occurs in the context of this broader consideration of self-and society. For example, there are examples of a broad community involvement in the development and continuation of local networks of palliative and end of life care services provided in partnership between non-governmental organizations, palliative care professionals, and community activists and volunteers trained to respond to the changing needs of individuals in Kerela in India and Kwazulu-Natal in South Africa (15, 46, 47). Wright's research on the development of hospice and palliative care in Southeast Asia (48) describes initiatives led by people who had first hand experience of treatment for cancer and who had identified shortcomings in services available, for example developments in Malaysia initiated by John Cardosa (48). Other developments relied on the input of volunteers, for example in the Philippines where a range of voluntary activity was closely linked to the Christian Church (48). We can see in the development of hospice and palliative care across the world similar factors to those that were key in its development in the west. These factors are the continuing importance of committed individuals driven by their experience of the gap between what is available and what is needed, and the impact of the encounter between civil and state activity which shapes the nature and importance of volunteer and community involvement. In this sense user and community involvement is a continuation of themes evident in the growth of the modern hospice movement.

Conclusions

In this chapter we have considered user and community participation at the end of life. Individuals, families and communities have always been concerned with end of life care. What we have identified as new is an interest by government and health professionals to develop a role for themselves not just in protecting from harm but in promoting good. This interest is consistent with the development of a public health focus in palliative care. Hospice and palliative care has always been concerned with the social—this approach just expands its scope. Expansion of palliative care into public health includes the possibility of the expansion of scrutiny and control but it also means opportunities for a more active citizenship. We have examined this by looking at a new subjectivity that can reform the relationship between the citizen and the state. User and community involvement fits into this.

To operationalize user and community involvement it is not enough to elicit the support of domains of power and authority, one also has to consider the inherent development and interaction of experiential and contextualized knowledges (9, 39, 41, 549) and develop skills (12, 35, 42) within service user, community and professional groups but also at the interfaces between them. It is likely that there will be challenges to overcome. Many of these are common to all user and community involvement. People are being asked to do new things at times when they may also be practically and emotionally stretched. Professionals are being asked to modify their practice in response to experiential knowledge, difficult for those in hierarchical organizations and especially difficult in the context of a commitment to (a narrowly defined) evidence-based health care. Policy makers are being asked to listen to a new sort of public voice, expressed continuously and contemporaneously as services are developed and delivered. But older people have an extra series of challenges. Some of these are practical, some are attitudinal, and, we argue, some are generational.

User and public involvement at the end of life has always been a part of the modern hospice movement. Continuing its trajectory of development might also see it as an indicator of a change from government to governmentality and from a passive to an engaged citizenry. It has to be seen as something that takes time, it's to be nurtured and grown not switched on and off. It will be significant it if makes system and attitudinal changes, for example in making thinking about death more evident in life. 'People often make the mistake of being frivolous about death and think, "Oh well, death happens to everybody. Its not a big deal, its natural. I'll be fine." That's a nice theory until one is dying' (50). If it is to make a real difference it has to challenge entrenched knowledges and established ways of doing things. If it feels cozy it probably isn't working!

References

1. Chadwick E (1842). *Report on the Sanitary Condition of the Labouring Population of Great Britain*. London: R. Clowes & Sons.
2. Foucault M (1979). On governmentality. *Ideology and Consciousness*, **6**: 5–22.
3. Rose N (1989). *Governing the Soul*. London: Free Association Press.
4. Reiff P (1966). *The Triumph of the Therapeutic*. Harmondsworth: Penguin.
5. Winslow C-EA (1920). The untilled fields of public health. *Science*, **51**(1306): 23–33.
6. Kellehear A (2005). *Compassionate Cities*. London: Routledge.
7. Kellehear A, O'Connor D (2008). Health-promoting palliative care: A practical example. *Critical Public Health*, **15**(1): 111–15.
8. Kellehear A (1999). *Health promoting palliative care*. Melbourne: Oxford University Press.
9. Barnes M (2005). The same old process? older people, participation and deliberation. *Ageing And Society*, **25**: 245–59.
10. Lister R (2003). *Citizenship: Feminist Perspectives*, 2nd revised edn. Hong Kong: Palgrave Macmillan.
11. Etzioni A (2009). Common good and rights: a neocomunitarian approach. *Law and Ethics* Winter/Spring, 113–19.
12. Help the Aged (2008). *On My Doorstep: Communities and Older People*. London: Help the Aged.
13. Help the Aged (2009). *Future Communities: Reshaping our society for older people*. London: Help the Aged.
14. Vincent J (2005). Understanding generations: political economy and culture in an ageing society. *British Journal of Sociology*, **56**(4): 579–99.
15. Conway S (2008). Public health and palliative care: principles to practice? *Critical Public Health*, **18**(3): 405–15.
16. Crigger N, Brannigan M, Baird M (2006). Compassionate nursing: professionals as good citizens. *Advances In Nursing Science*, **29**(1): 15–26.
17. NatCen (2010). *British Social Attitudes 26th Report*. London: Sage.
18. Munday B (2007). *Report on User Involvement in Personal Social Services*. Strasbourg: Council of Europe.
19. Small N (2005). User voices in palliative care. In C Faull, Y Carter, L Daniels (eds) *Handbook of Palliative Care*, 2nd edn, pp. 61–74. Oxford: Blackwell.
20. Department of Health (1999). *Patient and Public Involvement in the New NHS*. London: DH.
21. Department of Health (2000). *The NHS Cancer Plan*. London: DH.
22. Department of Health (2001). *Health and Social Care Act*. London: The Stationery Office Ltd.
23. Department of Health (2003). *Strengthening Accountability: Involving Patients and the Public*. London: DH.
24. National Council for Palliative Care (2004). *Listening to Users*. London: National Council for Palliative Care.
25. Black J (2008). User involvement in EOLC: How involved can patients/carers be? *End of Life Care*, **2**(4): 64–9.

26. Payne S, Gott M, Oliviere D, Small N, Sargeant A (2004). *User involvement in palliative care: a scoping study: final report to St Christopher's Hospice.* Available at: http://www.ncpc.org.uk/download/publications/ui_scopingstudy.pdf. (Accessed 1 December 2009.)

27. Arnstein S (1969). A ladder of citizen participation. *Journal of the American Institute of Planners,* **35**: 216–24.

28. INVOLVE (2003). *Involve Strategic Plan 2003–2006: Creating the Expert Resource.* Eastleigh: INVOLVE.

29. Tritter JQ, McCallum A (2006). The snakes and ladders of user involvement: moving beyond Arntein. *Health Policy,* **76**: 156–68.

30. Seymour J, Bellamy G, Gott M, Ahmedzai S, Clark D (2002). Using focus groups to explore older people's attitudes to end of life care. *Ageing and Society,* **22**: 517–26.

31. Seymour J, Gott M, Bellamy G, Ahmedzai S, Clark D (2004). Planning for end of life: the views of older people about advanced care statements. *Social Science and Medicine,* **59**: 57–68.

32. Gott M, Seymour J, Bellamy G, Clark D, Ahmedzai SH (2004). Older people´s views about home as a place of care at the end of life. *Palliative Medicine,* **18**(15): 460–7.

33. Sanders C, Seymour JE, Clarke A, Gott M, Welton M (2006). Development of a peer education programme for advance end-of-life care planning: an action research project with older adults. *International Journal of Palliative Nursing,* **12**(5): 216–23.

34. Seymour J, Almack K, Bellamy G, Clarke A, Crosbie B, Froggatt K, et al.(2009). *A Peer Education Programme for End of Life Care Education Among Older People and Their Carers. Final Report.* Nottingham: University Of Nottingham, Burdett Trust for Nursing.

35. Help the Aged (2008). *Learning For Living: Helping To Prevent Social Exclusion Among Older People.* London: Help the Aged.

36. Friere P (2000). *Pedagogy of the Oppressed,* 30th edn. London: Continuum International Publishing Group Ltd.

37. Cotterell P, Harlow G, Morris C, Beresford P, Hanley B, Sargeant A, et al. (2008). *Identifying the Impact of Service User Involvement on the Lives of People Affected by Cancer. Final Report.* London: Macmillan Cancer Support.

38. Abbot S, Fisk M, Forward L (2000). Social and democratic participation in residential settings for older people: realities and aspirations. *Ageing and Society,* **20**: 327–40.

39. Anderson J, Rodney P, Reimer-Kirkbam S, Browns A, Khan K, Lynam J (2009). Inequalities in health and healthcare viewed through the ethical lens of critical social justice. *Advances in Nursing Science,* **32**(4): 282–94.

40. Sargeant A, Payne S, Gott M, Small N, Oliviere D (2007). User involvement in palliative care: motivational factors for service users and professionals. *Progress in Palliative Care,* **15**(3): 126–32.

41. Clare L, Cox S (2003). Improving service approaches and outcomes for people with complex needs through consultation and involvement. *Disability and Society,* **18**(7): 935–53.

42. Comes M, Peardon J, Manthorpe J, The 3YO Project Team (2008). Wise owls and professors: the role of older researchers in the review of the National Service Framework for Older People. *Health Expectations,* **11**(4): 409–17.

43. Postel K, Wright P, Beresford P (2005). Older people's participation in political activity–making their voices heard: a potential support role for welfare professionals in countering ageism and social exclusion. *Practice,* **17**: 3:173–89.

44. Falk-Rafael A (2006). Globalisation and global health: toward nursing praxis in the global community. *Advances in Nursing Science,* **29**(1): 2–14.

45. Cook G, Klein B (2005). Involvement of older people in care, service and policy planning. *International Journal of Older People Nursing in Association with International Journal of Clinical Nursing,* **14**: A43–A47.

46. McDermott E, Selman L, Wright M, Clark D (2008). Hospice and palliative care development in India: a multimethod review of services and experiences. *Journal of Pain and Symptom Management*, **35**:583–93.
47. Wright M, Wood J, Lynch T, Clark D (2008). Mapping levels of palliative care development: a global view. *Journal of Pain and Symptom Management*, **35**: 469–85.
48. Wright M (2010). *Hospice and Palliative Care in Southeast Asia*. Oxford: Oxford University Press.
49. Branfield F, Beresford P, Andrews E, Chambers P, Staddon P, Wise G, et al. (2006). *Making User Involvement Work: Supporting Service User Networking and Knowledge*. York: Joseph Rowntree Foundation.
50. Rinpoche S (2008). *The Tibetan Book of Living and Dying*. London: Rider and Co.

Chapter 9

Advance care planning: international perspectives

Koen Meeussen, Lieve Van den Block, and Luc Deliens

Introduction

According to the United Nations' latest biennial population forecast, the median age worldwide is projected to increase from 29 to 38 years between 2009 and 2050. Today Europe has the oldest population in the world, with a median age of almost 40, which is expected to reach 47 by 2050. The population in developed regions aged 60 or over is growing at the fastest pace ever, and is expected to increase from 264 million in 2009 to 416 million in 2050 (1). The increase in life expectancy, in the proportion of elderly people and chronic diseases, and the consequent rise in health care costs, makes the provision of palliative care for older people one of the most important and urgent societal challenges for all developed countries (2, 3).

One key aspect of good palliative care is that it is in accordance with the wishes of the patient (4). Such wishes and preferences concerning treatment and care in the last few months of life can be ascertained at the time a decision needs to be taken; however, for many patients communication is difficult at this stage, especially in cases of urgency and for those suffering from mild or severe cognitive deficiencies. Therefore it is important to engage in advance care planning (ACP) to be able to shape future clinical care to fit each patient's wishes and values (5, 6).

ACP entails discussions with patients and/or their representatives about the goals and desired direction of care, particularly end of life care, in the event that the patient is or becomes incompetent to make decisions (7). In this chapter, we discuss the concept of ACP in an international context and describe its societal background, its prevalence, and the priority given to it by clinicians, health care organizations, and policy makers.

A societal meaning of advance care planning

Societal background

Several developments have contributed to making ACP an issue of great clinical and public health concern.

It is known that societies are ageing and that the number of older people is rapidly growing in many countries (8). Additionally, the pattern of disease is also changing: acute illnesses have been replaced as the major cause of death by more progressive and chronic diseases such as cancer and cardiovascular and neurological diseases requiring more long-term care at the end of life. Consequently, about two-thirds of all deaths do not occur totally unexpectedly leaving time for exploration and discussion of the patient's values and preferences towards the end of their life (9).

Additionally, one of the major challenges facing older people all over the world is dementia (10–12). In present Western society, dementia prevalence figures double about every 5 years after age 65 and it is expected that in the near future numbers will continue to increase owing to the rapid growth of the oldest age groups (13, 14). The median length of survival from diagnosis to death in dementia is 8 years, and during this time there is a prolonged decline in ability and awareness (3). At the end, most patients with dementia are not able to communicate their preferences, leaving them at an increased risk of symptom burden and prolonged suffering. Although there is growing recognition that people with dementia are entitled to appropriate palliative care, end of life care often remains suboptimal for these patients and their families (12, 15, 16). Engaging early in the exploration of their wishes and preferences is thus of particular importance in this population in order to improve the quality of life and death.

Also, over the past few decades, society has been moving away from traditional values towards more liberal moral attitudes which place increasing value on personal autonomy (17). ACP is, from an ethical perspective, an area where the principle of self-determination rather than medical paternalism is particularly evident. There is also an increasing recognition of the importance of focusing on patient-centred care rather than on the disease itself. While developments in diagnostic and therapeutic techniques have enabled an increase in the survival time of the terminally ill, there is an increasing awareness that care aimed at cure or at the prolongation of life might not always be in the best interests of the patient; quality of life may be considered a priority, even at the expense of survival time. In many models highlighting the domains of quality of palliative care, ACP takes a prominent position and is considered a key indicator for improving end of life care quality (18–23).

The importance of advance care planning in a palliative care framework

Palliative care was defined by the World Health Organization in 2002 as:

> . . . an approach that improves the quality of life of patients and their families facing the problem associated with life-threatening illness, through the prevention and relief of suffering by means of early identification and impeccable assessment and treatment of pain and other problems, physical, psychosocial and spiritual. (24)

Palliative care is patient-centred care and a core value of palliative care from its inception has been in enabling people to make genuine choices about their own care (3). A patient's inability to participate in decision-making can hinder the provision of good palliative care if their exact preferences remain unknown. Although not all seriously ill patients want to take part in decision-making, it is important that they have the choice of participating or being informed. Within a general population in the Netherlands, being able to decide about end of life care was ranked at the top of factors considered important for a good death (25, 26). ACP is a means of putting patients at the centre of their own care trajectory through exploring their preferences and identifying who they want to make important decisions for them if they are no longer competent. ACP is also reconcilable with the contemporary view of good palliative care as being a continuous, early-initiated, and ongoing process of exploration, communication, and discussion between the different actors involved. The potential for ACP discussions is to help people to prepare for death, which from the patient's perspective, tends to mean helping them to achieve a sense of control, relieving burdens on loved ones, and strengthening or reaching closure in relationships with loved ones (27).

The development of legislation concerning advance care planning

ACP is rooted in the USA where in the late 1960s consumer rights movements aimed to limit the amount of unwanted, aggressive medical interventions at the end of a patient's life. The concept of a 'living will' was initially proposed in 1969 in the USA, and was subsequently embedded in

US legislation which followed two high-profile cases of the 1970s and 1980s. These cases focused the public's attention on withdrawing life-sustaining treatments from vulnerable individuals who had lost decision-making capacity, and gave rise to pieces of legislation that enabled patients to record end of life treatment decisions in the form of living wills, do not resuscitate orders, or do not hospitalize orders (28).

Considerable effort has been made to unify the various state laws governing advance directives and to promulgate the use of advance directives. With the implementation of the Federal Patient Self-Determination Act in the USA in 1990, it became mandatory for all patients to be informed of their rights regarding decisions on their own medical care (29). Specifically, the rights ensured are those of the patient to dictate their future care should they become incapacitated. Patients are allowed to formulate their preferences which are then recorded in their medical records. The use of a written advance directive, such as a living will or a durable power of attorney, was thereby codified in law and has been widely promoted in the USA (30).

Ever since, there has been a growing awareness of the need to consider ACP in other countries as well. In Canada, since the mid-1990s almost all provinces and territories have enacted legislation concerning advance directives for health and personal care, following the US model (31). Also in Australia, the law has endorsed ACP by according statutory status to advance health directives and the appointment of substitute decision-makers, but with significant differences across the Australian states (32, 33).

Within the European Union advance directives have been formalized far less often compared with their original North American context *with a great variability across countries.* It was not until the European Charter of Patients' Rights of 2002 that 14 concrete patients' rights that *must be protected throughout the entire territory of the European Union* were declared (34) among which are:

- *The right to information*: 'every individual has the right of access to all information regarding their state of health, the health services and how to use them'.

- *The right to consent*: 'every individual has the right of access to all information that might enable him or her to participate actively in decisions regarding his or her death; this information is a prerequisite for any procedure and treatment'.

- *The right to freedom of choice*: 'each individual has the right to choose freely from among different treatment procedures and providers on the basis of adequate information'.

However, in 1997 the Convention on Human Rights and Biomedicine (35) had already stated that 'the previously expressed wishes relating to a medical intervention by a patient who is not, at the time of the intervention, in a state to express his or her wishes shall be taken into account', but the Convention was never ratified by the European Union in its entirety.

In 2008 a workshop was organized with the financial support of the European Science Foundation on the question of whether or not a common European position on advance directives is ethically required and practically feasible (36). However, no consensus was reached.

A review of the state of affairs on advance directives in Europe reveals that it is a complex matter with a great diversity of approaches between countries. In some, such as Belgium and the Netherlands, certain advance directives (e.g. the law on euthanasia) have a legal status. In others, such as Greece or Portugal, the concept of advance directives is practically unknown (37–39). In the UK, until recently no one was legally authorized to consent or refuse particular medical treatment on behalf of an adult lacking capacity and there was no statute directly governing the use of advance directives. In 2005, however, the UK parliament (England, Wales) approved the Mental Capacity Act 2005, which had as its primary purpose the provision of a statutory framework for acting on and making decisions for individuals who are unable to make decisions themselves (40). This Act came into force in April 2007. Advance decisions to refuse treatment that meet all the requirements of the Mental Capacity Act 2005 will be legally binding for health and social care professionals. This makes advance decisions to refuse treatment quite distinct from other aspects of advance care planning. The latter may include requests or other statements of wishes about future care and treatment which must be taken into account as part of an overall best interests judgement but are not legally binding (41).

Advance care planning: a definition

Definition

Although there is some variability between authors as to how ACP is defined, it refers in its broadest sense to the process of continuous communication between caregivers, patients and/or their representatives about the goals and desired direction of care, particularly end of life care, in the event that the patient is, or becomes, incompetent to make decisions.

Teno and colleagues formulate two important components required for a successful ACP (30):

1) Communication and negotiation with patients in order to facilitate their desired involvement in formulating preferences for current and future medical decisions (process)

2) The formulation of a contingency plan which facilitates the patient in achieving desired treatment goals (outcome).

Process of advance care planning

Several models of ACP, including recommendation at to when it should be initiated and how it can be maintained, have been proposed. Emanuel and colleagues state that it could be helpful to think of ACP as a process following a stepwise approach that can be integrated flexibly into routine clinical encounters by the physician or other health care providers. Their approach contains five steps for successful advance care planning (42):

Step 1. Introduce the topic

Whenever possible, physicians should routinely initiate the ACP process with every adult patient in their practice, regardless of age or current state of health.

Step 2. Engage in structured discussions

Convey the information patients need; involve the proxy decision-maker in the discussions; define key medical terms using words patient and proxy can understand; explain the benefits and burdens of various treatments; elicit the patient's values and goals; use a validated advisory document.

Step 3. Document the patient's preferences

Formalize the directives and check for inconsistencies and misunderstandings and enter them into the medical record. It is important to have these records wherever the patient may receive care.

Step 4. Review and update the directive

Revisit the subject of ACP on a periodic basis to review the patient's preferences and to update the document.

Step 5. Apply directives to actual circumstances

These steps are very similar to the three-step model proposed by Teno and colleagues (30):

Step 1 **Actively listen** to the patient about his or her understanding and current quality of life.

Step 2 Work with the patient to **create goals of care** that are based on mutual understanding of where the patient is in the disease trajectory.

Step 3 **Formulate contingency plans to honour those goals.**

Teno additionally proposes four periods that can be discerned in a patient's disease trajectory in which ACP should be initiated or reviewed (30, 43).

1. *Person has no serious illness:* focus is on naming a proxy, stating undesirable outcome states, and elicitation of atypical preferences.

2. *Person suffers from one or more chronic progressive illnesses:* focus is on understanding patient preferences regarding potential adverse outcome states.

3. *Person is at a critical turning point in which the treatment goals start to change:* this critical turning point is based on patient preferences and self-perceived quality of life rather than physiological futility of treatment.

4. *Person is dying:* the health care providers work with patient and family to achieve the patient's changing goals of care.

In the UK, a recent guideline highlighting the main issues and challenges of incorporating ACP into patient care also indicates that ACP can be initiated independently of the patient's own disease course at times, such as a life-changing event concerning another person, e.g. death of spouse or close relative (44). Other authors discern three clinical indications to start up ACP: urgent situations (e.g. diagnosis), routine situations (e.g. a general annual doctor's call), and casual indications (e.g. patients begin ACP themselves) (45).

Thus, ACP is a process that can be advantageous to all older people and which can be initiated at various times during a person's life, not only when they are facing a life-threatening disease.

Advance care planning documents

Positive and negative advance directives

As a potential outcome of advance care planning, advance directives might be a means of honouring a patient's expressed preferences in the near or distant future. Additionally, they could be an aid to stimulating or facilitating the process of ongoing end of life care communication.

A written advance directive or living will refers to a document in which a person indicates their health care preferences while he or she is cognitively and physically able to make decisions.

These preferences mostly relate to the withholding or withdrawal of certain potentially life-prolonging medical procedures such as artificial respiration, cardiopulmonary resuscitation, artificial food or fluid administration, transfer to a hospital, etc. People express preferences about treatments they would not want to receive; these documents might therefore be known as *negative* advance directives.

Alternately, patients can also express a preference to receive certain care or treatment rather than to have it withheld (a *positive* advance directive). The wish for adequate pain alleviation even with a potential life-shortening effect might be a case in point, as might an advance euthanasia directive.

Another example of a positive advance directive is the durable power of attorney for health care. In such a document one can assign a person as a decision-making proxy in the case of future incapacity.

Patient-orientated versus physician-orientated

Advance directives entail instructions set out by the patient themselves about their preferences at the end of life. Both positive and negative advance directives can be patient-orientated.

The most popular patient-orientated living will in the USA is a document called *Five Wishes* which is distributed by the national organization Ageing With Dignity. By means of the following five questions, people can express their preferences about the end of life:

- Who you want to make health care decisions for you when you can't make them
- The kind of medical treatment you want or don't want
- How comfortable you want to be
- How you want people to treat you
- What you want your loved ones to know.

Currently, more than 14 million copies of *Five Wishes* are in circulation across the nation, distributed by more than 15,000 organizations. *Five Wishes* meets the legal requirements in 42 states and is used in all 50 (46).

In Europe there are several organizations providing patient-orientated documents for people who want to state their wishes. In Belgium and the Netherlands, where euthanasia has been legal since 2002, organizations like the Belgian Life End Information Forum or the Dutch Association for Voluntary Euthanasia supply advance directive forms about euthanasia, but also about other aspects of end of life care, such as non-treatment, organ donation, or manner of burial (47, 48).

In the UK, the Preferred Priorities for Care form has been developed to record a patient's end of life preferences and states that:

> it can help you and your carers (your family, friends and professionals) to understand what is important to you when planning your care. If a time comes when, for whatever reason, you are unable to make a decision for yourself, anyone who has to make decisions about your care on your behalf will have to take into account anything you have written in your Preferred Priorities for Care form.(49)

It may be important to bear in mind that in the UK only preferences that relate to a refusal of specific medical treatment may become legally binding, and only if assessed as complying with the Mental Capacity Act 2005 and found valid and applicable (40, 44).

Apart from these patient-orientated forms, many health care organizations have also developed and implemented patient-specific treatment documents that contain instructions issued by a doctor and included in a patient's file. A DNR (do not resuscitate) code is a common example.

Other examples of treatment-codes in elderly care may refer to the artificial administration of food and fluids, medication, or the wish not to be transferred to a hospital.

Initiatives have been undertaken to develop guidelines for health and social care professionals to clarify the concept of ACP and related terms and on how best to manage ACP in clinical practice (44, 49–51). These guides are often practice-based and emphasize the process of continuous communication rather than merely the formalization of a written document.

Also health care organizations, such as hospitals or nursing homes, are more frequently outlining their own specific institutional policies and conventions on ACP, designed to guide doctors and nursing staff in their institutions. These guidelines might entail both general instructions on how to initiate ACP and patient-specific instructions that can be used in conversation with the patient and or family.

Prevalence of advance care planning

In 2007 the RAND Cooperation presented the results of a systematic review of the evidence published between 1990 and 2007 regarding the effectiveness of advance directives and advance care planning for improving end of life outcomes in the USA (28). One of the major conclusions of this 80-page report is that most Americans do not complete an advance directive and that when they are completed, these documents often do not affect care because they are narrow and legalistic. Most of the literature suggests that between 18% and 30% of Americans have completed an advance directive which may be considered as a low percentage in view of the widespread support for ACP from the public, government, and the medical community (28, 52). It seems that 15 years after the passage of the Patient Self-Determination Act, advance directives are still rarely available in the USA.

By comparison with the amount of research conducted in the USA, there have been relatively few empirical studies addressing the topic of advance directives and advance care planning in Europe. In the Netherlands, an interview study was conducted among relatives of a representative sample of deceased older persons (age 59–96) as part of the Longitudinal Ageing Study Amsterdam (53). Results showed that few older people had died with a written advance directive regarding medical end of life decisions (10%) or a written designated surrogate decision-maker (7%). About half had expressed a preference for or against one or more medical decisions at the end of life (54). Apparently, older people in the Netherlands are not inclined to plan in advance, at least not in a formal written way. However, among the younger Dutch population (20-60 years of age) even fewer were found to have formulated a living will (barely 3%) (55).

A recent cross-national study retrospectively investigated the prevalence of ACP in a terminally ill population in Belgium and the Netherlands via a representative network of general practitioners. In both countries ACP was discussed with patients in a third of cases, and a written advance care plan existed twice as often in the Netherlands (16%) as in Belgium (8%) (56). A study in Flemish nursing homes demonstrated that only 5% of residents had made a written advance directive which could be considered as a low proportion since almost all Flemish nursing homes have now implemented an ACP policy (57, 58).

In the UK, a study among the general public showed that only 8% in England and Wales had completed an ACP document of any kind (51, 59). A recent focus group study with health care professionals involved in the care of patients with chronic obstructive pulmonary disease revealed that discussions related to ACP were very rarely initiated (60).

Studies from outside Europe and the USA have shown similar results regarding ACP, with the general public, doctors, and nurses being strongly encouraged to engage in ACP, but with a generally low percentage of actual formal planning (61, 62).

In conclusion, although figures are not always easily comparable between countries, patient populations, and settings, several studies confirm the low prevalence of ACP and written advance directives, both among the general population and the terminally ill.

Challenges, pitfalls, and recommendations

Empirical evidence demonstrates that the implementation of ACP often fails and may be hampered by several barriers. In the following, we list these pitfalls briefly, and formulate recommendations for research, practice, and policy.

One of the key principles of ACP is that it must be a voluntary process. No pressure to take part in it should be brought to bear by professionals, the family, or any organization on the individual concerned (44); patients may feel uncomfortable addressing issues related to death, illness, and the end of life. If the patient does not want to confront these subjects, this reluctance should be respected. However, caregivers must not stand back but sensitively and proactively explore whether a patient is ready and willing to discuss their future care. For example, even though a patient does not want to discuss his or her prognosis, it may still be important to start up a conversation about other aspects or possibilities of care and treatment (45).

One major challenge is that the benefit of written advance directives is often questioned (63). Choices and preferences can change with time, age, and health status (64). As stated in the stepwise approach from Emanuel and colleagues, it is important to review and update the status of advance directives, and to ensure end of life care discussion is ongoing (42). Sometimes preferences may be unclear and vague which can be misleading; caregivers should clarify preferences if they do not seem clear to them or to the proxy (65). Also, questions are raised about the future applicability of a patient's preferences or about the way certain concepts should be interpreted in clinical practice, such as 'unbearable suffering', 'not competent to make own decisions' (66). Overall, large-scale empirical studies have uncovered additional problems related to advance directives. In the USA, the Study to Understand Prognoses and Preferences for Outcomes and Risks of Treatment (SUPPORT) showed that advance directives were often not completed, did not make it to the medical record, or did not influence medical care (52).

Nevertheless, there is also evidence that advance directives do have their benefits. Previous research in the nursing home setting demonstrated that a systematic implementation of a programme to increase the use of advance directives reduced use of health care services without affecting satisfaction or mortality (67). Data from the Asset and Health Dynamics Among the Oldest Old (AHEAD) study showed a lesser likelihood of dying in an acute hospital if an advance directive was in existence (68). Recently, Teno and colleagues examined whether or not advance directives were positively associated with the quality of end of life care as perceived by family members at all sites of medical care (63). Their study showed that a bereaved family member report of the completion of an advance directive was related to fewer concerns about physician communication and with more information about what to expect during the dying process.

Notwithstanding the controversial position advance directives hold in current research there is an unequivocal and growing awareness that they provide an important opportunity to improve the quality of end of life care for older people; in more recent years we have seen a shift to more emphasis being put on the process of communication and interaction rather than on a legal document (69). Written advanced directives are still acknowledged to be important but not sufficient to improve end of life care. Completing an advance directive form should be seen as a means to achieving desired goals, not an end in itself (70). They can be important results of an ACP process, but the communication underlying or preceding the formalization into a document is a prerequisite for high quality of care.

In an editorial Teno states that 'it is time to move from a focus on single interventions, such as a living will, to a focus on public policies that use multifaceted interventions to provide competent, coordinated, and compassionate end-of-life care' (71). ACP as an ongoing process of communication could be one way to achieve an integrated and holistic patient-centred approach.

In their recommendations to the US Department of Health and Services the RAND Cooperation stated that advance care planning in its broadest view holds great promise for the future, and that '. . . more flexible legal instruments and advance care planning education tools will aim the process toward the clinician-patient relationship where it belongs...' (28).

Once an advance directive has been formulated, the communication process has not come to an end. One pitfall may be to rely too much on these advanced statements while ignoring the views of competent patients at the time of the decision-making (65). A recommendation might be to invest in communicating with the patient as long as he or she is competent. Also, an impaired person may still be able to express wishes at some level.

Many health care providers, however, struggle to bring up conversations about end of life care and treatment preferences with their patient (6, 70). This may be because some feel constrained time-wise, or are uncertain about when to initiate end of life discussions (50, 72). Therefore the process of ACP should be time-effective by targeting its content in relation to the patient's disease trajectory, or with the patient's daily environment (43). Additionally, ACP might be a wise investment of time as future difficult and time-consuming decisions made in the absence of an advance care plan are minimized. Previous studies have shown that patients are more satisfied with their caregivers when ACP has been discussed (73). Moreover, it could be a satisfactory experience for the health professional as well (74). Caregivers may also proactively involve family and proxy decision-makers in the discussions from the outset; some families have already discussed the issues between themselves and would welcome the opportunity to share their conclusions.

Health professionals may rely on these proxy decision-makers to make end of life treatment decisions for incapacitated patients. However, the accuracy with which surrogates can predict patients' preferences is often questioned. Several studies indeed undermine the claim that reliance on surrogates is justified by their ability to predict a patient's preferences: it seems that surrogates project their own views and hopes onto what they predict the patient's preferences are as a result of which preferences of a patient and his/her family are often not in concordance (75–78). Therefore it is important to involve the patient's family in the process of ACP from the very beginning so as to provide care as much as possible in line with the patient's wishes in case of incapacity. In addition, drawing a patient's family into these end of life discussions is reassuring for both patients and family caregivers. Being a patient, it is a comforting thought to know that someone you love will take decisions on your behalf if you lose capacity. Being a patient's family, you may feel less stressed, anxious, or depressed at the time end of life decisions are required (79).

Another barrier may be the health professional's unwillingness to follow the patient's previously expressed preferences; they may assume they know what is in the advance directive without reading it (65). Specified preferences may also be overruled by the health professional's opinion of the clinical appropriateness of life-sustaining treatment or they may prefer to remain free to act according to their own judgment at the moment of decision-making, even if this is in conflict with the ACP (78, 80). However, sometimes patients themselves indicate that they prefer their family and health professionals to take decisions if they lose decision-making capacity instead of following their advance preferences (81). These things all exemplify the complexity of providing care in accordance with the patient's preferences at any given moment.

As ACP is emphasized to be a social process between the health professional, family, and patient, documenting it formally might sometimes be regarded as unnecessary which could result in patients not being given the opportunity or the information necessary to formulate their wishes in writing (55, 82). It is, however, recommended that people's preferences are also written down in their medical records, not only as the foundation for future updating and reviewing, but also so that they are available to inform later care. Continuity of care is valued as a core aspect of good end of life care by both patients and their healthcare providers and, more specifically, the continuity of advance directives and information collected during the process of ACP is considered a minimal standard of quality; it is burdensome for patients to have to explain their wishes all over again to different health care professionals in cases of a transfer to different care settings (83, 84). As end of life transitions are highly prevalent in some countries, especially to hospitals in the last week of life, the passing on of stated preferences and agreements to different health care providers should be a point of particular interest (85). An electronically-managed patient record which is used uniformly throughout the different care settings with the patient's consent would be a big step forward.

It may be clear that professionals engaging in ACP must acquire the appropriate skills to communicate effectively and to understand the legal and ethical issues involved (44). Organizations in many countries have now engaged in the development of guidelines about the importance and the meaning of ACP, providing practical guidance on core questions about when and with whom ACP discussions should be considered, how to raise delicate subjects, how to involve patients and proxies in difficult medical decision-making, and how to deal with patients who lose competence etc. (44, 49–51). Although such guidelines might be very useful, they may not be sufficient and interactive courses on palliative care and communication strategies to educate health and social care staff in medical and nursing schools may provide an additional step forward. Such training skills could be further maintained and developed by regular workplace-based education led by experts and expert patients (51).

Along with the growing awareness among health care organizations and professionals of the importance of end of life care communication, an important role in promoting ACP among the general public also lies with policy makers, who can set up information campaigns indicating the importance of ACP for all people, especially older people.

Conclusion

ACP refers to the process of continuous communication between healthcare providers, patients, and their family aimed at conveying the patient's wishes so that they can be taken into account at a future time when the patient has lost capacity. As a potential outcome of ACP, advance directives might be a means of honouring a patient's expressed preferences in the near or distant future and an aid to stimulating and facilitating the process of ongoing palliative care communication.

Despite its great value in the provision of high-quality palliative care, the implementation of ACP into practice is often limited and may be hampered by several barriers. However, the growing amount of attention ACP is receiving nowadays in terms of guidelines for care givers, information brochures, legislative initiatives, and institutional policy documents, is very promising.

References

1. United Nations Department of Economic and Social Affairs Population Division (2009). *World Population Prospects: The 2008 Revision. Highlights, Working Paper No. ESA/P/WP.210*. New York: UN.
2. World Health Organization (2004). *Palliative care: the solid facts*. Copenhagen: WHO.
3. World Health Organization (2004). *Better Palliative Care for Older People*. Copenhagen: WHO.
4. Institute of Medicine (IOM) (1997). *Approaching Death: Improving Care at the End of Life*. Washington, DC: National Academic Press.

5. Teno JM, Nelson HL, Lynn J (1994). Advance care planning. Priorities for ethical and empirical research. *Hastings Center Report*, **24**: S32–S36.

6. Gillick MR (2004). Advance care planning. *New England Journal of Medicine*, **350**: 7–8.

7. MeSH Database: the U.S. National Library of Medicine's controlled vocabulary used for indexing articles for MEDLINE/PubMed. Available at: http://www.ncbi.nlm.nih.gov/mesh.

8. Christensen K, Doblhammer G, Rau R, Vaupel JW (2009). Ageing populations: the challenges ahead. *Lancet*, **374**: 1196–208.

9. van der Heide A, Deliens L, Faisst K, Nilstun T, Norup M, Paci E, et al. (2003). End-of-life decision-making in six European countries: descriptive study. *Lancet*, **362**: 345–50.

10. Alzheimer Europe Report (2008). *End-of-life care for people with dementia*. Luxembourg: Alzheimer Europe.

11. Llibre Rodriguez JJ, Ferri CP, Acosta D, Guerra M, Huang Y, Jacob KS, et al. (2008). Prevalence of dementia in Latin America, India, and China: a population-based cross-sectional survey. *Lancet*, **372**: 464–74.

12. Mitchell SL, Teno JM, Kiely DK, Shaffer ML, Jones RN, Prigerson HG, et al. (2009). The clinical course of advanced dementia. *New England Journal of Medicine*, **361**: 1529–38.

13. Hebert LE, Scherr PA, Bienias JL, Bennett DA, Evans DA (2003). Alzheimer disease in the US population: prevalence estimates using the 2000 census. *Archives of Neurology*, **60**: 1119–22.

14. Lobo A, Launer LJ, Fratiglioni L, Andersen K, Di CA, Breteler MM, et al. (2000). Prevalence of dementia and major subtypes in Europe: A collaborative study of population-based cohorts. Neurologic Diseases in the Elderly Research Group. *Neurology*, **54**: S4–S9.

15. Hertogh CM (2006). Advance care planning and the relevance of a palliative care approach in dementia. *Age and Ageing*, **35**: 553–5.

16. Mitchell SL, Kiely DK, Hamel MB (2004). Dying with advanced dementia in the nursing home. *Archives of Internal Medicine*, **164**: 321–6.

17. Sepulveda C, Marlin A, Yoshida T, Ullrich A (2002). Palliative Care: the World Health Organization's global perspective. *Journal of Pain and Symptom Management*, **24**: 91–6.

18. Casarett DJ, Teno J, Higginson I (2006). How should nations measure the quality of end-of-life care for older adults? Recommendations for an international minimum data set. *Journal of the American Geriatrics Society*, **54**: 1765–71.

19. Emanuel EJ, Emanuel LL (1998). The promise of a good death. *Lancet*, **351**(Suppl 2): SII21–29.

20. Singer PA, Martin DK, Kelner M (1999). Quality end-of-life care: patients' perspectives. *Journal of the American Medical Association*, **281**: 163–8.

21. Steinhauser KE, Christakis NA, Clipp EC, McNeilly M, McIntyre L, Tulsky JA (2000). Factors considered important at the end of life by patients, family, physicians, and other care providers. *Journal of the American Medical Association*, **284**: 2476–82.

22. Stewart AL, Teno J, Patrick DL, Lynn J (1999). The concept of quality of life of dying persons in the context of health care. *Journal of Pain and Symptom Management*, **17**: 93–108.

23. Wenger NS, Rosenfeld K (2001). Quality indicators for end-of-life care in vulnerable elders. *Annals of Internal Medicine*, **135**: 677–85.

24. National cancer control programmes: policies and managerial guidelines. 2002. Geneva: WHO.

25. Pardon K, Deschepper R, Van der Stichele R, Bernheim J, Mortier F, Deliens L (2009). Preferences of advanced lung cancer patients for patient-centred information and decision-making: A prospective multicentre study in 13 hospitals in Belgium. *Patient Education and Counseling*, **77**: 421–9.

26. Rietjens JA, van der Heide, A, Onwuteaka-Philipsen BD, van der Maas PJ, van der Wal G (2006). Preferences of the Dutch general public for a good death and associations with attitudes towards end-of-life decision-making. *Palliative Medicine*, **20**: 685–92.

27. Martin DK, Emanuel LL, Singer PA (2000). Planning for the end of life. *Lancet*, **356**: 1672–6.

28. US Department of Health and Human Services. Assistant Secretary for Planning and Evaluation. Office of Disability Ageing and Long-Term Care Policy (2007). *Literature Review on Advance Directives*. Washington, DC: US Department of Health and Human Services.

29. Federal Law. Patient Self-Determination Act in Omnibus Budget Reconciliation Act of 1990.

30. Teno JM (2003) Advance care planning for frail, older persons. In RS Morrison, DE Meier (eds) *Geriatric Palliative Care*, pp. 307–13. New York: Oxford University Press.

31. Dunbrack J (2006). *Advance care planning: the Glossary project. Final report*. Ottawa: Health Canada.

32. Brown M (2003). The law and practice associated with advance directives in Canada and Australia: similarities, differences and debates. *Journal of Law and Medicine*, **11**: 59–76.

33. Parker M, Stewart C, Willmott L, Cartwright C (2007). Two steps forward, one step back: advance care planning, Australian regulatory frameworks and the Australian Medical Association. *Internal Medicine Journal*, **37**: 637–43.

34. Active Citizenship Network (2002). The European Charter of Patients' Rights. Rome, November, 2002.

35. Council of Europe. European Convention on Human Rights. Available at: http://conventions.coe.int/. (Accessed 1 April 2010.)

36. European Science Foundation. Available at: http://www.esf.org. (Accessed 1 April 2010.)

37. Belgisch Staatsblad 26 September 2002 [Belgian official collection of the laws Septembre 26 2002]. Wet betreffende de rechten van de patiënt 22 augustus 2002 [Law concerning patient rights in Belgium August 22, 2002] (in Dutch). Number bill 2002022737.

38. Staatsblad 1994:837. Act of 17 November 1994 amending the civil code and other legislation in connection with the incorporation of provisions concerning the contract to provide medical treatment (Medical Treatment Contract Act). 1994.

39. Alzheimer Europe. Available at: http://www.alzheimer-europe.org. (Accessed 1 April 2010)

40. Department of Constitutional Affairs (2007). *Mental Capacity Act 2005: Code of Practice*. London: The Stationery Office.

41. The National End of Life Care Programme (2008). *Advance decisions to refuse treatment. A guide for health and social care staff*. London: Department of Health.

42. Emanuel LL, Danis M, Pearlman RA, Singer PA (1995). Advance care planning as a process: structuring the discussions in practice. *Journal of the American Geriatrics Society* **43**: 440–6.

43. Teno JM, Lynn J (1996). Putting advance-care planning into action. *Journal of Clinical Ethics*, **7**: 205–13.

44. The National End of Life Care Programme (2008). *Advance Care Planning. A guide for health and social care staff*. London: Department of Health.

45. Keirse M (2009). *Het levenseinde teruggeven aan de mensen. Over vroegtijdige planning van de zorg*. Wemmel: Federatie Palliatieve Zorg Vlaanderen.

46. Ageing With Dignity (1997). *Five Wishes*. Available at: http://www.agingwithdignity.org/five-wishes. php. (Accessed 1 April 2010.)

47. Levenseinde Informatie Forum. Available at: http://www.leif.be. (Accessed 1 April 2010.)

48. Nederlandse Vereniging voor een vrijwillig levenseinde. Available at: http://www.nvve.nl (Accessed 1 April 2010.)

49. National End of Life Care Programme. Available at: http://www.endoflifecareforadults.nhs.uk/eolc/. (Accessed 1 April 2010).

50. Deschepper R, Vander Stichele R, Bernheim JL, De Keyser E, Van Der Kelen G, Mortier F, et al. (2006). Communication on end-of-life decisions with patients wishing to die at home: the making of a guideline for GPs in Flanders, Belgium. *British Journal of General Practice*, **56**: 14–19.

51. Royal College of Physicians (2009). *Concise guidance to good practice: A series of evidence-based guidelines for clinical management. Number 12: Advance Care Planning National Guidelines*. London: RCP.

52. Collins LG, Parks SM, Winter L (2006). The state of advance care planning: one decade after SUPPORT. *American Journal of Hospital Palliative Care*, **23**: 378–84.

53. Deeg D, Beekman A, Kriegsman D, Westendorp-de Serière M (1998) *Autonomy and well-being in the ageing population II: Report from the Longitudinal Ageing Study Amsterdam 1992–1996*. Amsterdam: VU University Press.

54. Klinkenberg M, Willems DL, Onwuteaka-Philipsen BD, Deeg DJ, van der Wal G (2004). Preferences in end-of-life care of older persons: after-death interviews with proxy respondents. *Social Science & Medicine*, **59**: 2467–77.

55. Rurup ML, Onwuteaka-Philipsen BD, van der Heide A, van der Wal G, Deeg DJ (2006). Frequency and determinants of advance directives concerning end-of-life care in The Netherlands. *Social Science & Medicine*, **62**: 1552–63.

56. Meeussen K, Van den Block L, Echteld M, Bossuyt N, Bilsen J, Van Casteren V, et al. (submitted). Advance care planning in Belgium and the Netherlands: a nationwide comparative study via sentinel networks of general practitioners.

57. De Gendt C, Bilsen J, Vander Stichele R, Deliens L (2010). Nursing home policies regarding advance care planning in Flanders, Belgium. *European Journal of Public Health*, **20**(2): 189–94.

58. Deliens L, De Gendt C, D'Haene I, Meeussen K, Van den Block L, vander Stichele R (2009). *Advance Care Planning: overleg tussen zorgverleners, patiënten met dementie en hun naasten*. Koning Boudewijnstichting Brussel.

59. ICM/Endemol/BBC Poll (2005). Survey of General Public.

60. Gott M, Gardiner C, Small N, Payne S, Seamark D, Barnes S, et al (2009). Barriers to advance care planning in chronic obstructive pulmonary disease. *Palliative Medicine*, **23**: 642–8.

61. Cartwright CM, Parker MH (2004). Advance care planning and end of life decision making. *Australian Family Physician*, **33**: 815–19.

62. Miyata H, Shiraishi H, Kai I (2006). Survey of the general public's attitudes toward advance directives in Japan: how to respect patients' preferences. *BMC Med Ethics* 7: E11.

63. Teno JM, Gruneir A, Schwartz Z, Nanda A, Wetle T (2007). Association between advance directives and quality of end-of-life care: a national study. *Journal of the American Geriatrics Society* **55**: 189–94.

64. US Department of Health and Human Services (2008). *Advance Directives and Advance Care Planning*: report to Congress.

65. Emanuel LL, von Gunten CF, Ferris FD (2000). Advance care planning. *Archives of Family Medicine*, **9**: 1181–7.

66. Seymour J, Gott M, Bellamy G, Ahmedzai SH, Clark D (2004). Planning for the end of life: the views of older people about advance care statements. *Social Science & Medicine*, **59**: 57–68.

67. Molloy DW, Guyatt GH, Russo R, Goeree R, O'Brien BJ, Bedard M, et al. (2000). Systematic implementation of an advance directive program in nursing homes: a randomized controlled trial. *Journal of the American Medical Association*, **283**: 1437–44.

68. Degenholtz HB, Rhee Y, Arnold RM (2004). Brief communication: the relationship between having a living will and dying in place. *Annals of Internal Medicine*, **141**: 113–17.

69. Cohen-Mansfield J (2006) Advance directives. In S Carmel, CA Morse, FMTorres-Gil (eds) *Lessons On Ageing From Three Nations*. Volume II: *The Art of Caring for Older Adults*, pp. 161–78. Amityville, New York: Baywood Publishing Company Inc.

70. Kolarik RC, Arnold RM, Fischer GS, Tulsky JA (2002). Objectives for advance care planning. *Journal of Palliative Medicine*, **5**: 697–704.

71. Teno JM (2004). Advance directives: time to move on. *Annals of Internal Medicine*, **141**: 159–60.

72. Brown M (2002). Participating in end of life decisions. The role of general practitioners. *Australian Family Physician*, **31**: 60–2.

73. Tierney WM, Dexter PR, Gramelspacher GP, Perkins AJ, Zhou XH, Wolinsky FD (2001). The effect of discussions about advance directives on patients' satisfaction with primary care. *Journal of General Internal Medicine*, **16**: 32–40.

74. Balaban RB (2000). A physician's guide to talking about end-of-life care. *Journal of General Internal Medicine*, **15**: 195–200.

75. Marks MA, Arkes HR (2008). Patient and surrogate disagreement in end-of-life decisions: can surrogates accurately predict patients' preferences? *Medical Decision Making*, **28**: 524–31.

76. Phipps E, True G, Harris D, Chong U, Tester W, Chavin SI, Braitman LE (2003). Approaching the end of life: attitudes, preferences, and behaviors of African-American and white patients and their family caregivers. *Journal of Clinical Oncology*, **21**: 549–54.

77. Shalowitz DI, Garrett-Mayer E, Wendler D (2006). The accuracy of surrogate decision makers: a systematic review. *Archives of Internal Medicine*, **166**: 493–7.

78. Tang ST, Liu TW, Lai MS, Liu LN, Chen CH (2005). Concordance of preferences for end-of-life care between terminally ill cancer patients and their family caregivers in Taiwan. *Journal of Pain and Symptom Management*, **30**: 510–18.

79. Detering KM, Hancock AD, Reade MC, Silvester W (2010). The impact of advance care planning on end of life care in elderly patients: randomised controlled trial. *British Medical Journal*, **340**: c1345.

80. Vezzoni C (2005). The legal status and social practice of treatment directives in the Netherlands. Dissertation, University of Groningen, The Netherlands. http://dissertations.ub.rug.nl/faculties/jur/2005/c.vezzoni/. 2005. (Accessed 6 May 2009.)

81. Puchalski CM, Zhong Z, Jacobs MM, Fox E, Lynn J, Harrold J, et al. (2000). Patients who want their family and physician to make resuscitation decisions for them: observations from SUPPORT and HELP. Study to Understand Prognoses and Preferences for Outcomes and Risks of Treatment. Hospitalized Elderly Longitudinal Project. *Journal of the American Geriatrics Society*, **48**: S84–S90.

82. Singer PA, Martin DK, Lavery JV, Thiel EC, Kelner M, Mendelssohn DC (1998). Reconceptualizing advance care planning from the patient's perspective. *Archives of Internal Medicine*, **158**: 879–84.

83. Borgsteede SD, Graafland-Riedstra C, Deliens L, Francke AL, van Eijk JT, Willems DL (2006). Good end-of-life care according to patients and their GPs. *British Journal of General Practice*, **56**: 20–6.

84. Walling A, Lorenz KA, Dy SM, Naeim A, Sanati H, Asch SM, et al. (2008). Evidence-based recommendations for information and care planning in cancer care. *Journal of Clinical Oncology*, **26**: 3896–902.

85. Van den Block L, Deschepper R, Bilsen J, Van Casteren V, Deliens L (2007). Transitions between care settings at the end of life in Belgium. *Journal of the American Medical Association*, **298**: 1638–9.

Chapter 10

New public health approaches to address diversity and end of life issues for older people

Jonathan Koffman

Introduction

Overall life expectancy is increasing in European and other developed countries, with more and more people living beyond 65 years of age. As part of population ageing, the pattern of diseases people suffer and die from is also changing. Given that many societies are now multicultural in nature, all health and social care professions working in hospital or community settings now require a different set of skills and knowledge to be able to ensure both quality and equality of health care provision. This situation is further amplified by growing numbers of older people from minority ethnic groups living in developed countries which will continue to increase in coming years (1). Older people from many minority ethnic groups are also now living with multiple morbidities until they die. Moreover, they can be poor, socially and emotionally marginalized, their expectations of culturally responsive care are frequently not realized, and sometimes they can face racism and ageism in care. Despite this, minority ethnic older people and their carers can resist and overcome some of these problems with the considered and active engagement of services. The aim of this chapter is therefore to examine public health 'differences that make a difference' (2) among older people when they negotiate institutions and practices for palliative and end of life care. This has particular resonance given that there is now increasing recognition of how multiple and simultaneous disadvantages can influence palliative care needs and end of life experiences (3). In this sense, this chapter also aims to foster debate with other complex approaches to manage inequality in palliative care for all service users.

Semantic confusion: making sense of understanding identity

Each year the number of published indexed under the headings of 'culture', 'race', and 'ethnicity' on Medline increases (4). All these terms have been used to explain patterns of disease, illness experiences, responses to treatment, and the use of services. However, substantial problems exist with this burgeoning body of research literature where semantic confusion is common. First, researchers rarely define the terms they use. Second, over the years, all terms have been used interchangeably, have been subject to misuse, or conflated with other social metrics, for example social class or education (5). Culture is but one of several typologies of difference that has been used to signify diversity among individuals and groups. Narrowly defined from an anthropological perspective, culture can be thought of as that which refers to the '. . . patterns, explicit and implicit, of and for behavior acquired and transmitted by symbols', language, and rituals (6).

Seen as a 'recipe' for living in the world, this conceptual framework for culture explains the means of transmitting these 'recipes' to the next generation (7). However, this is a limited understanding of culture that, if used here, risks minimizing discussions of cultural aspects of palliative medicine to an interpretive list of end of life beliefs and practices from a range of so-called 'cultural' groups. This has also been referred to as the 'fact-file' or 'checklist' (8) approach that, while informative in regards to interpreting behaviours, symbols, rituals, and other cultural practices of certain ethnic or religious groups that may be important and meaningful at the end of life, it runs the risk of encouraging generalizations about individuals and groups based on cultural identity. This in turn may then lead to the development of stereotypes, prejudices, and misunderstandings.

Culture is neither a static nor an intrinsic property of some cultural other. It is not static because identity, be it cultural, ethnic, religious, or other categories, is in a constant process of adaptation and change, often in response to interactions with yet 'others' who are different in multitudes of ways. Culture is not the sole possession of those who are considered 'ethnic' minority groups. All persons, the health or social care practitioner included, brings his or her own cultural self into the medical or social care encounter—a self that holds assumptions about the world and engages in practices and behaviours learned from their family and society of origin and, in the case of the health practitioner, from Western scientific and professional ideologies. Cross-cultural or intercultural interactions are not merely interpretative where each party needs only to translate language, signs, behaviours, or practices of the other. Ideally, these exchanges are also dialogic and relational. All parties enter into some transformational 'third space' (9) where meaning is negotiated and new understandings emerge. Therefore programs in 'cultural competency' that merely utilize an interpretive approach, emphasizing technical competencies utilized during the clinical encounter (such as communication skills) may miss the opportunity to teach skills needed for attitudinal transformations (such as sensitivity and humility) that are critical for 'developing mutually beneficial and nonpaternalistic . . . partnerships with patients and families' (10).

In addition to culture, self- or group identification may be based on race, ethnicity, tribal or clan affiliation, generational status, citizenship, gender, religion, politics, sexual orientation, social and economic class, and other categories (4). Race, a rather contentious category of identity, has its roots in social Darwinism, and relies heavily on an expectation of perceived (versus real) biological differences between people and populations (11). Historically, race has been used to describe geographically separated populations (such as the African race), cultural groups (Jews), nationality (the English race), and mankind in general (the human race). Racialized research in science has a long and inglorious history. In the mid-19th century, the cephalic index, a method for describing the shape of the skull, became a popular way of describing and dividing races. Under the influence of phrenology, a hierarchy of races was devised with white Europeans at the top and black Africans at the bottom. Intelligence, physique, culture, and morality were all placed in an order, the so-called 'Great Chain of Being' philosophy used to justify slavery, imperialism, anti-immigration policy, and the social status quo (12). Biological determinism also became prominent in medicine and medical practitioners frequently contributed to radicalized science (13) with the theory of racial hygiene in Nazi Germany being a horrific and notorious example. However, differences that do exist between peoples and populations are very minor and largely reflect superficial physical characteristics such as facial features, hair or skin colour. Many researchers have therefore now discredited race as being inaccurate and misleading (14).

Less controversial, but equally misunderstood is the concept of ethnicity. As a category of identity, it reflects the social grouping of persons on the basis of historical or territorial identity or by shared cultural patterns and traditions maintained between generations (15). One's ethnicity can be defined by language, such as Spanish language that unites Hispanic peoples in Central and South America and the Caribbean who are otherwise separated by geography, history, and politics. It can also be defined by shared ancestry, such as subgroups of diasporic black people who are descendants of slaves from West and Central Africa. There are also subcategories used in identifying certain ethnic groups. For example, among ethnic black populations, further delineations can be made by nativity and citizenship: African Americans who are descendants of slaves and of multiple generations born in and holding citizenship in the USA may be ethnically distinct (for example, in language or culture) from black Haitians, Cubans, Jamaicans, or other descendants of African slaves who reside in the Caribbean, South America, the UK, or other diasporic locations. Other ways in which people express their identity include kinship by tribal or clan affiliation which can be extremely influential (and potentially volatile) in intergroup dynamics.

Identity is both internally (self-) defined and externally (structurally) imposed (16) which has bearing not only in how an individual or group sees oneself but also in how they are treated by society. Needless to say, the politics and social science of identity is complex. Furthermore, semantic confusion is very common when the concepts of identity are used in clinical and research settings. The manner in which these concepts are used may change due to prevailing fashions and politics (17).

Structural factors, defined as rules, roles, and institutions derived from dynamic social, economic, political, and historical processes, may play an important role in creating and maintaining cultural, racial, and/or ethnic identities, themselves, or various aspects associated with those identities. An example can be seen with the conflation of ethnic identity with class: in places or situations where institutional racism or other forms of discrimination constrain freedom and development for certain segments of a population, say on the basis of racial or ethnic visibility, these structural factors may produce patterns (e.g. poverty, poor education, crime) that become erroneously attached to the identity of that group (16). The same can be said for structural factors that privilege other segments of the populations.

To compound the confusion, there is no uniformity in how persons are classified across national boundaries. For example, the National Health Service and census in the UK identify five different categories of 'ethnicity' (white, mixed, Asian, black, or Chinese) that are further broken down into different subgroups based on countries of origin (e.g. Indian, Pakistani, Bangladeshi, or other for Asian people; Caribbean, African, or other for black people, etc.) (18); while the USA census collapses many distinct populations into one dichotomous category of 'ethnicity' (Hispanic or non-Hispanic) and five single broad categories of 'race,' (white, black or African American, American Indian or Alaska Native, Asian, and Native Hawaiian or Other Pacific Islander) (19). The South African census uses five population categories based on self-classification (Black African, Coloured, Indian or Asian, White, or Other) (20). Canada collects census data based on ethnic origins (defined by ancestry) and on a category called 'visible minority' status, defined as 'persons other than Aboriginal persons who are not white in race or color' (21). Lastly, there is evidence that many people change their assigned identity over time, as is their prerogative. USA-based research has shown that at least 35% of respondents altered their self-assignment over a year and in the validation study following the 1991 British census 12% of 'black' people altered their ethnic group, as did 22% of 'other' category (22).

This mutability attests to the fact that persons inhabit multiple identities which are expressed or perceived differently as need and circumstance change (15, 16). The relevance of this discussion for palliative care is to caution the clinician and researcher to be mindful of the difficulties in interpreting events at the bedside or reports in the literature related to culture, race, ethnicity, or other identifiers. Employing clearly and rationally defined demographic categorizations of identity in studying epidemiological patterns of morbidity and mortality has usefulness for policy implications, such as determining what systems of care are needed or measuring inequities in quality of care delivered across population groups. However, employing 'essentialized' notions of preferences or behaviours at the patient's bedside runs the risk of compromising an individual's 'needs and concerns [that] may not conform to preconceived or stereotyped patterns'. (15). What best serves the needs of all patients is knowledge of the particular individual's beliefs, values, preferences, and practices—knowledge gained by asking the patient or family directly or by utilizing resources that promote patient-centred and relationship-centred care.

The special case of immigration: ramifications for services

Throughout human history, individuals, families, and groups have emigrated from their native homes to other places globally for many reasons: the prospect of education, economic, or social advantage; the need to escape war, political torture, or other conflicts; or the desire to reunite with other family members. Globalization has brought with it an unprecedented increase in the numbers of persons who have migrated to developed countries. In 2005, there was an estimated 191 million immigrants worldwide: approximately 64 million of these immigrants arrived in Europe and 44 million in North America—a tripling of the immigrant populations in these regions compared to 20 years earlier. This trend is expected to continue and to increase. In the USA, for example, it is estimated that by the year 2050, nearly two-thirds of the population will be immigrants.

The International Observatory on End of Life Care that monitors the global development of hospice and palliative care services around the world reports that such services are unavailable or are uneven at best in underdeveloped and medium developed countries as compared to Europe and English-speaking countries (23). Subsequently the immigrant may not have had much exposure to or knowledge of palliative care services provided by hospices or other health care institutions in their home countries. For example, the Observatory documented misperceptions about and stigmas regarding palliative care in Mexico. This finding has also been mirrored in the UK (24). As such, expectations for palliative care may thus be lowered among minority ethic groups who bring from their country of origin misperceptions or lowered priorities for this type of care (25). In addition, some immigrants may find accessing quality care and finding funds for hospice, palliative care, and other end of life heath services to be a complex and potentially confusing process that may be compounded by unfamiliarity with laws and regulations of the host country. The immigrant's knowledge of and preference for palliative or other health care may be influenced by factors related to immigration, itself. For example, refugees and asylum seekers who have experienced violence or who may have been exposed to torture or other state-sanctioned or war related trauma may be mistrustful of health care or social service institutions and authorities (26). They may also face fears and uncertainties that accompany their experiences as an immigrant within a polarized political climate. In a report on immigration issues and end of life care in California, investigators identified the unique concerns of *undocumented* immigrants—those who have entered the USA illegally or who have overstayed their visas (25).

Over 27% of the USA undocumented population reside in California, the most ethnically and culturally diverse state in that country. Greater than 25% of these undocumented persons are aged between 15–44 years and come to the USA primarily looking for work or other opportunities. While this younger, healthier cohort may not represent the typical patient in need of palliative care services, mortality data shows that a disproportionate number of these workers are at risk of dying from trauma and accidents. The implications of these patterns include the need to increase expertise in palliative care practices and services in emergency departments (including end of life decision-making and bereavement services for families and loved ones) and to support education and training programmes on unique issues of death and dying in emergency room settings for emergency personnel. This report also found that among patients for whom hospice would be appropriate (deaths following terminal illness or chronic disease trajectories), few immigrants and other ethnically diverse persons in California utilized hospice for their end of life care needs. The range of reasons included barriers due to lack of eligibility for state or federal funding benefits; lack of cultural acceptance of hospice and palliative care practices; and lack of referral by health providers. In addition, the 'salmon effect' where immigrants return home to their native countries to die, partially explained lower use of hospice (27). Immigration also impacts the workforce that provides caregiving for those who are dying. Foreign health care workers are motivated to leave their native countries for reasons general to all immigrants—education, economic, or social advantage; or they may leave due to inadequate health care infrastructures and technologies (28). The result in some receiving countries is a growing migrant workforce who brings with them their own unique cross-cultural issues to the health and social care delivery equation. Whilst on the one hand, an increasingly diverse health care workforce may help improve outreach to diverse communities, particularly in areas of language barriers and other access issues (these workers will represent a spectrum of acculturation or assimilation of the language, customs, values, and perspectives of the host country) there are also challenges; there can be those immigrant providers who lack these skills with native patients. Central to this issue is communication capability.

Differences that make a difference at the end of life

How we understand the influence of diversity in patterns of advanced disease, illness experiences, responses to treatment, and the use of specialist palliative care services is critical given increasing evidence that we are not all equal in death and dying (8, 29–8, 31). Race or ethnic-based disparities in mortality and in diagnosis, quality of care, referral patterns to specialist palliative care, and treatments for pain and other physical symptoms have been documented in many developed countries (15, 16, 32–37). In the USA, a comprehensive review of evidence of unequal treatment commissioned by the USA congress and produced by its Institute of Medicine (IOM) documented race- or ethnic-based inequities in pain and chronic disease management, cancer care, and other clinical care settings and suggested that inequities may be due to patient-level, provider-level, and/or health system-level variables, alone or in combinations (36). Patient-level factors would include ethnocultural, social or other beliefs, preferences, or knowledge about health options. According to the IOM study, patient-level factors were thought to be the *least* likely contributor to disparities. On the other hand, both provider stereotyping and bias and how health care systems are organized as well as the degree to which persons have access to care were shown to more likely influence on health outcomes for minority patients.

The existence of prejudice and stereotyping from the service provider's side of the exchange may be difficult for many non-minority providers to accept, as we all presume to consciously abhor such discriminatory attitudes and behaviours. The important contribution of the IOM report in thinking about this issue was its suggestion that it is not conscious attitudes that drive discrimination but rather those unconscious or implicit attitudes that may compel us when we are under duress.

Health system level factors such as poor access to health care services have been reported by black and minority ethnic groups in the USA and UK (38). This is also an issue for end of life care where the impact of ageing on the black and minority ethnic groups now means increasingly larger numbers of older members within these communities will require health services for advanced disease. A limited number of reports have levelled criticism of care at the end of life for these communities and poor access to appropriate care. Relatively lower rates of cancer have been advanced as one explanation to account for low uptake of services, but the figures may be inaccurate because of inadequate ethnic monitoring (39).

It could cautiously be concluded that 'some black and Asian patients and their carers are very disadvantaged, as they do not know what they are entitled to, and hence what to ask for by way of benefits and services' (40). A recent study in an inner London health authority demonstrated that older first-generation black Caribbean patients with advanced disease experienced restricted access to some specialist palliative care services compared to white British peers, yet an analysis of local provision revealed no lack of palliative care services (31). This example of underutilization of palliative care services by the black Caribbean community at the end of life supports other recent research among minority ethnic communities (32, 41). The explanations to account for this, all of which may operate in combination, are highlighted in Box 10.1 and have ramifications for wider public health policy. Identifying and eliminating health inequities in the delivery of quality palliative and related care therefore represents a critical mandate. Institutional standards for monitoring and insuring the cultural sensitivity and competency of the palliative medicine workforce should be employed, as should strategies to increase community-based partnerships.

Box 10.1 Black and minority ethnic social exclusion at the end of life: why does it occur?

Social and economic deprivation

Low socioeconomic status has been positively linked to an increased likelihood of hospital deaths although this would apply equally to all population groups

Knowledge of specialist palliative care services and poor communication

There is a growing body of evidence that black and ethnic minorities are not adequately aware of specialist palliative care services available to them

Ethno-centralism

Demand for services may be influenced by the 'ethnocentric' outlook of palliative care services, discouraging black and minority ethnic groups from making use of relevant provision

Attitudes to palliative care

Barriers to healthcare that the poor and the disenfranchised have traditionally encountered may influence their receptivity to palliative (47)

Dissatisfaction with health care

Uptake of health and social services among certain minority ethnic communities has revealed lower utilization of services due to dissatisfaction of services

Cultural mistrust

Evidence from USA to support the contention that black and minority ethnic groups as less likely than white patients to trust the motivations of doctors who discuss end of life care with them

Gatekeepers

Some health care professionals 'gatekeepers' to services among minority ethnic groups contributing to lower referral rates

Providing equitable, culturally appropriate palliative care

The World Health Organization definition of palliative care specifies two goals: (1) improving quality of life of patients and families and (2) preventing and relieving suffering. It identifies three strategies for meeting those goals: early identification; impeccable assessment; and (appropriate) treatment. Lastly, the definition addresses four domains of care: (1) problems related to pain, (2) physical conditions, (3) the psychosocial, (4) and the spiritual. The remaining section of this chapter addresses these public health goals, strategies, and domains in relation to the delivery of high quality palliative care in cross- or multicultural settings.

Information, information, information

Key demographic characteristics of the population that have been identified as influencing the need for palliative care are: age, gender, ethnicity/religion, socioeconomic status, and household composition (42, 43). Geographical areas with high proportions of older people in their locality have been recognized as having higher levels of need and as requiring more resources for palliative care (44). It has also been suggested that areas with high proportions of people from minority ethnic groups may need greater resources to train professionals to provide care to diverse who will require 'an understanding of the different approaches taken by different cultures to end of life issues' (43).

Despite the broad relationships between demographic characteristics and the need for palliative care, there are inherent difficulties in the availability of comprehensive and usable demographic data on ethnicity to assess the palliative care needs of minority ethnic older people and to monitor services. This is because there are a range of factors, many of which are not fully understood, which affect service needs and how people use services. Emerging research suggests that there are two main factors which are of particular importance:

- Ethnic differences in the patterning of diseases
- Culture and lifestyle differences and changes (which in turn have an effect upon disease and service needs).

Realizing the goals of palliative care in crosscultural contexts

Quality of life

The World Health Organization (WHO) defines quality of life (QOL) as 'an individual's perception of their position in life in the context of the culture and value systems in which they live and in relation to their goals, expectations, standards and concerns' (45). When applied to palliative care, the focus is on health gain—maximizing the quality versus the quantity of time remaining in a patient's life. Because quality should be subjectively defined by patients and their families, cultural factors relevant to the individual and their family need to be addressed when assessing their QOL preferences and requirements.

Many QOL assessment instruments include broad areas representing key domains such as physical symptoms, functional status, interpersonal relations, emotional well-being, and the experience of spiritual or existential transcendence. However, the subjective nature of the concept of QOL and instruments used to measure it must also consider variations in meanings of these domains across cultural groups. Recognizing the need to address cultural components in assessing quality, WHO initiated the WHOQOL project to 'develop an international cross-culturally comparable quality of life assessment instrument' (46).

The psychometric properties of the WHOQOL instrument were tested in several stages and across multicultural field sites to insure crosscultural validity including: agreement on the definition of QOL; standardization of questions or items and of scale construction; and field testing final instruments. Both the 100-item instrument (WHOQOL-100) and the shorter 26-item version (WHOQOL-BREF) are available in many languages and can be used clinically for individual patients and well as in crosscultural research for inter- and intragroup comparisons (45). The initial field sites, located in Australia, Croatia, France, India, Israel, Japan, the Netherlands, Panama, Russia, Spain, Thailand, the UK, the USA, and Zimbabwe, each adapted the standardized instrument to their population-based needs. To date there are now over 30 sites worldwide and more continue to field test and adapt the instrument to the unique cultural needs of their countries.

Preventing and relieving suffering and distress

Acknowledging that cultural factors influence the public health status of minority ethnic groups with advanced disease and the end of life has ramifications for preventing and relieving suffering This is because culture has been shown to mediate the ways in which symptoms associated with advanced disease are identified and interpreted, the appropriate modes of expression of pain and other symptoms and associated suffering, whether an illness and symptoms are stigmatized, and whether the dependency needs that accompany advanced disease are considered an acceptable part of the normal life cycle or marginalized (Figure 10.1). The evidence of the influence of cultural and ethnic factors on symptom interpretation is fascinating and frequently raises more questions than it answers. In the 1950s, Zborowski demonstrated differences among old American, Irish, and other migrant communities' perceptions of their pain (47). Most recently, Koffman et al. observed significantly higher levels of symptom related-distress among African Caribbean compared with native-born white UK patients with advanced cancer living in south London. This finding was only partly explained by simple variations in treatment levels between the two groups (34). Along with other researchers (48, 49) the authors have identified that the language of expressing symptom-related distress may possibly be reinforced by symptom attributions shaped and patterned by culture that, when present, assist the patient to comprehend the inexplicable.

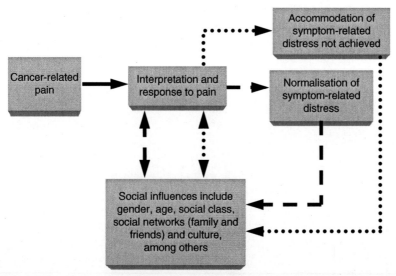

Fig. 10.1 Relationship between the experience of cancer-related pain, construction of meaning, and patients' culture.
Reproduced from Koffman et al., 2008 (58); **22**: 350–9. Reprinted by permission of SAGE.

In other communities the actual language used to describe distress and suffering has implications for the delivery of palliative and end of life care. Krause revealed that the expression in Punjabi, 'dil me girda hai' used by Panjabis in Bedford often translates as the 'sinking heart' to reflect a range of psychological and somatic conditions (50). In addition, she suggests that the 'generalized hopelessness' which characterizes depressive disorders in women living in London would not be regarded as abnormal among Hindu, Muslim, and Buddhist women who would regard 'hopelessness' as an aspect of life which can only be overcome on the path to salvation. Ahmed takes the view that while South Asian patients may be well aware of their own psychosomatic symptoms, general practitioners (including Asian general practitioners) tend only to acknowledge physical symptoms but do not recognize psychological distress (51). The ongoing challenge is for health care professionals to explore and acknowledge culturally determined understandings and expressions associated with advanced disease that do not mirror their own.

Public health strategies of palliative care in crosscultural settings

Early identification

Problems with late referrals to hospice or for palliative care in general are a concern for many populations (3). To avoid the appearance of medical abandonment, it is important to integrate the goals of hospice and of palliative care early in the disease process, particularly for those illnesses that are predictably fatal. This is particularly important for immigrants or members of ethnic or cultural communities who may already feel marginalized or vulnerable due to their minority status. Myths or misunderstandings about the goals of palliative care should be addressed early on through culturally effective communication—which can also enable the palliative care team to learn about and incorporate the unique perspectives of the patient into the multidisciplinary management of their care. Recent research would suggest that low awareness of palliative care and related services among materially deprived minority ethic communities contributes to perpetuating this knowledge void (24).

Identifying preferences for medical care in advance of untoward or terminal circumstances can be a difficult and emotional process. The decision-making model of advance care planning derived from bioethics practices assumes that choices made by the individual can be arrived at through rational processes that are unchanged by time, shifting social consequences, or disease and illness progression. Such a model may only appeal to certain subsets of groups, thus limiting the utility of instruments used for advance planning (living wills or durable powers of attorney for health care). For some groups, speaking about the dying process or planning for death may represent a transgression of a strong cultural taboo and could create additional distress. Other patients, unfamiliar with or mistrustful of the legal system may misconstrue the purpose, or nature of formal advance care planning documents. In all cases, rather than abandon the goals of anticipatory or advance care planning, strategies should be sought that facilitate understanding. For example, a generic discussion to identify a health care proxy need not be cast as a discussion of death, but rather an opportunity to determine desired roles of various family members and support persons. Discussions about patient preferences for end of life care should be culturally and linguistically appropriate and reflect sensitivity to patient values and beliefs.

Impeccable assessment

Critical to assessing and monitoring palliative care needs is the ability to communicate clearly and effectively. The inability to do so not only affects access to palliative care services but has been shown to be a source of serious problems in clinical consultations and the cause of misunderstandings among patients, family members, and health care providers (31).

Important communication difficulties arise where there is an over-reliance on patient's relatives acting on their loved one or dependants' behalf. While this may well be simpler than accessing an interpreter, it can potentially disadvantage both the doctor and the patient (30).

The family interpreter may filter, abbreviate, or omit very important information, or inform the doctor or the patient what he or she thinks the doctor and patient needs to know. Important medical information may not be understood adequately or conveyed in full. Further, the use of children as interpreters is considered inappropriate. Details about an illness may be very intimate and it places an unfair burden on them, who, depending on their age, may be less likely to understand adult conversations in English, or even their own language. Using friends or untrained lay interpreters from the local community can be even more problematic since there can be issues of confidentiality and fear of gossip in the wider community (52). Moreover, communication is not only an issue of spoken language. It also involves body language, cultural rules as to what is courteous (such as not looking the professionals—especially opposite gender—in the eye) and appropriate behaviours in an unequal gender and power relationship (29). People who speak English with a different accent or dialect, can also judged to be less intelligent or fail to be understood or understand what is being said to them (52).

Appropriate treatment

It is widely acknowledged that management of physical and psychological symptoms associated with advanced disease can be difficult in monocultural interactions between clinicians and patients because of differences in perspective between Western biomedicine and lay health beliefs and practices. However, the design and assessment of effective health care for culturally diverse patients, both long-term residents and new immigrants and refugees, is even more complicated. New immigrants increasingly come to the USA and the UK among other countries from regions such as Southeast Asia, Latin America, and Africa, and are even more heterogeneous than their European predecessors (48). Within the same ethnic group, individuals come from all walks of life with differing educational, occupational, and economic status, ties to their country of origin, and geographical background. All these factors affect their ethnic identity and their cultural responses to health and illness. Understand and controlling patients' symptoms in a health care system where the dominant imperative is for economic efficiency represents an overwhelming challenge. When clinicians look to published research to acquaint themselves with the ways in which ethnicity or culture may impinge upon the experience of symptoms, their expression, pain behaviours, or coping responses, they find a vast array of disciplinary lenses, diverse theoretical approaches that are often not made explicit, inconsistent findings, and methodological weaknesses. Upon closer reading, however, one can see that varied disciplines are starting to speak to each other and that a biological and social model of pain is attainable.

Domains of palliative care for culturally diverse populations

Pain and other symptoms

Investigators in a range of health care settings in the USA have reported on disparities in the assessment and management of pain in ethnic minority groups as compared to white patients. In a qualitative study of nursing home residents, black residents consistently reported more incidents of prolonged and untreated moderate to severe pain as compared to white residents. Studies in emergency room settings similarly found inequities in pain treatment of Hispanic and black patients as compared to white patients (53). Surprisingly, studies in cancer centres documented similar patterns (54, 55). These disparities can not be explained by cultural differences in the expression of pain, although such differences do exist.

Pain and other physical symptoms are experienced, understood, and expressed by patients in ways that are mediated by culture, gender, age, social role, personality, and other factors. One's learned response for the expression and reactions of pain or other physical distress may range from the vocally or physically demonstrative to the passive or quietly stoic, with all possible forms between. Studies that explore different meanings, that can be defined as perceived relationships between the individual and his/her world that is developed within the context of specific events (56), and forms of expression across cultures may be useful for increasing awareness of variability in patient presentation of pain and for assessment of its subjective manifestations. For example, meanings ascribed to pain could be viewed positively as a challenge to overcome or negatively as the accompaniment to profound loss (57). In a recent study exploring and comparing cancer-related pain among African Caribbeans and white British patients, pain was understood by both ethnic groups as a challenge and an enemy, and by African Caribbean patients as a test of religious faith or as a divine punishment (58). These findings are supported by others who suggest that enduring pain is encouraged within African American where struggle and survival are considered noble (30).

Comparative studies on pain thresholds across populations groups—identifying which group experiences more or less pain under given conditions—are potentially racist and without clear clinical value. However, what would be clinically relevant is individual patient assessment of pain levels. Like quality of life measures, a range of crossculturally validated instruments for assessing pain can be employed at the bedside. Pain intensity scales and multidimensional tools have been translated into several languages; however, mere translation of standardized instruments into the language of a given patient may not ensure its efficacy for that patient's cultural group. The selection of a scale or tool should be based on the patient's literacy and ability to understand numerical ratings, images, or sensory, affective and evaluative descriptors used in numerical rating, visual analogue, or multidimensional scales.

Symptoms of anxiety, depression, and delirium, common in the advanced and terminal stages of death, may be expressed and understood differently across various ethnic and cultural groups. Symptom formation can be influenced by sociopolitical factors in conjunction with biological and environmental variables. For example, paranoia expressed by persons from oppressed groups may actually represent a healthy, protective response. Other behaviours considered normative within the psychospiritual belief systems of a given culture (e.g. spirit possession, visions of spirits or ghosts, etc.) may be considered delusional or otherwise pathological within a Western biomedical model. Conversely, certain culture specific patterns of anxiety or distress that do not fit medical classifications (so-called culture bound syndromes) may be missed in evaluating the mental health of patients and their families.

Psychosocial and spiritual domains

Social support networks are crucial factors in the psychological well-being of the seriously ill and the dying patient (59). Within those networks, informal caregivers perform an essential role for both the patient and for the health delivery system. The emphasis on care in the community rather than institutions, and the growing awareness that in some communities, people would prefer to die at home given the choice means that informal caregivers are indispensable partners of health and social care professionals. Many assume responsibilities of care that were previously confined to specialist inpatient settings and community hospitals (60). Caring for family members is regarded as an important obligation in many ethnic communities (61). Further, for many ethnic minority families, caring for dying relatives at home when possible is considered a matter of honour and integrity as well as a means of ensuring the death occurs in a holy place. Karim et al. refer to the stigma and loss of face from not caring for close family relatives (62). In the Hindu tradition, the concepts of karma and sacred duty may place the family of a loved one or dependant under additional stress in order to do the right thing (52). Spruyt found that east London Bangladeshi children became actively involved in the care of dying patient and in interactions with professionals, and had to act as interpreters. This had a negative impact on them subsequently. A number of children were required to give up formal schooling and older sons gave up work to help with care of their dependants. When there is home care the burden often falls upon one person, but without ready access to outside support. For example, in the UK, multigenerational Pakistani and Bangladeshi families who wish to provide traditional support may also be in situations with high unemployment and poverty, and large families of young children (63). Home care is also not without problems when outside help is needed, because many ethnic minorities would regard this as a sense of failure in the eyes of the community, and it may also be regarded as an invasion of privacy (29). Smaje and Field also point out the tensions which can arise when an elderly person needs and demands care from a female relative who may have quite different expectations, especially if the carer also has children born in the host country (64). However, it is important to bear in mind that expectations of care from family relatives may change in coming years as patterns of family life and social networks evolve through a process of acculturation.

The experience of advanced disease can have a profound effect on patients and their family and friends. Indeed, during their illness many patients may raise questions that relate to their identity and self-worth as they seek to find the ultimate meaning in their life. Some patients attempt to answer these questions by examining their religious or spiritual beliefs. Formal religion is a means of expressing an underlying spirituality, but spiritual belief, concerned with the search for existential or the ultimate meaning in life, is a broader concept and may not always be expressed in a religious way.

Most of the published literature on role of religious faith at the end of life are descriptive and focus on 'factfile' approaches to manage the experience of death and dying across different faiths (65, 66). As discussed above, this approach is not without criticism as it has a tendency to over-categorize religious and cultural groups (8). The lack of serious study of the religious and spiritual needs of ethnic minority communities may be partly due to an assumption that faith communities will provide their own religious and spiritual care. Anecdotal evidence from specialist palliative care nurses suggests that it is often assumed that ethnic minority patients have no spiritual problems because 'they have their own beliefs and rituals', and once again, 'they look after their own.' (29). While some models of palliative and supportive care have not included mention of the role of spiritual care at the end of life others have begun to acknowledge the important role of spirituality (67). Dein and Stygall suggest the lack of interest by health care professionals in patients' religious concerns may be due to the discomfort created by the discussion of personal matters, that they associate religion with 'superstition, intolerance and persecution', or that 'religion may be seen as a kind of consolation, a last resort, which is offered when all else fails' (68).

Conclusions

The palliative care movement has assumed a leading role in addressing the health and social care needs of patients and families facing the inevitability of death. It has only been recently that attention has focused on the importance of providing care for increasingly diverse societies that include those in the USA, UK Australia, and New Zealand, among others. This has now become an increasingly important demographic imperative. This chapter has shown that the language of understanding difference is complex yet fascinating. When considering its influence in the provision of care at the end of life and during bereavement, perhaps we should hold a double lens: one that applies a framework of equity to understand and serve population needs of specific communities; and another that never loses sight of the individuals and families before us—those with clinical, psychosocial, and spiritual needs and concerns that may not conform to preconceived or stereotyped patterns. And always we should be mindful that an individualized approach to palliative care with a focus on quality is paramount for any patient, regardless of their ethnic or cultural background.

References

1. WHO (2004). *Better Palliative Care for Older People: the Solid Facts*. Milan: The World Health Organisation Regional Office for Europe.
2. Parens E (1998). What differences make a difference? *Cambridge Quarterly of Healthcare Ethics*, **7**(1): 1–6.
3. Koffman J, Camps J (2008). No way in: including the excluded at the end of life. In S Payne, J Seymour, J Skilbeck, C Ingelton (eds) *Palliative Care Nursing: Principles and Evidence for Practice*, 2nd edn, pp. 362–82. Maidenhead: Open University Press.
4. Koffman J (2006). The language of diversity: controversies relevant to palliative care research. *European Journal of Palliative Care*, **11**(1): 18–21.
5. Hillier S, Kelleher D (1996). Considering culture, ethnicity and the politics of health. In S Hillier, D Kelleher (eds) *Researching Cultural Differences in Health*, pp. 1–10. London: Routledge.
6. Kroeber AL, Kluckholn C (1952). *A Critical Review of Concepts and Definitions. Vol 47*. Cambridge, MA: The Peabody Museum of Archaeology and Ethnology, Harvard University.
7. Donovan J (1986). *We Don't Buy Sickness, It Just Comes*. Aldershot: Gower.
8. Gunaratnam Y (2003). Culture is not enough. In D Field, J Hockey, N Small (eds) *Death, gender and ethnicity*, 1st edn, pp. 166–86. London: Routledge.
9. Bhabha HK (1988). The commitment to theory. *New Formations*, **5**: 5–23.
10. Tervalon M, Murray-Garcia J (1998). Cultural humility versus cultural competence: a critical distinction in defining physician training outcomes in multicultural education. *Journal of Health Care for Poor Underserved*, **9**(2): 117–25.
11. Stepan N (1982). *The Idea of Race in Science*. London: Macmillan Press.
12. Singh SP (1997). Ethnicity in psychiatric epidemiology: need for precision. *British Journal of Psychiatry*, **171**: 305–8.
13. Ahmad WIU (1993). *'Race' and Health in Contemporary Britain*. London: Open University Press.
14. Karlesen S, Nazroo JY (2002). Relation between discrimination, social class and health among ethnic minority groups. *American Journal of Public Health*, **92**(4): 624–31.
15. Crawley LM (2005). Racial, cultural, and ethnic factors influencing end-of-life care. *Journal of Palliative Medicine*, **8**(1): ss58–ss69.
16. Karlsen S, Nazroo JY (2002). Agency and structure: the impact of ethnic identity and racism on the health of ethnic minority people. *Sociology of Health and Illness*, **24**(1): 1–20.
17. Gunaratnam Y (2003). *Researching 'Race' and Ethnicity: Methods, Knowledge and Power*. London: Sage.
18. Office of National Statistics (2003). *Ethnic group statistics: A guide for the collection and classification of ethnicity data*. Newport: Her Majesty's Stationery Office.
19. Federal Register Notice (2004). *Revisions to the Standards for the Classification of Federal Data on Race and Ethnicity*. Washington, DC: National Archives and Records Administration.
20. Lehohla P (2003). *Census 2001: Census in Brief*. Pretoria: Statistics South Africa.

21. Statistics Canada (2001). *Census Dictionary: Visible Minorities*. Ottawa: Statistics Canada.

22. Pringle M, Rothera I (1995). *Ethnic group data collection in primary care: problems and solutions*. Nottingham: University of Nottingham Medical School.

23. *International Observatory on End of Life Care* (2006). *Global Development*. Lancaster: School of Health and Medicine, Lancaster University.

24. Koffman J, Burke G, Dias A, Ravel B, Byrne J, Gonzales J, et al. (2007). Demographic factors and awareness of palliative care and related services. *Palliative Medicine*, **21**(2): 145–53.

25. Crawley LM, Chaudhary S (2006). *The State of the Knowledge of the Impact of Racial, Cultural, and Ethnic Factors on Quality of End-of-Life Care in California: Immigrant Issues at the End of Life*. Oakland, CA: California Healthcare Foundation.

26. Gavagan T, Brodyaga L (1998). Medical care for immigrants and refugees. *American Family Physician*, **57**(5): 1061–8.

27. Palloni A, Arias E (2004). Paradox lost: explaining the Hispanic adult mortality advantage. *Demography*, **41**(3): 385–415.

28. Crawley LM, Kagawa-Singer M, Rutman LE, Chaudhary S (2007). *Racial, Cultural, and Ethnic Factors on Quality of End-of-Life Care in California: Findings and Recommendations*. Oakland, CA: California Healthcare Foundation.

29. Firth S (2001). *Wider horizons: Care of the Dying in a Multi-Cultural Society*. London: National Council for Hospices and Specialist Palliative Care Services.

30. Crawley L, Payne R, Bolden J, Payne T, Washington P, Williams S (2000). Palliative and end-of-life care in the African American community. *Journal of the American Medical Association*, **284**: 2518–21.

31. Koffman J, Higginson IJ (2001). Accounts of carers' satisfaction with health care at the end of life: a comparison of first generation black Caribbeans and white patients with advanced disease. *Palliative Medicine*, **15**(4): 337–45.

32. Farrell J (2000). *Do disadvantaged and minority ethnic groups receive adequate access to palliative care services?* Glasgow: Glasgow University.

33. Department of Health (1998). *Inequalities in Health: Report of an Independent Inquiry Chaired by Sir Donald Acheson*. London: The Stationery Office.

34. Koffman J, Higginson IJ, Donaldson N (2003). Symptom severity in advanced cancer, assessed in two ethnic groups by interviews with bereaved family members and friends. *Journal of the Royal Society of Medicine*, **96**(1): 10–16.

35. Koffman J, Donaldson N, Hotopf M, Higginson IJ (2005). Does ethnicity matter? Bereavement outcomes in two ethnic groups living in the United Kingdom. *Palliative and Supportive Care*, **3**: 183–90.

36. Smedley BD, Stith AY, Nelson AR (2003). *Unequal Treatment: Confronting Racial and Ethnic Disparities in Healthcare*. Washington DC: National Academies Press.

37. Mooney G (2003). Inequity in Australian health care: how do we progress from here? *Austalian and New Zealand Journal of Public Health*, **27**(3): 267–70.

38. O'Neill J, Marconi K (2001). Access to palliative care in the USA: why emphasize vulnerable groups? *Journal of the Royal Society of Medicine*, **94**: 452–4.

39. Aspinall PJ (1999). Ethnic groups and our healthier nation: whither the information base? *Journal of Public Health Medicine*, **21**: 125–32.

40. Hill D, Penso D (1995). *Opening doors: Improving access to hospice and specialist palliative care services by members of the black and ethnic minority communities*. (Report No.: Occasional Paper 7.) London: National Council for Hospice and Specialist Palliative Care Services.

41. Skilbeck J, Corner J, Beech N, Clark D, Hughes P, Douglas HR, et al. (2002). Clinical nurse specialists in palliative care. Part 1. A description of the Macmillan Nurse caseload. *Palliative Medicine*, **16**(4): 285–96.

42. Higginson IJ, Koffman J (2004). Public health and palliative care. *Clinics in Geriatric Medicine*, **21**: 45–55.

43. Tebbit P (2004). *Population-Based Needs Assessment for Palliative Care—A Manual for Cancer Networks*. London: National Council for Hospice and Specialist Palliative Care Services.

44. Grande GE, Addington-Hall JM, Todd CJ (1998). Place of death and access to home care services: are certain patient groups at a disadvantage? *Social Science & Medicine*, **47**(5): 565–79.

45. World Health Organization (2006). *WHO Quality of Life-BREF (WHOQOL-BREF)*. Gebeva: WHO.

46. Murphy B, Herrman H, Hawthorne G, Pinzone T, Evert H (2000). *Australian WHOQoL instruments: User's manual and interpretation guide*. Melbourne: Australian WHOQoL Field Study Centre.

47. Zborowski M (1952). Cultural components in response to pain. *Journal of Society Issues*, **8**: 16–30.

48. Lasch KE (2002). Culture and pain. *Pain Clinical Updates*, X(5).

49. Koffman J, Morgan M, Edmonds P, Speck P, Higginson IJ (2008). Cultural meanings of pain: a qualitative study of Black Caribbean and White British patients with advanced cancer. *Palliative Medicine*, **22**: 350–9.

50. Krause I (1989). The sinking heart, a Punjabi communication of distress. *Social Science & Medicine*, **29**(4): 563–75.

51. Ahmed T (1998). The Asian experience. In R Salman, V Bahal (eds) *Assessing Health Needs in People from Minority Ethnic Groups*, pp. 319–328. London: Royal College of Physician.

52. Firth S (1997). *Dying, Death and Bereavement in the British Hindu Community*. Leuven: Peeters.

53. Todd KH (2001). Influence of ethnicity on emergency department pain management. *Emergency Medicine*, **13**: 274–8.

54. Cleeland CS, Mendoza TR, Wang XS, Chou C, Harle MT, Morrissey M, et al. (2000). Assessing symptom distress in cancer patients: the M.D. Anderson Symptom Inventory. *Cancer*, **89**(7): 1634–46.

55. Bernabei R, Gambassi G, Lapane K, Landi F, Gatsonis C, Dunlop R, et al. (1998). Management of pain in elderly patients with cancer. SAGE Study Group. Systematic Assessment of Geriatric Drug Use via Epidemiology. [see comment][erratum appears in *Journal of the American Medical Association* 1999; 281(2): 136]. *Journal of the American Medical Association*, **279**(23): 1877–82.

56. Fife B (1994). The conceptualization of meaning in illness. *Social Science &. Medicine*, **38**(2): 309–16.

57. Lipowski ZJ (1983). Psychosocial reaction to illness. *Canadian Medical Association Journal*, **128**: 1069–73.

58. Koffman J, Morgan M, Edmonds P, Speck P, Higginson IJ (2008). Cultural meanings of pain: a qualitative study of Black Caribbean and White British patients with advanced cancer. *Palliative Medicine*, **22**: 349–59.

59. Gomes B, Higginson IJ (2006). Factors influencing death at home in terminally ill patients with cancer: systematic review. *British Medical Journal*, **332**: 515–21.

60. Rhodes P, Shaw S (1999). Informal care and terminal illness. *Health and Social Care in the Community*, **7**: 39–50.

61. Koffman J, Higginson IJ (2003). Fit to care? A comparison of informal caregivers of first-generation black Caribbeans and white dependants with advanced progressive disease in the UK. *Health & Social Care in the Community*, **11**(6): 528–36.

62. Karim K, Bailey M, Tunna K (2000). Non white ethnicity and the provision of specialist palliative care services: factors affecting doctors referral patterns *Palliative Medicine*, **14**: 471–8.

63. Blakemore K (2000). Health and social care needs in minority communities: an over problemitized issue? *Health and Social Care in the Community*, **8**(1): 22–30.

64. Smaje C, Field D (1997). Absent minorities? Ethnicity and the use of palliative care services. In J Hockey, N Small (eds) *Death, gender and ethnicity*, pp. 142–65. London: Routledge.

65. Neuberger J (1994). *Caring for Dying People in Different Faiths*. London: Mosby.

66. Shanmugasundaram S, O'Connor M, Sellick K (2010). Culturally competent care at the end of life. *End of Life Care*, **4**(1): 26–31.

67. Ellershaw J, Smith C, Overhill S, Aldridge J (2001). Care of the dying: setting standards for symptom control in the last 48 hours of life. *Journal of Pain and Symptom Management*, **21**: 12–7.

68. Dein S, Stygall J (1997). Does being religious help of hinder coping with chronic illness? A critical literature review. *Palliative Medicine*, **11**: 291–8.

Chapter 11

Loss and bereavement in older age: developing community-based bereavement support

Amanda Roberts, Sinead McGilloway, and Orla Keegan

Introduction

Bereavement is often the province of the older person, as the experience of loss in older age is statistically more common (1). For example, there are 900,000 adults widowed each year in the USA, almost three-quarters of whom are aged over 65 (2). A similar pattern exists in western and central Europe (3). There are also some important gender differences in the exposure to loss in old age because women typically tend to outlive men; it is estimated that 51% of women and 14% of men will be widowed, at least once, by the age of 65 (4). Societies are also ageing more rapidly to the extent that, by 2025, it is estimated that the number of people aged over 60 will exceed one billion worldwide, whilst by 2050, there will be more people in the world over 60, than children under 14 (5). It is likely that these demographic trends will have significant implications for the provision of health and social care support services including those involving bereavement support. Furthermore, the growing secularization of society has led to an increased use of professional bereavement services over and above the more traditional forms of support, such as families, the general community, and members of the clergy (6).

Bereavement studies, in general (and across all age groups), have been conducted mainly within the Western world. Whilst some authors have highlighted cultural differences in the experience and impact of bereavement across different contexts (e.g. the expression of grief), little if anything, is known about the experience of older bereaved people from ethnic minorities. Nonetheless, early studies throughout the world have identified the negative effects of bereavement in older members of the population including: poorer mental health (7), lower morale (7), lower life satisfaction (8), increased mortality (9), and greater use of health services (10). However, findings from a recent US-based study (Changing Life of Older Couples (CLOC)) (11) indicate that older spouses are a heterogeneous group. Thus, while some people in this study experienced depression and grief symptoms as a result of loss, a substantial proportion were psychologically resilient and successfully managed the emotional and practical strains of bereavement. In addition, those who experienced some bereavement-related depressive symptoms, 'bounced back' within 18 months of the death. Available evidence from the USA and Canada also indicates that the effects of widowhood on psychological, social, physical and financial well-being, may be more severe for men than women (11, 12). However, there are relatively few widower studies due to the challenges of accessing and researching this population; for example, there are higher re-marriage rates amongst men when compared to women, whilst men also tend to die earlier from illnesses such as cancer and heart disease (2).

If life is characterized as a series of losses, we can hypothesize about grief and bereavement in two directions; that is, either we become accustomed to loss and more adept at coping with it during the course of our lives, or we come to struggle with the cumulative effect of loss and bereavements. However, bereavement is a complex, albeit common, life event and each encountered death deprives us of a different relationship, whilst creating a new set of challenges for adaptation. Age is one of a complex interplay of factors involved in the experience and process of bereavement and, in this chapter, we examine what is known about bereavement in older age and what may mediate outcomes and maximize more positive experiences, particularly within the context of community-based bereavement support.

Bereavement-related issues for the older person

Bereavement is a particularly significant life event amongst older people because it may lead to a number of far-reaching emotional and practical changes in their lives including, for example, living alone, dealing with new tasks for the first time (e.g. household bills or particular household chores) and/or coming to terms with living on a lower income (13). The specific effects of bereavement include: social isolation and loneliness, depression, disenfranchised grief, bereavement overload, mortality and suicide, and resilience. A full discussion of these often complex issues is beyond the scope of this chapter. However, each is briefly mentioned below (with reference to the international literature from the UK/Europe, USA, and Canada), as they are important considerations when designing and delivering appropriate and effective support services and structures to meet the needs of older people who have been bereaved.

Firstly, those older people who have been recently bereaved are considered to be an 'at-risk' group for social exclusion and bereavement has been found to be one of the main reasons why people become increasingly isolated in later life (14). Likewise, depressive symptoms have been identified in 8%–17% of the general population of older people (15, 16), although detection rates are poor and the effectiveness of treatments are modest (14, 17). A need for further research in this area is indicated.

Another important issue relates to the concept of 'disenfranchised grief' which refers to the experience of grief amongst those whose bereavement may be perceived to represent little social loss—as is often the case when an older person dies (18). According to Doka (19), 'disenfranchised grief' refers to grief that is experienced when the bereaved person incurs a loss 'that is not, or cannot be openly acknowledged, publicly mourned, or socially supported'. Furthermore, the impact of multiple and sequential loss in old age may lead to 'bereavement overload' (18). The effects of this may be compounded by other types of loss experienced by older people, such as losses in: cognitive ability, physical health, functional ability, independence, financial resources, and work roles. Studies in the USA and New Zealand that have incorporated multivariate analyses, have also identified a number of significant risk factors for suicide in older people including: depression, marital status (widowhood or divorced), psychiatric admission within the previous year, poor social networks, substance misuse, and family discord (20, 21). Numerous UK- and US-based studies also show typically high mortality rates amongst bereaved people and, in particular, older persons (22).

Whilst widowed people frequently report the death of their spouse to be one of the most stressful events of their lives, there is much evidence to suggest that they may also demonstrate considerable resilience. For example, older widows have been found to make a conscious effort to adjust and adapt to widow(er)hood. Whilst this transition is frequently difficult and stressful and is often accompanied by loneliness and a pervasive sense of loss and confusion about the meaning of life, most people tend to adapt successfully over time (23).

Bereavement support services

Bereavement support is an umbrella term that encompasses a large number of activities and which, according to the international literature, ranges from phone calls, home visits (e.g. from the hospice nurse), memorial rituals, and the provision of written or educational materials (e.g. on coping), to one-to-one counselling, therapeutic groups, social activities, mutual-help groups and other forms of therapies and interventions (e.g. cognitive restructuring and behavioural skills programmes, brief group psychotherapy, behaviour therapy, and family therapy (24–26)). Such diversity reflects the varying levels of need amongst those who have been bereaved including a need for: information about loss and grief, additional support to deal with the emotional and psychological impact of the loss, and, in a small number of cases, a need for formal mental health service intervention (27). Internationally, services are offered by a variety of providers, such as voluntary organizations (e.g. Cruse Bereavement Support), parish-based supports, public services (e.g. hospitals and health centres), and private individuals and organizations. However, in the UK, it has been estimated that 80% of bereavement support is undertaken by voluntary groups and 90% by volunteers (28). Furthermore, most volunteers are female (86%), as are the majority of those who use bereavement support services (75%) (6).

Current evidence from the international literature suggests that a tiered/component model of bereavement support service provision is required to meet varying levels of need (26, 27, 29, 30). This involves the provision of information about the experience of bereavement and how other forms of support may be accessed. For those who require more support, a formal opportunity to review and reflect on the loss experience should be made available (e.g. a listening service) and a process put in place to refer people with complex needs to appropriate health and social care professionals. Finally, specialist interventions such as mental health and psychological support services, and specialist counselling/psychotherapy services, should be available for those who require these more intensive forms of support (25, 29).

The effectiveness of bereavement interventions and services

Most people adjust to bereavement without professional intervention (31) and longitudinal studies of bereavement show naturally occurring declines in bereavement symptoms over time (e.g. 32, 33). Thus, most mourners are able to work through their grief and adjust well with the help and support of family and friends. However, a significant minority tend to require more dedicated and intensive forms of bereavement intervention. Unfortunately, little is known, to date, about the effectiveness of services that provide dedicated bereavement support, either to the older person, or to the bereaved population in general (34).

Recent reviews of the international literature coupled with meta-analyses in this area, suggest that bereavement interventions may have only limited effectiveness (26, 30, 35). For example, interventions targeted at the general population of the bereaved would appear to be less effective than for those in high-risk categories (e.g. bereaved mothers, suicide survivors), or amongst those who show increasing or unrelenting levels of distress. Indeed, the available evidence suggests that interventions are only needed by, and effective for, a minority (10–20%) of bereaved people (36, 37). Furthermore, these studies (including those which focus on the older bereaved) tend to be characterized by a number of important methodological limitations, including small sample sizes, unreliable measures and a focus on interventions which tend to be delivered in controlled rather than 'real world' clinical settings (38).

Community-based bereavement support services for the older person

Whilst a wide range of service providers offer different forms of bereavement support, a key question in the context of this chapter, relates to which specific services and supports are available to older people within their community. Undoubtedly, there is a wide variety of *generic* community-based services targeted at this group and these tend to be quite similar across a number of geographical contexts including countries, such as Ireland, the UK, and the USA. For instance, services aimed at meeting practical needs might include 'Meals-on-Wheels', home help, handyman schemes, transport services and medical and personal care. Other forms of community-based provision have a greater focus on meeting social needs and might include: visitation programmes, day care centres, social clubs, and friendly phone-call programmes. These services, which tend to be located in a variety of settings, including hospice- and hospital-based day centres, local community centres, and health centres, play an important role in maintaining social contact with older people who have become house-bound or isolated, although in some cases (e.g. Meals-on-Wheels and home help), this contact may be minimal (39).

Despite the relatively wide availability of general community-based services, little is known about specific community-based services for bereaved older people (40). For example, in one recent Irish study, a sample of community dwelling older people (n=205) identified bereavement counselling as a service that was lacking within their community (39). Furthermore, whilst some community-dwelling older people have access to community-based bereavement supports, these services tend to be targeted at the general population and may, therefore, not meet the specific needs of vulnerable older people. This is of particular concern given that the great majority of those who are affected by bereavement tend to be older and are often multiply bereaved (28). Nonetheless, there are some general community-based bereavement services to which the older person has access (e.g. mutual help groups), whilst other services may provide low-level bereavement support as part of their overall service provision (e.g. day or community centres for the older person or primary health care teams).

Some variability in general bereavement service provision exists across different countries. For example, in studies of hospice and palliative care, group support would appear to be more typically provided in the USA and UK than other countries, such as Spain, although one-to-one support tends to be the most common form of service provision overall (41–43). Similar survey-based studies have not yet been conducted on the provision of community services. However, descriptions of individual services such as Cruse (UK) and Compassionate Friends (International), incorporate various forms of service provision, including literature, online support, one-to-one befriending/counselling, group support and community workshops, and/or information sessions. Some of the general community-based bereavement services to which older people have access, are discussed in more detail below, primarily with reference to research conducted in the UK, USA, and New Zealand.

Voluntary services

Voluntary agencies

Voluntary agencies, such as Cruse (UK) and parish-based bereavement services, offer important support to the bereaved, although they are not specifically targeted at older people. It is estimated that 300,000 people in the UK work as voluntary counsellors, as opposed to only 8000 who work in a professional (paid) capacity (44). Voluntary agencies tend to offer similar services across different countries and these typically include information/education, phone support/information, newsletters, support groups and counselling/befriending schemes (e.g. Cruse (UK)). More specifically, it is interesting to note that a number of large voluntary organizations have emerged in locations as diverse as Hong Kong (Comfort Care Concern Group), Australia (the Australian Centre for Grief and Bereavement) and Canada (the BC Bereavement Helpline). However, the range of services that are available across different contexts may vary considerably, whilst some agencies may also specialize in providing only one or two particular forms of support. For example, the Canadian BC Bereavement Helpline provides telephone support and referral as well as community-based grief support.

In addition, bereavement support is becoming an integral component of palliative and hospice care. However, many volunteer-based services tend to vary in terms of the level of support provided (e.g. a listening service or one-to-one counselling) and the training offered. Interestingly, volunteer service providers also tend to be older adults; for example, a survey of bereavement volunteers based at 26 hospices in New Zealand, showed that over half were aged over 60 (34). Whilst voluntary services would appear to play an important role in bereavement support, they have received very little attention in the empirical literature. Nonetheless, studies which have included an assessment of clients' views have, for the most part, reported positive findings (44).

Mutual-help groups

Mutual-help groups (or self-help groups), such as the internationally-based Compassionate Friends, are a common form of community-based bereavement support. These may be time-limited and involve discussion, role plays, guest lectures, social events, and/or education (45). In one early study (USA), older adults who attended bereavement support groups, reported a greater reduction in depression and grief than controls without access to such support (46). These kinds of supports are important because they can address loneliness and social isolation, as well as strengthening informal support networks and encouraging a sense of belonging (47).

Statutory/public services

Community resource centres

Community centres or 'senior centres' are in existence in many countries (e.g. the UK, Ireland, and the USA) and help older people to remain independent in their communities by providing a range of supports, such as recreational opportunities and social and community action opportunities (48). Whilst these types of centres may not specifically offer bereavement support to their clients, some do offer *indirect* bereavement support through the provision of social activities and programmes. Some individual centres, particularly in the USA, also list bereavement support groups as one of their services, whilst those that do not, may often refer those who require bereavement support to the appropriate service.

Primary health care teams

Bereavement is also an important issue for health and social care professionals, due to its often negative impact on overall health and well-being (28). Typically, at least within an Irish and UK context, the key members of the primary health care team are the General Practitioner (GP) and the public or district health nurse. The older person is likely to see their primary care physicians regularly and many bereaved people tend to visit their GP for help (49). Studies in the USA and UK have reported that GPs are an important resource, not only in providing medical support, but also in informing the bereaved about relevant community-based bereavement supports (44).

Main (2000) reported that it is also important to bereaved people that their GP acknowledges the death (50). Indeed, GPs are well placed to respond to a bereaved person's need for support and counselling by noting any increase in frequency of attendance and the nature of the symptoms presented, as well as being aware of any bereavement services and supports that might be available. Notwithstanding, many bereavement counselling organizations report that those who could benefit most from their services are rarely referred to them by their family doctor (51).

Other community-based staff, such as nurses, may often be unsure of how to deal with the bereaved (52). Nonetheless, district nurses in primary care teams are ideally placed to offer bereavement care because they are often in the right place (client's home) at the right time (at the time of death). Therefore, they have an opportunity to assess and observe the needs of the bereaved and to offer necessary advice, support and information. Unsurprisingly perhaps, Birtwistle et al. (52) found that most district nurses, in a large UK-based study, would like to offer some sort of bereavement support to the families of their patients and acknowledged that they can play an important role in supporting the bereaved. However, they also found that district nurse-led bereavement support services vary considerably in terms of overall structure and rationale, whilst there are also important inter-individual differences amongst staff. More specialist nursing services, such as Clinical Nurse Specialists (CNSs) who deliver palliative care in the community, may also constitute an important source of support early in the bereavement period, as most hospices offer some form of bereavement support. Thus, the CNS may be able to provide initial support and information about, and appropriate referral to, more specific hospice-based bereavement supports.

The way forward

This chapter has highlighted some of the specific issues facing older bereaved people and the types of generic and specialist bereavement services available to them. These are important considerations when developing or improving specialist community-based bereavement supports for this population. However, there are other important factors to consider with respect to charting a way forward in this area, each of which is discussed below.

Targeting those most at-risk

In general, bereavement support interventions have been found to be most effective for those who are considered to be 'at risk,' or who are experiencing a complicated (or prolonged) grief reaction[1] (35, 38). Thus, targeting those most 'at risk' is recommended, both in bereavement support provision and in the delivery of services to meet the many other needs (e.g. social isolation) of the older person. For example, a recent report by Age Action (UK) (53) proposed that local services should be re-designed to target the needs of older people who are at risk of social exclusion, as opposed to solely funding community services that benefit the wider population. Furthermore, little formal risk assessment of the bereaved exists in either primary care or the voluntary sector, although assessment protocols have been incorporated routinely into hospice services in the UK (54). The question, then, is how to target those groups of older people who are most in need of bereavement support? One way is to ensure that there is effective signposting of the services within the community; this is examined in the following section.

---

[1] Complicated/prolonged grief reaction 'constitutes a persistently elevated set of specific symptoms of grief identified in bereaved individuals with significant difficulties adjusting to the loss' (56).

In general, older widowed persons are at a lower risk of poor bereavement outcomes than younger persons. However, whilst the former may have less intense grief than their younger counterparts, their levels of emotional and physical distress tend to decline more slowly (55). Thus, family, friends, and professionals should make a concerted effort to provide appropriate support and recognition, where needed (18), for their older bereaved relatives and friends. Similarly, there is a greater need to focus more clinical work and research on older people who tend to be neglected in favour of younger members of the population, such as children and their families. In addition, most of the voluminous research on widows has tended to focus on those aged under 65 years (18).

Certain groups may also be disadvantaged in terms of their access to appropriate bereavement care; for example, a large proportion of older people die in nursing homes and community hospitals. Although, for many, these settings represent 'home' and a community, the extent of bereavement care provision and support tends to be negligible. For example, a large national survey of all residential and acute care settings in Ireland, found that less than 30% of private care facilities and fewer (4%) state facilities had formal structures to follow-up relatives or friends after a death (57). Most facilities (over 80%) did not have a bereavement officer, or family liaison nurse, whilst just over half (55%) of statutory settings held memorial services for residents who had died (57). The lack of support for other subgroups of older people (e.g. widowers and older bereaved people with dementia) has also been highlighted in studies conducted elsewhere (58, 59).

Another important question relates to the extent to which older people have differential access to bereavement support when compared to their younger counterparts. In general, bereavement support services are not aimed at older people *per se*, but focus instead, on specialist forms of support that target specific types of loss (e.g. suicide), or which focus on the nature of the relationship to the deceased (e.g. widow/widower). Services also tend to be divided broadly into those aimed at children/teenagers and those catering for the needs of adults, without a specific focus on the older person. These service structures/divisions, coupled with the possible presence of disenfranchised grief, may pose significant barriers to service provision for those older people most in need of bereavement support.

Widowers are another potentially disadvantaged subgroup amongst the older bereaved. Whilst widowhood is more common in women than men, it has been found to have a greater impact on men. For instance, research conducted in the UK has shown a significant decline, amongst widowers, in their mental health, social functioning and morale, as well as lower rates of participation in outdoor activities and an attendant increase in indoor activities (60). Another more recent study from the USA, reported that the majority of older widowers feel that they do not have support when they are depressed (58). Thus, it is crucial to identify the needs of this vulnerable subgroup and link them to appropriate services, particularly in view of the fact that older men, and men in general, have been found to have fewer social supports. As noted earlier, voluntary services are primarily provided by female volunteers and tend to be based largely on a 'counselling-type' approach and may not, therefore, be entirely suited to many male clients.

Signposting of services

The role of the GP would appear to be central to signposting relevant services for the older bereaved person, although GPs should, ideally, be closely linked to community-based services for older people. Interestingly, GPs who keep a death register and/or who have a special interest in palliative care are more likely to offer routine bereavement support (61). However, their knowledge of social services and community programmes can often be poor, with many highlighting a lack of information about services as the reason for non-referral (62).

Melis and her colleagues (63) found that the involvement of GPs in the referral of older people to a community-based intervention in the UK, was an effective way of targeting their service. Others have also highlighted the value of strengthening primary care as a gateway to alternative sources of bereavement support (e.g. befriending, self help groups etc.), particularly for those vulnerable and at-risk groups, such as the recently bereaved (64). This might involve awareness-raising initiatives designed to promote a greater understanding amongst GPs of how to address the challenges faced by older widows/widowers (11) and to ensure that they are appropriately informed of local supports (e.g. through a local directory) and happy to provide patient information leaflets/notice boards etc. (64). It is critical that older people receive proper information, advice, and advocacy in order that they can make informed choices about the support that they require (14).

Additionally, due to varying levels of need, information about services at different levels should be provided (e.g. telephone support, mutual help groups, one-to-one volunteer support, counselling etc.). As outlined earlier in this chapter, current evidence from the international literature suggests that a tiered/component model of bereavement support service provision is required to meet varying levels of need (26, 27, 29, 30). This may range from the provision of information about the experience of bereavement and how other forms of support may be accessed, to services that allow the bereaved to review and reflect on the loss experience (e.g. a listening service), or more intensive supports or specialist interventions, such as mental health and psychological support services, and specialist counselling/psychotherapy services (27, 29). This multi-tiered approach should be underpinned by a number of significant activities including: targeting those most at-risk, signposting services, providing integrated services, addressing barriers to access, and ensuring the provision of a holistic range of service provision (see Figure 11.1).

Integrated/joined-up care

Although general bereavement care activities are provided in health and social care settings throughout the developed world, a lack of consistency in the overall approach to bereavement

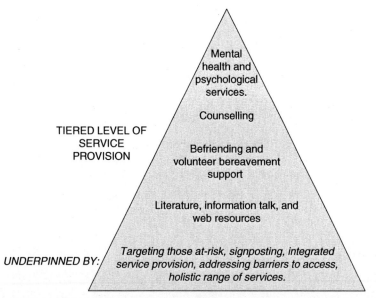

Fig. 11.1 An integrated tiered approach to service provision—based on a number of tiered conceptualizations of bereavement care (27, 29, 35, 65, 66).

support provision has been noted (67). This may be due, at least in part, to poor coordination between statutory and voluntary sectors. This, in turn, presents an obstacle to knowing what services are available, who should be providing care and at what stage, and who communicates with whom about the bereaved (68). It is interesting to note, in this context, that Irish service providers for the elderly in the community have identified a need to set up a formal structure and closer communication links between the various voluntary and statutory providers at local level, in order to better coordinate service delivery (39).

A recent report by Age Concern (UK)—a voluntary organization—recommends the re-modelling of local services around the needs of the most excluded, in order to ensure that services are joined up, user-friendly, rooted in the community, and sufficiently flexible to reach out to the vulnerable in the community. The report goes on to recommend targeted initiatives for the recently bereaved, as well as counselling and support services and the identification and follow-up of those bereaved people who are most at risk of exclusion. A coordinated approach to community-based bereavement support for the older person is needed, but there are some important unanswered questions. For example, who is responsible for informing older people about the community services available? How can this best be achieved? How are 'at-risk' or struggling individuals identified or targeted? To what extent is a reactive or proactive approach adopted in the provision of care and is there a range of supports available to meet the varying levels and potential complexity of need (e.g. from information to one-to-one counselling)? Should services be solely dedicated to the older bereaved person? Thus, the development of responsive bereavement support services may be less about an additional investment of resources and more about linking networks together, creating appropriate referral pathways and perhaps reconfiguring existing services, all of which should be underpinned by coordinated attempts to ensure that people are aware of the services that are already available (28).

Timing and location of services

The timing and location of community-based bereavement services are additional sources of concern for older bereaved people, many of whom do not have the support they require during the critical 6–8 weeks after the death. Additionally, it has been shown that, if support services are not offered in a timely and effective manner, this group can quickly become lonely, isolated, and excluded. Some existing evidence indicates that bereaved individuals appreciate and value follow-up contact shortly after the death (69, 70). However, other authors argue, at the same time, that early intervention can be detrimental as it can reduce the support received within an individual's natural support network and deter them from finding their own way of coping with their loss (35).

The duration of support is another important consideration. For example, Age Concern advocates that both public services and voluntary organizations should experiment with short-term, intensive forms of post-bereavement support, such as practical initiatives designed to address skills deficits (e.g. managing household finances). The location of services is an additional important factor as inaccessibility may pose a further barrier to service use. Thus, older people should be able to access services that are tailored to meet their needs and at a time and place that is convenient for them (14).

Barriers to service use

Research from the USA has shown that older adults engage with health- and community-based services, either to supplement and complement the support provided by informal networks, or to receive care when such networks are either unavailable, or unable to assist them (71).

However, several factors, other than physical accessibility, have been shown to prevent, or hinder access to formal services amongst older people living in the community. For instance, those who are better educated (72) tend to be more aware of services and their need for them and are, therefore, more likely to access services. Additional barriers to service utilization may include the older person's contact with family, the cost of the service and cultural antagonism (73). However, these may be addressed through the provision of more information on services, as well as through GPs and family members and friends, who should be encouraged to promote the more frequent use of formal support services amongst older members of the general population (71).

Offering a holistic range of services

As indicated earlier, there are a number of community programmes that offer social opportunities, accessible transport, home repairs, and befriending schemes for older people living in the community (14). For example, the National Health Initiative in the UK (74) recognizes the benefits of physical activity in later life and recommends increasing the opportunities for older people to engage in a range of activities, such as free swimming and organized walks. Thus, the provision of a wide range of services for older people (e.g. attending social clubs, accessing befriending schemes, using home help) may mean that many of the social and practical needs arising from a bereavement (and other losses), may be effectively met, thereby reducing the need for subsequent bereavement-specific support. However, for those who do require such support, accessing available physical and social supports may be an important first step.

Conclusion

According to the international research literature, older people are not a homogenous group; they have multiple diverse needs which ought to be addressed in order that they can experience as good a quality of life as possible. Thus, it is important to consider a range of factors in the provision of community-based bereavement support for this important (and growing) segment of the population including: health, functional status, relationships, social contacts/support, autonomy, dignity, privacy, security, and spiritual well-being. This chapter has highlighted many of the key issues facing older bereaved people (in many different countries) following the death of a spouse, family member, or close friend. In particular, it has examined the kinds of bereavement services that are currently available across different geographical contexts and, more specifically, the community-based bereavement services to which older people have access, as well as some salient issues that should be considered when developing or enhancing bereavement support services for older people who are living in the community.

Although service provision may differ within and across geographical regions and countries, it is possible to identify a number of key common elements that may be helpful in enhancing community-based bereavement support throughout the developed world. These include: developing integrated service provision, providing bereavement services to meet all levels of need, ensuring that these services are appropriately signposted and accessible, and promoting an awareness amongst key 'frontline' health and social care professionals of the kinds of support services that are available and, more importantly, ensuring that they understand the need for such services.

In conclusion, it is also important to give a voice to the older person and to remember that:

Ageing is a privilege and a societal achievement. It is also a challenge, which will impact on all aspects of 21st century society. It is a challenge that cannot be addressed by the public or private sectors in isolation: it requires joint approaches and strategies. (75)

References

1. Catalano G (2005). Bereavement, depression and our growing geriatric population. *Southern Medical Journal*, **98**(1): 3–4.
2. Federal Interagency Forum on Ageing-Related Statistics (2004). *Older Americans 2004: Key indicators of well-being*. Washington, DC: US Government Printing Office.
3. de Jong-Gierveld J, de Valk H, Blommedteijn M (2002). Living arrangements of older persons and family support in more developed countries. *Population Bulletin of the United Nations*, **42–43**: 193–217.
4. Sadock BJ, Sadock VA (2003). *Kaplan and Sadock's synopsis of psychiatry: Behavioural Sciences Clinical Psychiatry*. Philadelphia, PA: Williams & Wilkins.
5. United Nations (2007). *World population prospects: The 2006 Revision*. New York: UN.
6. Walter T (1999). *On bereavement*. Buckingham: Open University Press.
7. Bennet KM, Morgan K (1992). Health, social functioning, and marital status: stability and change among the elderly recently widowed women. *International Journal of Geriatric Psychiatry*, **7**: 813–17.
8. Mouser NF, Powers EA, Keith PM, Goudy WJ (1985). Marital status and life satisfaction: A study of older men. In WA Peterson, J Quadagno (eds), *Social bonds in later life*, pp. 71–90. London: Sage.
9. Bowling A (1988). Who dies after widow(er)hood? A discriminant analysis. *Omega Journal of Death and Dying*, **19**: 135–53.
10. Tudiver F, Permaul-Woods JA, Hilditch J, Harmina J, Saini S (1995). Do widowers use the health care system differently? *Canadian Family Physician*, **41**: 392–400.
11. Carr D (2008). Factors that influence late-life bereavement: Considering data from the changing lives of older couple study. In M Stroebe, R Hansson, W Stroebe, H Schut (eds) *Handbook of bereavement research and practice: Advances in theory and intervention*, pp. 417–40. Washington, DC: American Psychological Association.
12. Fry PS (2001). The unique contribution of key existential factors to the prediction of psychological well-being of older adults following spousal loss. *The Gerontologist*, **41**(1): 69–81.
13. Daly M, O'Connor J (1984). *The world of the elderly: The rural experience. A study of the elderly person's experience of living alone in a rural area*. Dublin: The National Council for the Aged.
14. Harrop A, Jopling K (2009). *One voice shaping our ageing society*. London: Age Concern & Help the Aged.
15. Denihan A, Kirby M, Bruce I, Cunningham C, Coakley D, Lawlor B (2000). Three-year prognosis of depression in the community dwelling elderly. *British Journal of Psychiatry*, **176**: 453–7.
16. Copeland, JRM (2002). EURODEP-Prevalence of depression in Europe. In JRM Copeland, MT Abou-Saleh, DG Blazer (eds) *Principles and Practice of Geriatric Psychiatry*, 2nd edn, p. 393. Chichester: Wiley.
17. Cole MG, Bellavance F, Mansour A (1999). Prognosis of depression in elderly community and primary care populations: a systematic review and meta-analysis. *American Journal of Psychiatry*, **156**: 157–61.
18. Moss M, Moss S (2003). Doubly disenfranchised grief in old age. *Grief Matters*, Autumn: 4–6.
19. Doka KJ (1989). Disenfranchised grief. In KJ Doka (ed) *Disenfranchised grief: Recognising hidden sorrow*, pp. 3–11. Lexington, MA: Lexington Books.
20. Conwell Y, Lyness JM, Duberstein P, Cox C, Seidlitz L, DiGiorgio A, et al. (2000). Completed suicide among older patients in primary care practices. A controlled study. *Journal of the American Geriatric Society*, **48**: 23–9.
21. Beauttrais AL (2002). A case control study of suicide and attempted suicide in older adults. *Suicide and Life-Threatening Behavior*, **32**: 1–9.
22. Bowling A (1994). Mortality after bereavement: An analysis rates and associations with mortality 13 years after bereavement. *International Journal of Geriatric Psychiatry*, **9**: 445–59.

23. Fry P (1998). Spousal loss in late life: A 1-year follow-up of perceived changes in life meaning and psychosocial functioning following bereavement. *Journal of Personal & Interpersonal Loss*, 3(4): 369–91.

24. Demmer C (2003). A national survey of hospice bereavement services. *Omega*, 47(4): 327–41.

25. Forte A, Hill M, Pazder R, Feudtner C (2004). Bereavement care interventions: A systematic review. *BMC Palliative Care* 3(3): 1–14.

26. Schut H, Stroebe M (2005). Interventions to enhance adaptation to bereavement. *Journal of Palliative Medicine*, 8(1): 140–7.

27. National Institute for Clinical Excellence (NICE) (2004). *Services for families and carers. Improving supportive and palliative care for adults with cancer. The manual*. London: NICE.

28. Stephen AI, Wimpenny P, Unwin R, Work F, Dempster P, MacDuff C, et al. (2009). Bereavement and bereavement care in health and social care: Provision and practice in Scotland. *Death Studies*, 33: 239–61.

29. National Advisory Committee in Palliative Care (2001). *The report of the national advisory committee on palliative care*. Ireland: Department of Health and Children.

30. Currier M, Neimeyer R, Berman J (2008). The effectiveness of psychotherapeutic interventions for bereaved persons: A comprehensive quantitative review. *Psychological Bulletin*, 134(5): 648–61.

31. Stroebe M, Folkman S, Hansson R, Schut H (2006). The prediction of bereavement outcome: Development of an integrative risk factor framework. *Social Science and Medicine*, 63: 2440–51.

32. Stroebe M, Schut H (2001). Risk factors in bereavement outcome: A methodological and empirical review. In M Stroebe, R Hansson, W Stroebe H Schut (eds) *Handbook of bereavement research: Consequences, coping and care*, pp. 349–71. Washington, DC: American Psychological Association.

33. Ott C, Leuger R (2002). Patterns of change in mental health status over 2 years of spousal bereavement. *Death Studies*, 26: 387–411.

34. Payne S (2002). Dilemmas in the use of volunteers to provide hospice bereavement support: evidence from New Zealand. *Mortality*, 7(2): 139–54.

35. Schut H, Stroebe M, Van Den Bout J, Terheggen M (2001). The Efficacy of Bereavement Interventions: Determining who benefits. In M Stroebe, R Hansson, W Stroebe H Schut (eds) *Handbook of bereavement research: Consequences, coping and care*, pp. 705–38. Washington, DC: American Psychological Society.

36. Parkes C (2001). A historical overview of the scientific study of bereavement. In M Stroebe, R Hansson, W Stroebe H Schut (eds) *Handbook of bereavement research: Consequences coping and care*, pp. 25–46. Washington, DC: American Psychological Society.

37. Prigerson H (2004). Complicated grief: When the path to adjustment leads to a dead-end. *Bereavement Care*, 23: 38–40.

38. Jordan J, Neimeyer R (2003). Does grief counselling work? *Death studies*, 27: 765–86.

39. Doyle M (2007). *Older people's perceptions on services and activities in the Marino and Fairview area: a participatory project*. Dublin: Social Policy and Ageing Research Centre, Trinity College.

40. Reif LV, Patton MJ, Gold PB (1995). Bereavement, stress, and social support in members of a self-help group. *Journal of Community Psychology*, 35: 292–306.

41. Foliart D, Clausen M, Siljestrom C (2001). Bereavement practices among California hospices: Results of a statewide survey. *Death Studies*, 25: 461–7.

42. Field D, Reid D, Payne S, Relf M (2004). A national postal survey of adult bereavement support in hospice and specialist palliative care services in the UK. *International Journal of Palliative Nursing*, 10(12): 569–76.

43. Yi P, Barreto P, Soler C (2006). Grief support provided to caregivers of palliative care patients in Spain. *Palliative Medicine*, 20: 521–31.

44. Gallagher M, Tracey A, Millar R (2005). Ex-clients' evaluation of bereavement counselling in a voluntary sector agency. *Psychology and Psychotherapy: Theory, Research and Practice*, 78: 59–76.

45. Hamilton HB (2004). Widow to widow: How the bereaved help one other. Conclusion. In PR Silverman (ed) *Widow to widow: How the bereaved help one other*, pp. 193–204. New York: Brunner & Routledge.

46. Caserta MS, Lund DA (1996). Beyond bereavement support group meetings: Exploring outside social contacts among the members. *Death Studies*, **20**: 537–56.

47. Stewart MJ, Craig D, MacPherson K, Alexander S (2001). Promoting positive affect and diminishing loneliness of widowed seniors through a support intervention. *Public Health Nursing*, **18**(1): 54–63.

48. Skarupski KA, Pelkowski JJ (2003). Multipurpose senior centers. Opportunities for community health nursing. *Journal of Community Health Nursing*, **20**(2): 119–32.

49. Birtwistle J, Kendrick T (2001). The psychological aspects of bereavement. *Primary Care Psychiatry*, **7**: 91–5.

50. Main J (2000). Improving management of bereavement in general practice based on a survey of recently bereaved subjects in a single general practice. *British Journal of General Practice*, **50**: 863–6.

51. Wiles R, Jarrett N, Payne S, Field D (2002). Referrals for bereavement counselling in primary care: A qualitative study. *Patient Education and Counselling*, **48**(1): 79–85.

52. Birtwistle J, Payne S, Smith P, Kendrick T (2002). The role of the district nurse in bereavement support. *Journal of Advanced Nursing*, **38**: 467–78.

53. Demakakos P (2008). *Being socially excluded and living alone in old age: findings from the English Longitudinal Study of Ageing (ELSA)*. London: Age Concern.

54. Relf M, Machin L, Archer N (2008). *Guidance for bereavement needs assessment in palliative care*. London: Help the Hospices.

55. Sanders CM (1981). Comparison of younger and older spouses in bereavement outcome. *Omega*, **11**: 217–32.

56. Prigerson HG, Vanderwerker LC, Maciejewski PK (2008). A case for inclusion of prolonged grief disorder in DSM-V. In M Stroebe, R Hansson, H Schut, W Stroebe (eds) *Handbook of bereavement research and practice: Advances in theory and intervention*, pp. 165–86. Washington, DC: American Psychological Association.

57. O' Shea E, Murphy K, Larkin P, Payne S, Froggatt K, Casey D, et al (2008). *End-of-life care for older people in acute and long-stay care settings in Ireland*. Dublin: Hospice Friendly Hospice Programme and National Council on Ageing and Older People.

58. Balaswamy S, Richardson V, Price C (2004). Investigating patterns of social support use by widowers during bereavement. *Journal of Men's Studies*, **13**(1): 67–84.

59. Rentz C, Krikorian R, Keys M (2005). Grief and mourning from the perspective of the person with a dementing illness: Beginning the dialogue. *Omega*, **50**(3): 165–79.

60. Bennett KM (1998). Longitudinal changes in mental and physical health among the elderly, recently widowed men. *Mortality*, **3**(3): 265–73.

61. Harris T, Kendrick T (1998). Bereavement care in general practice: A survey in South Thames Health Region. *British Journal of General Practice*, **46**: 1560–4.

62. Craven MA, Kates N, Raso P (1990). Assessment of family physicians' knowledge of social and community services. *Canadian Family Physician*, **36**: 443–7.

63. Melis R, Van Eijken M, Borm G, Wensing M, Adang E, van de Lisdonk EH, et al. (2005). The design of the Dutch EASY care study: A randomised controlled trial on the effectiveness of a problem-based community intervention model for frail elderly people. *BMC Health Services Research*, **5**(65): 1–11.

64. Friedli L (2005). Private minds in public bodies: The public mental health role of primary care. *Primary Care Mental Health*, **3**: 41–6.

65. Petrus Consulting, Bates U, Jordan N, Malone K, Monahan E, O'Connor S, et al. (2008). *Review of general bereavement support and specific services available following suicide bereavement*. Dublin: National Office for Suicide Prevention.

66. Walsh T, Foreman M, Curry P, O'Driscoll S, McCormack M (2008). Bereavement support in an acute hospital: An Irish model. *Death Studies*, **32**(8): 768–86.

67. Payne S, Relf M (1994). The assessment of need for bereavement follow-up in palliative and hospice care. *Palliative Medicine*, **8**: 197–203.

68. Nucleus Group (2004). *Review of specific grief and bereavement services: Final report*. Melbourne: Department of Human Services Victoria.

69. Milberg A, Olsson E, Jakobsson M, Olsson, Friedrichsen M (2008). Family members' perceived needs for bereavement follow-up. *Journal of Pain and Symptom Management*, **35**(1): 58–69.

70. Roberts A, McGilloway S (2008). The nature and use of bereavement support services in a hospice setting. *Palliative Medicine*, **22**: 612–25.

71. Blieszner R, Roberto KA, Singh K (2001). The helping networks of rural elders: Demographic and social psychological influences on service use. *Ageing International*, **27**(1): 89–119.

72. Lave J, Traven N, Ives D, Kuller L (1995). Participation in health promotion programs by the rural elderly. *American Journal of Preventive Medicine*, **11**: 6–53.

73. Crawley B (1988). The social service needs of black elderly women. *Affilia*, **3**: 6–16.

74. Department of Health (2009). *Be active, be healthy: A plan for getting the nation moving*. London: Department of Health.

75. World Health Organization (2007). The world is ageing fast–Have we noticed? Available at: http://www.who.int/ageing/en/. (Accessed 21 December, 2009.)

Section 3

Family and professional carers as partners in care-giving
Introduction

Merryn Gott and Christine Ingleton

Rising palliative care populations, coupled with economic constraints on health service expansion internationally, mean that the already significant role of family caregivers in providing palliative and end of life care can only increase in importance in the future. This section begins by considering some of the challenges of ensuring that family caregivers receive the support they require. In Chapter 12, Sheila Payne discusses the changing profile of family caregivers of older people, contextualizing her analysis by defining family in its broadest sense as encompassing any relationship with 'strong emotional and social bonds'. She identifies key social, economic, and demographic changes in Europe that are going to result in a decline in the number of available family carers, but a concomitant increase in people dying with complex care needs. As she recognizes, this poses significant challenges for ensuring high-quality care, particularly for certain subgroups of older people such as those living alone. Payne concludes that central to future policy development in this area must be a 'stronger recognition of care as a partnership between families and professionals'.

In Chapter 13, Grande and Keady take up this theme, exploring the specific support needs of older carers in more detail. They identify that older carers provide 'longer hours of care, have worse health, and may have fewer financial and social resources to cope than younger carers', but at the same time receive less formal support. The impact of caring upon older carers would therefore be expected to be significant and we learn that this is indeed the case; however, at the same time the need for a more nuanced understanding of caring as an activity that can bring reward as well as burden is identified. The authors go on to outline the specific support needs of older carers and finish by discussing the inadequacies of the current evidence base in terms of being able to identify specific interventions with the potential to enhance the caregiving experience.

Mike Nolan and Tony Ryan further develop this argument in Chapter 14, drawing on the wider gerontology and sociology literature to identify how family carers can be supported in providing good palliative care. Again, achieving effective partnership working between carers and paid staff is seen to be critical. Paid staff are argued to have a particular role to play in helping family carers achieve an appropriate balance between the negative experiences of loss and the potentially positive outcomes of caring. The authors conclude by proposing a framework that could be used with the person being cared for, family carers, and staff teams, as a means to improving outcomes for 'all stakeholders in the short, medium, and longer term'.

Barbara Hanratty turns the spotlight onto the economics of family caregiving in Chapter 15. She identifies that, whilst the evidence base in this area is very limited, what we do know is that caring costs families a significant amount in financial terms: 'illness is one of the most potent causes of poverty'. In England and Wales, it has been estimated that the total cost of care provided by family members amounts to between 50–160% of gross expenditure on personal social services for all age groups. Supporting this unpaid workforce of carers is obviously in the interests of statutory service providers. However, as Hanratty argues, too little is known about how to identify, and appropriately support, those carers in greatest need. A need for significant new research in this area is very apparent.

In the final chapter in this section, Philip Larkin and Meg Hegarty consider the need to support the paid workforce providing care to older people at the end of life. They argue that the expanded remit of specialist palliative care to all diagnoses and 'upstream' in terms of time from diagnosis, has blurred lines of responsibility; 'who provides care remains a grey area', something which complicates workforce development activities. The need for integration is again highlighted, particularly between gerontology, geriatric medicine, and specialist palliative care. As the authors identify, joint education and training initiatives provide opportunities to share expertise and models of good practice. Key to ensuring success must be a more informed understanding of 'how to embed palliative care principles into the language and practice of older people caring'. They close by arguing that ensuring a skilled and motivated health care workforce that includes family carers as integral members, 'is the greatest challenge for palliative aged care at this time'; an apt conclusion for this section as a whole.

Chapter 12

The changing profile of the family caregivers of older people: a European perspective

Sheila Payne

Introduction

This chapter reflects on some of the realities to be encountered in the care provided by family and friends to very sick and dying older people. Roy (1) highlights the ambiguities inherent in palliative care situations where differences, contradictions, and tensions are balanced with desire for unity, harmony, love, and compassion. These are themes that, in my view, are ever present in familial and friendship relationships but they take on a special significance in the period before the end of life. This chapter aims to present an analysis of the changing profile of family caregivers of older people and identify the implications this has for end of life care. Consideration will also be given to research undertaken with older people that indicates that many of them, including those from minority ethnic groups, are fearful of becoming dependent on family members. The chapter starts with offering definitions of key terms and highlighting where such definitions are problematic. It goes on to address the evidence about contemporary changes in family structure and the nature and patterns of relationships that may or may not support older people in the final phase of life. Drawing upon examples of specific research conducted with older people, there will be an examination of the needs, access, and support available to carers of older people, who may themselves be older.

Definitions of terms

At the outset it is helpful to offer some definitions of key terms, although most of the words used are contested (2). There are a number of different definitions of carers including those that focus primarily on 'hands-on' or task-driven care provision, but the one used in this chapter will encompass a more inclusive and extended role. In the UK the National Institute for Health and Clinical Excellence (NICE) (3) defines carers as follows:

> Carers, who may or may not be family members, are lay people in a close supportive role who share in the illness experience of the patient and who undertake vital care work and emotional management.

The notion of what constitutes a family is historically, culturally, and economically situated. Functional accounts of family tend to emphasize their role in procreation and childrearing, and mutual social and economic welfare. Contemporary accounts emphasize mutually supportive relationships but a romantic idealization of the family should be resisted as they can also be the focus of abusive, exploitative, and damaging relationships. Within palliative care, the following broad definition is drawn from NICE (3).

Family includes 'those related through committed heterosexual or same sex partnerships, birth and adoption, and others who have strong emotional and social bonds with a patient'.

Who provides care for older people?

In the context of caregiving for older people, it is possible to identify the following categories of people who may be involved in delivering unpaid care:

◆ Family

◆ Friends and neighbours

◆ Peers in institutional contexts such as care homes (nursing and residential homes) and prisons.

This chapter will not deal with care provided by volunteers, self-help groups, or paid workers. Grande et al. (2) have pointed out that there is difficulty in identifying actual numbers of carers as health services either do not record this information or only identify people as next-of-kin who may or may not occupy a caregiving role. It is well reported in the literature that people may not recognize themselves as 'carers' and may also resist the label (4). Health and social care professionals may not recognize that family caregiving is largely hidden work that is often taken for granted yet it is crucially important if dying people are to receive good care and eventually achieve 'a good death'. Moreover, bereaved family members occupy a number of current and previous roles with respect to end of life care, in that they can function as proxies for patients' end of life care experience, and have their own retrospective experience of being a caregiver of a dying person and a current experience of being a bereaved person.

The heterogeneity of the older population is rarely acknowledged, even with a growing awareness of the role of individual factors in determining how end of life is understood and experienced. A comprehensive review of the academic, policy, and practice literature suggests that there is evidence of both under- and overtreatment for older people, and less adequate support for their carers (5, 6). While cancer care for older people may be excellent in some hospitals and hospices, previous research from the USA has identified that people over 65 diagnosed with cancer are less likely to receive appropriate therapies (7) and, in particular are more likely to be offered non-curative treatments due to unfounded assumptions that aggressive treatments are both less acceptable and more poorly tolerated. Older carers may therefore have an advocacy role in mediating between older patients and the assumptions and stereotyping of health and social care professionals providing care (for a fuller discussion see Grande and Keady, Chapter 13, this volume).

Family caregiving

It is important to examine in greater depth what 'family' means in the context of end of life care for older people and how that notion is changing in contemporary society. There is consistent evidence that the majority of care for dying people is provided by spouses who themselves may be older people (8). During the latter part of the 20th century trends in family and household composition became less predictable as established family patterns began to change with increasing divorce rates even in older age, reductions in numbers of offspring, and longevity increasing opportunities for grandparenting and great grandparenting (9). In many developed countries family size has declined to one or two children per partnership following declines in the overall birth rate, and in the UK approximately 10% of women remain childless (10). In many European Union (EU) countries, rapidly rising divorce rates with over one million divorces annually, have led to more complex family configurations including remarriage, single-parent households, cohabiting couples, and stepfamilies becoming commonplace (11). Similarly in Japan, there have been marked changes in the composition of households where people over 65 years live, with growing proportions of single-person households and couples both over 65 years and reductions in three-generation households which were the norm in 1975 (12). The important point is that it cannot be assumed that people who are no longer in stable family relationships such as ex-partners and stepchildren will provide care. Contemporary complex family relationships and evolving family roles may leave older people, particularly men following divorce or women following bereavement, living alone and isolated. Alternatively, the diversity of family relationship may open up new opportunities for intergenerational care in both directions, for example by greater involvement by grandparents in providing childcare and for young adults caring for their grandparents or great-grandparents. These facets of changing family structures have not been adequately explored in the context of dying older people.

Across the world demographic patterns indicate that in most countries people are living longer, and that dying typically occurs in later life, and these demographic trends are predicted to continue (13). Continuing developments in medical technology alongside improving living conditions have resulted in changed patterns of mortality. One of the challenges now facing European countries and many resource-rich regions is that of ageing populations. As more people live longer there are now growing numbers of the 'old old' (people over 85 years) and these numbers will increase over the next 20 years. It is estimated that by 2050 the total population of Europe will have dropped by 1% and half the population will be aged over 50 years. As an example it is predicted that in the UK the percentage of deaths amongst those aged 85 and over will rise from 32% in 2004 to 44% in 2030 (14). As the demand for palliative care rises, the overall decline in the population will mean that there will be fewer adults available to provide paid and unpaid care. This will have the potential to considerably compromise the quality of care to patients requiring palliative care. However, there is evidence from a systematic review that suggests that older people are less likely to access specialist palliative care services, although it was not clear if this results from having needs that are judged to be less amenable to palliative care interventions, less demand from older people and their carers, lower rates of referral, or less uptake of offered services (15).

Financial implications of caregiving for family carers

Caring for a person with a chronic or life-limiting illness places heavy demands upon the financial resources of all families. When that person is older, they and their spouse are likely to be living on fixed retirement incomes, which may result in considerable hardship. For example, there are costs associated with treatment and management of their condition including physician fees, medication, hospitalizations, and medical investigation costs. Even in countries, where medical expenses are covered by statutory or individual insurance schemes, there are associated costs such as transport to clinics. For example, an evaluation of transport problems for patients and family carers utilizing specialist palliative care services, indicated the value of a dedicated ambulance funded by Marie Curie Cancer Care (a UK-based cancer charity) (16). Family carers were confident in the role of the specially trained ambulance personnel to safely and without delay transfer patients from hospital to home, especially when very near the end of life (as demonstrated in Chapter 15 by Hanratty in this volume).

The majority of costs in providing home care of dying people relate to increased domestic expenditure and these may well be greater for frail older people who may require more heating, laundry, special foods and clothing. For example, a Swedish study of advanced home care (a type of multidisciplinary team-supported home care programme for older people, offered as an alternative to institutional care) demonstrated that informal care constituted a considerable part of the overall costs (17). If a calculation for the cost of leisure time was included, the informal carers' costs were twice as high as those for professional carers. This study indicates that if informal carers' costs are excluded, there is a considerable underestimation of the true costs of providing care at home. These hidden costs include forgone work time and leisure time; in other words, the opportunity costs of providing care within the family are rarely calculated or acknowledged within policy initiatives that seek to promote home care near the end of life (14), thus perpetuating the impression that they are cheaper, when in fact they are shifting costs on to patients and families. There is an urgent need to undertake more rigorous health economic research to appraise the real costs of end of life care at home and establish methodologies that allow comparisons to be made across countries.

Family carers provide end of life care in the wider context of the uncertainties of the changing global economy. Writing this chapter at the end of the first decade of the 21st century, it has been a remarkably economically volatile period with global 'boom and bust'—a period of affluence closely followed by recession. The impact of this on family carers will largely depend upon their country of residence and their particular circumstances. However, there may be wider changes in society such as reductions in carers' support services or welfare allowances. Changes in the employed workforce, and varying patterns of employment such as increases in part-time working and less employment stability, have seen increasing numbers of women employed outside the home leaving fewer people available to undertake a full-time caring role for older family members. Relaxations in restrictions on the retirement age mean that increasing numbers of older people continue to be employed, either for reasons of economic necessity as their pensions become less adequate or because they find employment socially and intellectually fulfilling. The EU is currently concerned about increases in the workforce and EU polices and current economic pressures mean that more women have paid jobs, and people work longer hours and for more years before retirement, than in the past (18). The demand for a geographically mobile workforce has led to higher levels of migration within and into European societies resulting in household disruption and changed family constellations (9). For example, in many Eastern European countries, high levels of economic migration amongst younger people leave older family members without practical and social support towards the end of life (19).

Many countries rely on migrant labour to provide paid care workers in health and social care. For example, a study conducted in Ireland about end of life care for older people in institutions including hospitals, nursing and welfare homes, indicated that care workers from other parts of Europe or Asia, often had difficulties in understanding the cultural and spiritual needs of older people and their family members. While these misunderstandings were compounded by language difficulties, these alone did not account for the reported problems (20). In research conducted with older Chinese people resident in the UK (21, 22), it was found that their attitudes to cancer and end of life were strongly shaped by experiences of migration and change, and personal experiences of caregiving. These views were expressed in the contexts of personal biographical narratives of migration, transition, resilience, and adaptation which accords with research on older migrants in Europe (23, 24) and finds expression in anthologies such as those of older Chinese people who have migrated to live in the South West of England (25). These sources of data all point to the expectations that are embedded in many cultures that older people, especially those facing the end of life, will be sustained by extended family relationships and that care will be provided by younger or middle generation adults. Migration for whatever reason, removes those wider social supports and extensive relationships that may make it possible for families to provide care. Therefore, there needs to be more research focused at understanding how migrant communities sustain family care provision, both in their countries of origin and in their current country of residence. Changing patterns of global economic and political (asylum-seekers) migrant workers may ultimately shape the availability and opportunities to care for older people in the last period of their lives in a number of countries.

The impact of these developments means that fewer people are likely to be available to provide unpaid care at home. These changes in the employment sector are likely to increase the tensions between work and caring responsibilities (18). While providing care for the people near the end of life is a time-limited activity associated with progressive losses, it may entail focusing solely on the patient for the duration of their illness, in the knowledge that it is a temporary situation because the patient will die (2, 26). Consequently family carers may stop paid work or reduce working hours to care for their relatives. Economic pressures on families are likely to impact on their ability to provide care at home, for the reasons highlighted above. Moreover, migrant workers and others with less secure employment may have fewer options. A review of the literature on family carers and the impact on their employment indicated a dearth of research that focused on this topic (27) largely because it is difficult to identify carers from records (2) and arguably because there is an assumption that women within families will be available to provide care.

In summary, there have been significant social, economic, and demographic changes in Europe during the last few decades. These changes have affected all aspects of social life and therefore also impacted heavily on areas of health and social care related to end of life. As a consequence it is likely that in the future there will be fewer carers yet more people dying with complex care needs (28). This will have implications for maintaining high standards of care across the range of settings in which care occurs.

Environments of care: caregiving at home

Throughout the world the majority of older people live at home during the last few months and years of their life, although there have been increasing trends in some countries for people to move into institutions before their death (29, 30). This may or may not be in accord with their preferences for place of care or the preferences of their family carers, and there is some evidence to suggest that for older people dying at home may not be regarded as realistic or feasible as they seek to reduce the 'burden' on family carers and maintain their independence (31). Most patients receiving specialist palliative care services are in middle or later life and as a result, many carers themselves are older people who may have health problems of their own. It should be recognized that 'home' is a heterogeneous concept and that it represents both the physicality of place and 'space', encompassing locality (e.g. safety), environment, and domestic facilities such as access to electrical appliances, clean water, heating; and perhaps of equal importance, 'home' may also represent private 'space', status, ownership, wealth, and be imbued with emotional attachments and links to ancestors and family history (as discussed by Chaudhury et al., Chapter 17, this volume). Globally, there are large differences in what constitutes a home, from one room to a mansion. Economic pressures mean that purchasing or renting homes consume a considerable proportion of domestic income. For older people, maintaining a large 'family' home may be difficult on a fixed pension, and some people choose special accommodation options specifically designed for their needs such as 'retirement apartments'. The suitability of delivering end of life care in homes that are architecturally or environmentally challenging has largely not been considered in the academic literature. However, there is a widespread assumption in current policy directives, for example from the UK (14), that enabling more people to die at home is both desirable and feasible, despite criticisms that this fails to acknowledge the special needs of older people and their carers (32).

The majority of the literature on home care near the end of life comes from the perspectives of those delivering palliative care or hospice programmes in the home (33). For example, in the UK, there have been important initiatives led by charitable organizations to pioneer more effective solutions to providing home care near the end of life (34, 35) and offer more support to family carers (36). Likewise, there is evidence from a British hospice that providing palliative care at home is challenging because of difficulties in defining and responding to the complex needs of patients and ensuring that staff are competent to deliver appropriate care, especially for older people and those with advanced dementia (37). Internationally there is a diversity of responses to delivering home care but virtually all are based on the assumption that there are family carers able and willing to contribute to care (38–42). This assumption will be challenged in the final section.

Enabling people to die at home requires more than mere access to specialist palliative care services or primary health care services (43). Older people and their carers may also need social care provision, such as help with cleaning, shopping, and personal care. Evidence from a large study of older people with end-stage heart failure and their family carers conducted in the UK indicates that less than a quarter received support from social services, despite high levels of apparent need in terms of symptom distress and carer burden (44). The increasing numbers of older people and the complexity of their health and social care needs are placing financial pressures on statutory organizations such as local councils to deliver appropriate services to sufficient numbers of older people (45).

Living alone

It is also salutatory to note that some older people are very isolated as they are living alone without contacts from family or friends. Increasing numbers of older patients are living and dying alone in the UK which presents a challenge to health and social care services striving to offer equitable care (46). A survey of 116 local councils in England and Wales indicated that 4900 funerals in 2007–2008 were paid for by public funds because there was no family or friends able or willing to pay, a 10% rise on the previous year (47). This suggests that in these cases there were unlikely to be family carers available to provide end of life care. Older women are more likely than older men to live alone and the percentage increases with advancing age. In 2007 in Great Britain, 30% of women aged 65 and over lived alone compared to 20% of men in this age group; and for those aged 75 and over this increases to 61% and 34% respectively (48). It is therefore proposed that we need to consider a wider group of people, outside conventional family structures, as potential carers for those approaching the end of life in future. For example, for older people living in care homes or extra care housing, peers may take on important emotionally and practically supportive roles, in addition to, or instead of family members (49). In many countries such as the UK, the prison population is also ageing, raising issues about appropriate care as more prisoners face the end of life within the penal system and there is a possible role for peers in providing informal care (50).

Conclusion

In conclusion this chapter has reviewed the changing profile of family caregivers of older people. It has offered working definitions to guide readers and provided a framework for the subsequent chapters. It has considered the impact of demographic change on the availability and expectations placed on family carers, especially on economic welfare and home care. Finally, there is a recognition that increasing numbers of older people will be dying without close family to provide care and other sources of support will be required. The implications for these social and demographic changes are inadequately incorporated into strategic planning for health and social care in many countries. Future policies, while being steadfast in their determination to ensure the delivery of high-quality care to older patients and their family carers, need to address priorities of matching service provision, financial support, and expanding the engagement of additional non-kin carers. The next 10 years will provide many opportunities for carers' role development, crossing or blurring of boundaries between care sectors, and advancing a stronger recognition of care as a partnership between families and professionals.

References

1. Roy DJ (2009). Ambiguity in palliative care? (Editorial.) *Journal of Palliative Care*, 25(4): 243–4.
2. Grande G, Stajduhar K, Aoun S, Toye C, Funk L, Addington-Hall J, et al. (2009). Supporting lay carers in end of life care: current gaps and future priorities. *Palliative Medicine*, 23(4): 339–44.
3. National Institute for Clinical Excellence (2004). *Guidance on Cancer Services: Improving Supportive and Palliative Care for Adults with Cancer: The Manual*. London: NICE.
4. Hudson P, Payne S (eds) (2008). *Family Carers in Palliative Care*. Oxford: Oxford University Press.
5. Seymour J, Witherspoon R, Gott M, Ross H, Payne S (2005). *Dying in Older Age: End-of-Life Care*. Bristol: Policy Press.
6. Bee PE, Barnes P, Luker KA (2008). A systematic review of informal caregivers' needs in providing home-based end-of-life care to people with cancer. *Journal of Clinical Nursing*, 18: 1379–93.
7. Terret C, Zulian G, Droz JP (2004). Statements on the interdependency between the oncologist and the geriatricians in geriatric oncology. *Critical Reviews in Oncology and Hematology*, 2: 127–33.
8. Help the Hospices (2009). *Identifying carers' needs in the palliative setting. Guidance for professionals*. London: Help the Hospices.
9. Allan G, Hawker S, Crow G (2001). Family diversity and change in Britain and Western Europe. (2001). *Journal of Family Issues*, 22(7): 819–37.
10. Payne S, Hudson P (2008). Assessing the family and caregivers In D Walsh, R Fainsinger, K Foley, P Glare, C Goh, M Lloyd-Williams, et al. (eds) *Palliative Medicine*. New York: Elsevier.
11. Dugan E (2008). Solitary lives in Europeans leading continent into old age. *The Independent*, 8 May.
12. Kawagoe I, Ito M, Matsuura S, Kawagoe K (2009). Home hospice care for the lung cancer patient living alone: a case report from Japan. *Journal of Palliative Care*, 25(4): 289–93.
13. Davies E, Higginson I (eds) (2004). *Better palliative care for older people*, Copenhagen: World Health Organization Europe.
14. Department of Health (2008). *End of life care strategy: promoting high quality care for all adults at the end of life*. London: Department of Health.
15. Burt J, Raine R (2006). The effects of age on referral to and use of specialist palliative care services in adult cancer patients: a systematic review. *Age and Ageing*, 35: 469–76.
16. Ingleton C, Payne S, Sargeant A, Seymour J (2009). Barriers to achieving care at home at the end of life: transferring patients between care settings using patient transport services. *Palliative Medicine*, 23(8): 723–30.
17. Andersson A, Carstensen J, Levin L-A, Emtinger BG (2003). Costs of informal care for patients in advanced home care: a population-based study. *International Journal of Technology Assessment in Health Care*, 19(4): 656–63.
18. Eurocarers: European Association for Working Carers (2008). *Family Care in Europe: the contribution of carers to long term care, especially for older people* (Eurocarers factsheet). Available at: http://www.eurocarers.org (Accessed 3 November 2008.)
19. Kellehear A (2008). Understanding social and cultural dimensions of family carers. In P Hudson, S Payne (eds) *Family Carers and Palliative Care*, pp. 21–36. Oxford: Oxford University Press.
20. O'Shea E, Murphy K, Larkin P, Payne S, Froggatt K, Casey DC, et al. (2007). *End-of-Life Care for Old People in Acute and Long-Stay Care Settings in Ireland. Final Report to the National Council on Ageing and Older People and The Irish Hospice Foundation*. Dublin: Irish Hospice Foundation and National Council on Ageing and Older People.

21. Payne S, Seymour J, Chapman A, Holloway M (2008). Older Chinese people's views on food: implications for supportive cancer care. *Ethnicity and Health*, **13**(5): 497–514.

22. Seymour J, Payne S, Chapman A, Holloway M (2007). Hospice or home? Expectations of end-of-life care among white and Chinese older people in the UK. *Sociology of Health and Illness, Special Edition on Ethnicity and Health*, **29**(6): 872–90.

23. Warnes T (2004). *Older Migrants in Europe: Essays, Projects and Sources*. Sheffield: Sheffield Institute for Studies on Ageing.

24. Hoeksma J (2004). The care needs of elderly Chinese migrants in Rotherham. In T Warnes (ed) *Older Migrants in Europe: Essays, Projects and Sources*. Sheffield: Sheffield Institute for Studies on Ageing.

25. Wong SL, Frances L (2007). *Sweet and Sour: Recollections of the Chinese Elder Communities in the South West of England*. Plymouth: Plymouth and District Racial Equality Council.

26. Harding R, Higginson I (2003). What is the best way to help caregivers in cancer and palliative care? A systematic literature review of interventions and their effectiveness. *Palliative Medicine*, **17**: 63–74.

27. Smith P, Payne S, Ramcharan P (2006). *Carers of the Terminally Ill and Employment Issues: a comprehensive literature review. Final report for Help the Hospices, January 2006*. Lancaster: Lancaster University.

28. Seale C (2000). Changing patterns of death and dying. *Social Science and Medicine*, **51**: 917–30.

29. Gomes B, Higginson IJ (2006). Factors influencing death at home in terminally ill patients with cancer: a systematic review. *British Medical Journal*, **332**: 515–21.

30. Gomes B, Higginson IJ (2008). Where people die (1974–2030): past trends, future projections and implications for care. *Palliative Medicine*, **22**: 33–41.

31. Gott M, Seymour JE, Bellamy G, Clark D, Ahmedzai S (2004). How important is dying at home to the 'good death'? Findings from a qualitative study with older people. *Palliative Medicine*, **18**: 460–7.

32. Gott M (2008). At odds with the end of life care strategy. *Nursing Older People*, **20**: 16–17.

33. Baines M (2010). The origins and development of palliative care at home. *Progress in Palliative Care*, **18**(1): 4–8.

34. Agelopoulos N, Tate T (2009). The Marie Curie Delivering Choice Programme. *European Journal of Palliative Care*, **16**(6): 290–4.

35. Addicott R, Dewar S (2008). *Improving choice for end of life: a descriptive analysis of the impact of costs of Marie Curie Delivering Choice Programme*. London: King's Fund.

36. Payne S, Ingleton C, Nolan M and O'Brien T (2009).*Evaluation of the Help the Hospices Major Grants Programme for Carers of those who are terminally ill. Final Report to Help the Hospices, July 2009*. Lancaster: Lancaster University.

37. Monroe B, Hansford P (2010). Challenges in delivering palliative care in the community–a perspective from St Christopher's Hospice, London, UK. *Progress in Palliative Care*, **18**(1): 9–13.

38. Sallnow L, Kumar S, Numpeli M (2010). Home-based palliative care in Kerala, India: the Neighbourhood Network in Palliative Care. *Progress in Palliative Care*, **18**(1): 14–17.

39. Merriman A (2010). Going the extra mile with the bare essentials: home care in Uganda. *Progress in Palliative Care*, **18**(1): 18–22.

40. Landon A, Mosoiu D (2010). Hospice 'Casa Sperantei'–pioneering palliative home care services in Romania. *Progress in Palliative Care*, **18**(1): 23–6.

41. Murphy S (2010). Territory palliative care–a model for remote area palliative care provision. *Progress in Palliative Care*, **18**(1): 27–30.

42. Devi BCR, Tang TS, Corbex M (2010). A model of palliative care programme integrating rural with hospital care: Sarawak, Malaysia. *Progress in Palliative Care*, **18**(1): 31–6.

43. Burt J, Shipman C, Addington-Hall J, White P (2008). Nursing the dying within a generalist workload: a focus group study of district nurses. *International Journal of Nursing Studies*, **45**: 1470–8.

44. Gott M, Barnes S, Payne S, Parker C, Seamark D, Gariballa S, et al. (2007). Patient views of social service provision for older people with advanced heart failure. *Health and Social Care in the Community*, **15**: 333–42.

45. The Audit Commission (2010). *Under pressure: tackling the financial challenges for councils of an ageing population.* London: The Audit Commission.

46. Office for National Statistics; Babb P, Burkner H, Church J, Zealey L (eds) (2006). *Social Trends No. 36. 2006 Edition.* Basingstoke: Palgrave Macmillan.

47. Bennett R, Bowers M (2009). Life in solitary: silent epidemic sweeping through modern society. *The Times*, 31 December, p. 18.

48. National Statistics Online. Available at: http://www.statistics.gov.uk/cci (Assessed 8 January 2010.)

49. Froggatt K (2004). *Palliative Care in Care Homes for Older People.* London: National Council for Palliative Care.

50. Her Majesty's Chief Inspector of Prisons (2008). *Older prisoners in England and Wales: A follow-up to the 2004 thematic review.* London: Her Majesty's Inspectorate of Prisons.

Chapter 13

Needs, access, and support for older carers

Gunn Grande and John Keady

Introduction

Family carers play a pivotal role in supporting and caring for older people towards the end of life. However, in addition to the rewards that such a role can afford, caring can also bring about considerable physical, emotional, financial, practical, and social costs which may affect the family carer's quality of life. It is therefore important that health, social care, and third-sector providers are aware of such issues and how to best support carers in performing this role.

In this chapter we will consider

◆ The context of caregiving in old age

◆ Adverse effects and rewards from caregiving

◆ The influence of older carers' life situation and perspectives

◆ Supporting older carers.

In doing so we need to keep in mind that caring occurs at all ages and between all generations, although older carers may well face additional age-related challenges, such as the onset of arthritis and/or other long-term conditions. Furthermore, whilst some broad trends may apply, older carers are not one homogenous group and it is important to consider the particular circumstances that affect the caregiving experience and the associated needs in each individual case. Throughout the chapter we have defined older carers as carers who are 65 years and above and who are likely to be retired.

Context of caregiving in old age

Overall the number of older carers is increasing (1), an outcome which reflects the global ageing population and the fact that older people are the greatest consumers of health and social care. As an illustration, *The State of Ageing and Health in America* (2007) suggests that at least 80% of older Americans are living with at least one chronic condition (e.g. cancer, coronary heart disease, Alzheimer's disease, diabetes, stroke) and '50% have at least two' (2). The report highlights that the three main causes of death for older Americans are heart disease, cancer, and stroke and that improved end of life care is a key issue that could significantly improve the quality of life for older adults (2). On this last point, it is difficult to obtain a clear indication of the numbers of older people receiving end of life care provided by older carers. However, it is well-known that older carers are likely to be looking after someone of the same generation who is also likely to be old; this will predominantly be their spouse (1, 3, 4) although other caregiving relationships also exist, such as adult child to parent and neighbour to older person, for instance (1). Younger carers are comparatively more likely to be looking after someone of a different generation to them and/or someone living in a different household (5) (although, as before, many will be looking after a child, spouse, or older parents or in-laws who live in the same household).

Typically, there are a higher proportion of carers among women than among men. Furthermore, given women's longer life expectancy (in the developed world), married women can normally expect that their husbands will predecease them (5) and that they, rather than their husband, will provide spousal end of life care. However, once men live past 70, there are a higher proportion of carers among men than among women, so that numbers of female and male carers become more similar in older age (6). Again, it is not known how much of this comprises end of life caregiving, but it raises the importance of considering gender in caregiving and that male and female carers may well construct the meaning, act, and tasks involved in the performance of care differently. For instance, in dementia care, it has been known for some time that older male spousal carers predominantly view their role as a 'job' (7) and find moments of greater satisfaction in the caregiving process than female carers (8).

In general, older carers have worse health and provide longer hours of care than younger carers, yet they have fewer financial and social resources to support them. The older the carer, the more likely they are to spend long hours providing care. Of those aged 60–64 years, 22% of men and 26% of women provide 50 hours of care per week. Of those aged 85–89 years this increases to 54% of men and 48% of women (4). In the oldest age groups, male carers are more likely than female carers to provide long hours of care (6). Older carers are furthermore more likely to provide higher levels of personal and physical care than younger carers (1) and to provide the nursing tasks associated with terminal care (3).

At the same time, older carers are themselves more likely to suffer from serious health conditions. Milne et al. (1) report that over half of older carers have a long standing illness or disability. At all age bands over 60, a higher proportion of those caring for more than 50 hours per week are in poor general health compared to those caring for fewer hours (4). Furthermore, older carers who coreside with their care recipient spend more hours on care and do heavier tasks (9), whilst those caring outside the home care for fewer hours per week, offer more practical support and are involved on a more limited basis (1). Financially, older carers are amongst the least well-off groups in the UK (1). Carers aged 65 and above are unlikely to be in paid work with Buckner and Yeandle (4) reporting in 2005 that only 12% of male and 8% of female carers are in paid work (compared to 15% and 8% of non-carers, respectively). Whilst, on the one hand, this could be seen as making more time available for older carers to simply deliver 'care', on the other hand the limitations of post-retirement incomes, statutory disqualification from some carer's allowances, and failing health status combine to result in a deprived group. In short, fewer economic resources and low incomes limit the options for easing caregiving tasks and increase the practical demands on older carers (10).

Older carers may also increasingly have fewer social resources available to support them in caregiving which is of itself a concern as social networks can act as a buffer to the potential stressors of caregiving (11). While the carer role itself may lead to greater isolation, the extended family appears to play a decreasing role in supporting older carers (1). Those who live with a spouse, who often will be the care recipient, increasingly live with the spouse alone (4, 5) and families generally are more dispersed (1). However, friends and neighbours may play an increasing role in supporting older carers (1).

Although older carers provide longer hours of care, have worse health, and may have fewer financial and social resources to cope than younger carers, at the same time they and their care recipients receive less formal support than younger carers. There is clear evidence that specialist palliative care can improve quality of life both for patients and carers (12, 13) and that such care may even reduce mortality among older carers (14). However, older patients and their carers are less likely to have specialist palliative care (see discussion in Chapter 5 by Gott et al. in this volume) and also are less likely to have generalist care towards the end of life than younger patients (15, 16). Milne et al. (1) report that three-quarters of older carers living with the cared-for person receive no regular visits from health or social services, although it is not clear how many of these provide end of life care. These differences in formal care provision do not appear to be related to differences in need among the patients looked after by older carers towards the end of life (16).

Recent work suggests that when it comes to age biases in access to specialist palliative care, the age of the carer may be more important than the age of the care recipient, at least for home-based care, with access being worse for older carers (17). We therefore need to understand more about the context of older carers, how this shapes their own view of their situation and role, sense of empowerment, and ability to act as patient advocates, and in turn how they may be viewed by providers.

Adverse effects and rewards from caregiving

This section will first review the adverse effects and rewards from caregiving in end of life care which will apply to all carers. Next, it will consider specifically how older carers may differ from younger carers in terms of adverse effects. The section will mainly draw on two recent comprehensive international reviews of the quantitative and qualitative family care research literature in end of life care 1998–2008 (18, 19). These reviews contrast with the general caregiving literature which has focused on care for frail older people and those with chronic conditions. The reviews included carers of patients of all diagnoses and considered peer reviewed studies in English that addressed a palliative, terminal, or otherwise advanced or end-stage phase of care, and that focused on home-based caregiving. Home is where most end of life care is likely to take place, as most of the last year of life is spent at home (20), although death itself may not take place at home.

Caring stress, rewards, and coping: a general context

In order to better understand this context in caregiving, Morrissey et al. (21) suggested that stress is an important factor in determining coping and that stress can be viewed as resulting from a transaction between an individual and his/her environment, in accordance with Lazarus' (1966) transactional model of stress (22). Here stress is only said to result when demands of a situation or event is perceived to pose a potential threat, harm, or challenge and there is a perceived mismatch between the demands posed and the individual's ability to respond effectively to reduce the threat, harm, or challenge. Using this approach the crucial determinant is not the objective nature of the demand (stressor) itself, but its appraised impact. Hence carers may be able to tolerate the seemingly stressful event of their dependent's incontinence at the end of life, but less well able to manage the social embarrassment that such actions evoke. In other words, events only become stressors when the mind identifies them as such. This distinction is important as it allows for the possibility of the same event being differentially stressful for different people, or even for the same person at different points in time.

The quantitative review by Stajduhar et al. (18) included 123 papers and found that a considerable number of studies identified moderate to high levels of emotional and psychological difficulties among carers, specifically depression and anxiety. However, feelings of low self-esteem, powerlessness and helplessness, emotional stress, and psychosocial difficulties were also reported. Many studies in the review also found caregiving to be associated with physical health impacts, including fatigue and sleep disturbance. In addition to health impacts, caregiving was associated with financial strain, need for financial support and advice, and/or occupational disruption, as well as general activity restrictions. Some research has also identified that carers had reduced quality of life and life satisfaction, experienced general caregiver burden or strain, as well as social dysfunction and relationship challenges. The qualitative literature review by Funk et al. (19) involved 105 studies and allowed more in-depth exploration of carers' perspectives. It reports strong, conflicting, and difficult emotions associated with caregiving. Accounts of negative emotions are predominant, including fear, dread, anger, disillusionment, guilt, grief, helplessness, and hopelessness. However, accounts also highlight the physical demands of the carer role and its impact on physical health (19). While carers of all patients will share many of these challenges, those who care for someone towards the end of life have been found to have poorer quality of life and worse physical, but not mental, health compared to other carers (23).

However, adverse effects are not the whole story, as several studies have reported that caregivers also find the experience of caregiving towards end of life rewarding and/or meaningful (24, 25). For instance, Hudson (25) found that 60% of carers report positive aspects of caring, including being able to give, growing closer, and increased confidence. Other positive dimensions of caregiving include: a sense of pride, esteem, and mastery (25–27); being able to demonstrate love and fulfil reciprocity (27); gaining satisfaction and sense of accomplishment (27); development of closer relationships (25–27); and personal growth (27, 28). These positive aspects of care may partly explain the importance of finding meaning in caregiving (25), a cognitive process necessary to conduct care in a humanistic, sensitive, and person-centred way.

The above studies focused on home care, while some patients will spend an extended period in care homes towards the end of life. The evidence suggests that when patients go into care homes, the caregiving role does not become easier, just different, and it has been known for some time that a family role in care home decision-making has benefits on a number of relational and interpersonal dimensions. For example, Rowles and High (29) Author query: please check that new ref 29 I have inserted is the one you wanted when discussing Rowles and High (1996)found that family involvement in the ongoing care for their relative served as a biographical link between the previous life 'at home' and the newly acquired identity of care home resident. This biographical link was crucial in ensuring care home staff intervened on a person-to-person basis, rather than from the inherent power imbalance of staff member to resident. Moreover, these authors also revealed that families preserved special tasks during their time with their loved one, such as performing comforting, pampering, and monitoring roles during their visits to the care home. The families' ongoing ability and opportunity to perform such intimate and personalized caregiving tasks was seen by Gaugler et al. (30) to strengthen the need for family involvement in care homes, and to enrich the lives of residents. Accordingly, barriers to family involvement in care homes, such as a lack of information or encouragement to participate in daily decision-making (31), should be challenged if the resident's positive sense of well-being is to be maintained or, ideally, raised (32).

Families also perform a monitoring role within the care home (33), a process that can be constructed as an act of 'keeping', such as through 'keeping an eye' on the situation (33). Arguably, this process of 'keeping' is heightened at the time of the admission into the care home when the expectations of family involvement are raised. As Davies and Nolan (34) report, family involvement in a care home is enhanced if family members view themselves as working in partnership with care home staff. An 'inclusive' organizational care philosophy, therefore, becomes crucial determinants to the perceived success, or otherwise, of family involvement and togetherness within a care home setting (1, 35).

Studies of those who have provided care over an identifiable palliative phase report both positive and negative outcomes in bereavement. Caregivers report a high rate of post-traumatic stress symptoms (35) and experience increases in loneliness, sadness, depression, sleeplessness, loss of appetite, and general low mental health after the death (37–40). However, authors also report, often within the same study, positive effects post-bereavement such as high rates of post-traumatic growth (36), reduced distress and anxiety (40), higher self-acceptance, closure, and gain, better health and lower burden (37–41), commonly report that they are coping well (38), have a fairly positive outlook, and low negative reactions to caring (39).

Age and adverse effects

As older carers typically have a higher care burden and may have fewer physical, financial, social, and formal resources to support them in this task, it would be natural to assume that older carers would experience more adverse effects from caregiving than their younger counterparts. However, the picture that emerges is more complex than it first may appear. For instance, the review of the end of life care literature by Stajduhar et al. (18) found that, compared to older carers, younger care givers experience greater levels of: emotional strain and psychological distress, task difficulty, impact of stressors, and caregiving burden and strain more generally. In contrast, one study by Kwak et al. (42) found that younger carers report more comfort, closure and satisfaction from caring than older carers. Pinquart and Sorensen (43) conducted a literature review of the impact of caregiving on carers of frail elderly compared to non-carers, some of whom would be involved in end of life care. They found that while younger carers were more likely to report increased stress than older carers, older carers were more likely to report high levels of depression. They also report that older carers had lower levels of self-efficacy than younger carers, which relates to their sense of mastery and perceived control. The differences between carer and non-carers were more pronounced in samples with a higher proportion of spouses.

Compared to caregiving at younger ages, caregiving at an older age is associated with premature mortality (44). Furthermore, older carers generally experience worse outcomes in bereavement (37, 45–47). However, research by Bernard and Guarnaccia (48) and Brazil et al. (38) did not find this association (5) and additional studies are required to help develop a knowledge and evidence base.

The influence of older carers' life situation and perspectives

In general, caregiving in old age is less likely to conflict with demands of paid work and caring for young children compared to caregiving at a younger age. Role adjustments for spousal carers may also be fewer, whereas at younger ages the loss of a spouse or partner's ability to do paid work or share childcare responsibilities may lead to dramatic life changes and role adjustments (49). While the level of care provided is associated with unmet need and burden (19, 50), research suggests that it is not so much the patient's level of care dependency that increases burden and emotional distress, but the disruption and restriction of carers' own activities (11, 51). Therefore, long hours of care and level of physical assistance may be less burdensome if they are not perceived to interfere with other activities. Possible evidence for this is found in research that suggests that retired caregivers may have better quality of life and lower burden (52), whereas those of working age may have higher levels of depression in attempting to juggle many conflicting demands (53); however, Grov et al. (54) reported in 2006 that employment was associated with higher quality of life.

Insofar as the care recipients of older carers may contain a larger proportion of patients with long-term conditions, dementia, and/or general comorbidity, older carers may have provided care for longer by the time the patient reaches end of life. They may therefore be more likely to be 'expert carers' (55), which would imply both greater confidence in caring task and more reluctance to accept outside help. Nolan et al. (55) cite evidence from the general carer literature that suggest that the more competent carers feel in their role, the less stress and burden they may feel. The qualitative literature on end of life caregiving correspondingly suggests there is a connection between lack of preparedness for caregiving and carers' accounts of fear and anxiety associated with the role (19).

Where the care recipient is the spouse, caregiving is more likely to be perceived as a natural extension of the existing relationship (56) and caring between older spouses an expression of expectations underpinning marriage (15). Conversely, when a child becomes the carer for a parent, this probably represents a greater role adjustment both for the child and parent (5), especially around the provision of personal, intimate care (57). Although increased deterioration, dependency, and symptoms in the patient are associated with more adverse carer outcomes, personal appraisals of the situation may be more important (18, 21). Carers experience better outcomes if there are perceived benefits of caregiving, greater comfort with tasks, acceptance and sense of meaning, role esteem, sense of control, and confidence (18).

Old age is often associated with loss of social and citizenship status in general (57) and older people's own negative images of 'oldness' may include being unimportant, irrelevant, and having no role (59). Caregiving may be more likely to offer an opportunity for retention of purpose and worth for older carers and may therefore be associated with more positive appraisals in older carers compared to younger carers. Being able to display resourcefulness in face of difficulties and giving the appearance of being able to manage may also be crucial in maintaining positive identity and sense of self in old age and may be particularly important for those in a caring role (60). From a more negative perspective, dying in old age may be disproportionately associated with a period of 'social death' prior to the death itself, which may render the patient and their carers more 'invisible' to health professionals (58, 59). One of the key tasks and rewards of caring involves preservation of the patient's value and personhood (25, 55), which may therefore become a more acute concern for older carers as they mainly care for older people. This may preclude acceptance of external support or institutional support which may be seen to be impersonal and involve depersonalization of the patient (55). Also, while caregiving can pose considerable restrictions and demands on the lives of older carers, they may be more likely to regard these as unexceptional and part of the general limitations/expectations of old age (61).

Whilst caregiving may be seen as a natural extension of the spousal relationship, this may be an externally imposed 'norm' that the carer feels hard to reject. This is an invidious position especially when past/present interpersonal relationships are poor and there is a transcending expectation—from family, society, the local community—to care. If the carer role is imposed, and carers feel unable to exercise genuine choice, caregiving is likely to be associated with greater burden (62). Research also suggests that the older person's natural expectation towards their spouse is that care will be provided, a duty that is not automatically bestowed on their adult children (63). Older people worry more about being a burden to their adult children than to their spouse (57) and are more likely to see assisted living, or care home entry, as a more preferable outcome under these circumstances (59).

These factors may help explain why older carers express less distress from caring and are less likely to accept or receive formal support in end of life care. On the one hand, caring may be something seamlessly taken on by older carers because it fits with their role, life situation, wishes, and vows. On the other hand, caring in old age may be something that is laden with expectation, performed by someone who is available but fairly invisible to service providers, with fewer resources to bear, less inclination to express needs, and little power to decline the role. Caregiving may therefore involve resigned acceptance, a coping strategy more likely to be associated with old age (64) which is less likely to be expressed in terms of stress and distress, but perhaps more likely to manifest itself in depression.

The evidence that older carers suffer more in bereavement is a cause for concern here. The cost of caregiving to older carers may be more likely to manifest itself at this stage. Other risk factors for negative outcomes in bereavement that may relate to old age are being a spousal carer, the intensity of the pre-bereavement level of care, having low social support, and coping by accepting responsibility (18). It can also be hypothesized that carers who attain a sense of purpose and role satisfaction from caring, may also feel the greatest loss when it comes to an end (65). Alternatively, detrimental outcomes have also been associated with greater pre-loss emotional distress, burden, and caregiving problems, which are more likely to be reported by younger carers (18).

Supporting older carers

There is considerable research literature on carers' support needs in end of life care. In broad outline the main support needs are (18, 66–68):

- Psychological support
- Information, including information about the patient's illness and help available
- Help with caring for the patient, including personal care, nursing care, medical care
- Access to support out of hours
- Respite
- Practical help, e.g. with household tasks
- Finance
- Transport.

A recent qualitative study (69) involving focus groups and interviews with 75 bereaved carers explored carers' support needs when caring for someone at home in the last 2 months of life. This sample mainly consisted of older carers, although some younger carers also participated. Carers were found to feel that the responsibility for the patient's care and well-being rested with them, and their main focus was on support that enabled them to provide care for the patient. Support that enabled them to provide care included

- Knowing who to contact when concerned
- Understanding the patient's illness
- What to expect in the future
- Managing symptoms and medicines
- Talking to the patient about their illness
- Equipment to help care for the patient
- Help with personal care.

They placed less emphasis on support for themselves. Nevertheless, this is important in enabling carers to continue to care. Such support included help with:

- Own physical health concerns
- Dealing with their own feelings and worries
- Beliefs or spiritual concerns
- Practical help in the home
- Financial and work issues

- Day time respite
- Overnight break from caring.

While these support needs are common to carers of all age groups, some support areas may require specific attention for older carers. This includes financial support in light of the potential poverty of older carers, including improved carer allowances and help with accessing these (1). Given the higher prevalence of ill health among older carers, they need support to look after their own health needs (1). Older carers have less support from specialist palliative care and formal care in general, and ways of facilitating access need to be identified (17). Given potential isolation in old age (1) it may be important to identify ways of facilitating social networks and support from other carers. Milne et al. (1) also note the specific needs of older carers in rural communities, where mobility and lack of access to transport may be an issue, an issue in dementia care that has been known for some time (70). Furthermore, although the heterogeneity of ethnic minority groups precludes broad statements about their support needs, older carers in such communities may specifically need help with communication and language difficulties.

Older carers may also require more support with transitions to institutional care. Admission to institutional care may often be a period of turmoil and guilt, and while not exclusive to older carers, this may be a particularly difficult transition for older spousal carers who have cared for the patient over a prolonged period, e.g. when the patient suffers from dementia (1). Moreover, research suggests that older carers may suffer disproportionately in bereavement, and providers of bereavement care may need to focus more on this client group (19).

When considering the manner in which we may support carers, it is important to recognize both their role as care providers and as 'experts' on how to care for the patient. Carers will normally feel that it is their responsibility to provide care, will put the patient's needs first (69), and will have in-depth knowledge of the patient's needs and preferences (55, 71). This will particularly be the case for older spousal carers who have provided care for a prolonged period. One implication is that carers may only accept help that they feel will help them provide care for the patient (68, 69), and support that is sensitive to the preferences of both carer and patient. It is furthermore important to recognize the potential benefits derived from caregiving (25). This suggests that service provision should seek to complement rather than replace carer's input (71) and poses particular challenges for the delivery of respite, a key element of carer support. Respite that takes the patient out of the home may be difficult for carers to accept. While respite delivered in the home may be preferred, this also needs be sensitive to the above issues and delivered on carers' own terms. The above issues are also very pertinent in relation to admission to institutional care where carers experience a substantial change from being in charge of care to having a secondary role (1). Carers will often still feel a strong need to play a part in the patient's care and preserve their relationship with the patient, while struggling with feelings of guilt and potential loss of companionship (1, 55).

There has been limited research into interventions to support carers. A recent review by Lorenz et al. (72) into palliative care interventions for carers suggests that individual and/or multicomponent interventions may be most likely to yield benefits. This implies that interventions that are tailored to the individual and that address several aspects of support may be the most promising. However, while there is moderate evidence that carer interventions in dementia care lead to benefits, palliative care for other conditions only shows moderate evidence for carer satisfaction and weak evidence for actual carer benefits. The vast variety of different types of support evaluated, and the lack of outcome measures relevant to carers furthermore makes it difficult to learn from existing evidence. Evidence relating to psychological interventions for bereavement suggests that these may lead to improvements, but their benefit to carers have not been specifically investigated (73).

While some broad patterns have been outlined in this chapter, older carers are a heterogeneous group, and the circumstances and needs of each individual will be different. Appropriate targeting of support requires appropriate assessment of individual need, and there is increased recognition of the importance of carer needs assessment in end of life care (20). Such assessment should ideally be made separately from the patient, as carers' needs and concerns may be quite different, they may have difficulty expressing their own needs particularly in front of the patient, and separate assessment may help carers acknowledge that their needs are legitimate.

References

1. Milne A, Hatzidimitriadou E, Chryssanthropoulou C, Owen T (2001). *Caring in later life: reviewing the role of older carers*. London: Help the Aged.

2. Centers for Disease Control and Prevention and The Merck Company Foundation (2007). *The State of Ageing and Health in America* [Internet]. Whitehouse Station, NJ: The Merck Company Foundation. Available from: http://www.cdc.gov/ageing and http://www.merck.com/cr.

3. Wenger GC (1990). Elderly carers: the need for appropriate intervention. *Ageing and Society*, **10**: 197–219.

4. Buckner L, Yeandle S (2005). *Older Carers in the UK* [Internet]. UK: Carers UK. Available at: http://www.carersuk.org/Professionals/ResearchLibrary/Profileofcaring/1207234833.

5. Victor C (2005). *The social context of ageing: a textbook of gerontology*. Abingdon: Routledge.

6. Dahlberg L, Demack S, Bambra C (2007). Age and gender of informal carers: a population-based study in the UK. *Health and Social Care in the Community*, **15**(5): 439–45.

7. Fitting M, Rabins P, Lucas MJ, Eastham J (1986). Caregivers for dementia patients: a comparison of husbands and wives. *The Gerontologist*, **26**(3): 248–59.

8. Nolan M, Keady J (2001). Working with carers. In Cantley C (ed) *A handbook of dementia care*, pp. 160–72. Buckinghamshire: Open University Press.

9. Arber S, Ginn J (1991). *Gender and later life: a sociological analysis of resources and constraints*. London: Sage.

10. Seymour JE, Witherspoon R, Gott M, Ross H, Payne S (2005). *End of life care: promoting comfort, choice and well being among older people facing death*. Bristol: Policy Press.

11. Goldstein NE, Concato J, Fried TR, Kasl SV, Johnson-Hurzeler R, Bradley EH (2004). Factors associated with caregiver burden among caregivers of terminally ill patients with cancer. *Journal of Palliative Care*, **20**(1): 38–43.

12. Hearn J, Higginson IJ (1998). Do specialist palliative care teams improve outcomes for cancer patients? A systematic literature review. *Palliative Medicine*, **12**: 317–32.

13. Grande GE, Todd CJ, Barclay SIG, Farquhar MC (2000). A randomised controlled trial of a hospital at home service for the terminally ill. *Palliative Medicine*, **14**(5): 375–85.

14. Christakis NA, Iwashnya TJ (2003). The health impact of health care on families: a matched cohort study of hospice use by decedents and mortality outcomes in surviving, widowed spouses. *Social Science and Medicine*, **57**: 465–75.

15. Cartwright A (1993). Dying when you're old. *Age and Ageing*, **22**: 425–30.

16. Seale C, Cartwright A (1994). *The year before death*. Aldershot: Avebury.

17. Grande GE, Farquhar MC, Barclay SIG, Todd CJ (2006). The influence of patient and carer age in access to palliative care. *Age and Ageing*, **35**: 267–73.

18. Stajduhar KI, Funk L, Toye C, Aoun S, Grande G, Todd C (2010). Part 1: Home-based family caregiving at the end of life: a comprehensive review of published quantitative research (1998–2008). *Palliative Medicine*, **24**: 573–93.

19. Funk L, Stajduhar KI, Toye C, Grande G, Aoun S, Todd C (2010). Part 2: Home-based family caregiving at the end of life: a comprehensive review of published qualitative research (1998–2008). *Palliative Medicine*, **24**: 594–607.

20. Department of Health (2008). *End of life care strategy: promoting high quality care for all adults at the end of life* [Internet]. Available at: http://www.dh.gov.uk/en/Publicationsandstatistics/Publications/PublicationsPolicyAndGuidance/DH_086277 (Accessed 5 February 2009.)

21. Morrissey E, Becker J, Rupert, MP (1990). Coping resources and depression in the caregiving spouses of Alzheimer patients. *British Journal of Medical Psychology*, **63**: 161–71.

22. Lazarus RS (1966). *Psychological stress and the coping process*. New York: McGraw Hill.

23. Weitzner MA, McMillan SC, Jacobsen PB (1999). Family caregiver quality of life: differences between curative and palliative cancer treatment settings. *Journal of Pain and Symptom Management*, **17**(6): 418–28.

24. Addington-Hall J, Walker L, Jones C, Karlsen S, McCarthy M (1998). A randomised controlled trial of postal versus interviewer administration of a questionnaire measuring satisfaction with, and use of, services received in the year before death. *Journal of Epidemiology and Community Health*, **52**(12): 802–7.

25. Hudson P (2004). Positive aspects and challenges associated with caring for a dying relative at home. *International Journal of Palliative Nursing*, **10**(2): 58–65.

26. Aoun SM, Kristjanson L, Hudson P, Currow DC (2005). The experience of supporting a dying relative: reflections of caregivers. *Progress in Palliative Care*, **13**(6): 319–25.

27. Koop PM, Strang VR (2003). The bereavement experience following home-based family caregiving for persons with advanced cancer. *Clinical Nursing Research*, **12**(2): 127–44.

28. Hoppes S (2005). Meanings and purposes of caring for a family member: an autoethnography. *American Journal of Occupational Therapy*, **59**(3): 262–72.

29. Rowles GD, High DM (1996). Individualizing care: family roles in nursing home decision-making. *Journal of Gerontological Nursing*, **22**(3): 20–5.

30. Gaugler JE, Anderson KA, Zarit SH, Pearlin LI (2004). Family involvement in nursing homes: effects on stress and well-being. *Ageing and Mental Health*, **8**(1): 65–75.

31. Hertzberg A, Ekman S-L, Axelsson K (2001). Staff activities and behaviour are the source of many feelings: relatives' interactions and relationships with staff in nursing homes. *Journal of Clinical Nursing*, **10**: 380–8.

32. Brown Wilson C, Davies S, Nolan MR (2009). Developing relationships in care homes—the contribution of staff, residents and families. *Ageing and Society*, **29**: 1–23.

33. Sandberg J, Lundh U, Nolan MR (2001). Placing a spouse in a care home: the importance of keeping. *Journal of Clinical Nursing*, **10**: 406–16.

34. Davies S, Nolan MR (2004). 'Making the move': relatives' experiences of the transition to a care home. *Health and Social Care in the Community*, **12**(6): 517–26.

35. Woods B, Keady J, Seddon D (2007). *Involving families in care homes: a relationship-centred approach to dementia care*. London: Jessica Kingsley.

36. Cadell S (2003). Trauma and growth in Canadian carers. *Aids Care*, **15**(5): 639–48.

37. Brazil K, Bedard M, Willison K (2002). Correlates of health status for family caregivers in bereavement. *Journal of Palliative Medicine*, **5**(6): 849–55.

38. Brazil K, Bedard M, Willison K (2003). Bereavement adjustment and support among caregivers. *Journal of Mental Health and Ageing*, **9**(3): 193–204.

39. Wyatt GK, Friedman L, Given CW, Given BA (1999). A profile of bereaved caregivers following provision of terminal care. *Journal of Palliative Care*, **15**(1): 13–25.

40. Waldrop DP (2007). Caregiver grief in terminal illness and bereavement: a mixed-methods study. *Health and Social Work*, **32**(3): 197–206.

41. Salmon JR, Kwak J, Acquaviva KD, Brandt K, Egan KA (2005). Transformative aspects of caregiving at life's end. *Journal of Pain and Symptom Management*, **29**(2): 121–9.

42. Kwak J, Salmon JR, Acquaviva KD, Brandt K, Egan KA (2007). Benefits of training family caregivers on experiences of closure during end-of-life care. *Journal of Pain and Symptom Management*, **33**(4): 434–45.

43. Pinquart M, Sörensen S (2003). Differences between caregivers and non-caregivers in psychological health and physical health: a meta-analysis. *Psychology and Ageing*, **18**(2): 250–67.

44. Schulz R, Beach SR (1999). Caregiving as a risk factor for mortality. The caregiver health effects study. *Journal of the American Medical Association*, **282**(23): 2215–9.

45. Hunt Raleigh E, Robinson JH, Marold K, Jamison MT (2006). Family caregiver perception of hospice support. *Journal of Hospice and Palliative Nursing*, **8**(1): 25–33.

46. Rossi Ferrario S, Cardillo V, Vicario F, Balzarini E, Zotti AM (2004). Advanced cancer at home: caregiving and bereavement. *Palliative Medicine*, **18**(2): 129–36.

47. Ringdal GI, Jordhoy MS, Ringdal K, Kaasa S (2001). Factors affecting grief reactions in close family members to individuals who have died of cancer. *Journal of Pain and Symptom Management*, **22**(6): 1016–26.

48. Bernard LL, Guarnaccia CA (2003). Two models of caregiver strain and bereavement adjustment: a comparison of husband and daughter caregivers of breast cancer hospice patients. *Gerontologist*, **43**(6): 808–16.

49. Bull MA (1998). Losses in families affected by dementia: coping strategies and service issues. *Journal of Family Studies*, **4**(2): 187–99.

50. Abernethy AP, Currow DC, Fazekas BS, Luszcz MA, Wheeler JL, Kuchibhatla M (2008). Specialized palliative care services are associated with improved short- and long-term caregiver outcomes. *Supportive Care in Cancer*, **16**(6): 585–97.

51. Cameron JI, Franche RL, Cheung AM, Stewart DE (2002). Lifestyle interference and emotional distress in family caregivers of advanced cancer patients. *Cancer*, **94**(2): 521–7.

52. Meyers JL, Gray LN (2001). The relationships between family primary caregiver characteristics and satisfaction with hospice care, quality of life, and burden. *Oncology Nursing Forum*, **28**(1): 73–82.

53. Given B, Wyatt G, Given C, Sherwood P, Gift ADD, Rahbar M (2004). Burden and depression among caregivers of patients with cancer at the end of life. *Oncology Nursing Forum*, **31**(6): 1105–17.

54. Grov EK, Dahl AA, Fossa SD, Wahl AK, Moum T (2006). Global quality of life in primary caregivers of patients with cancer in palliative phase staying at home. *Supportive Care in Cancer*, **14**(9): 943–51.

55. Nolan M, Grant G, Keady J (1996). *Understanding family care: a multidimensional model of caring and coping*. Buckinghamshire: Open University Press.

56. Finch J (1995). Responsibilities, obligations, and communities. In I Allen, E Perkins (eds) *The future of family care for older people*, pp. 51–64. London: HMSO.

57. Thomas C, Morris SM, Clark D (2004). Place of death: preferences among cancer patients and their carers. *Social Science and Medicine*, **58**: 2431–44.

58. Lloyd L (2004). Mortality and morality: ageing and the ethics of care. *Ageing and Society*, **24**: 235–56.

59. Minichiello V, Browne J, Kendig H (2000). Perceptions and consequences of ageism: views of older people. *Ageing and Society*, **20**: 253–78.

60. Tanner D (2001). Sustaining the self in later life: supporting older people in the community. *Ageing and Society*, **21**: 255–78.

61. Twigg J, Atkin K (1994). *Carers perceived: policy and practice in informal care*. Milton Keynes: Open University Press.

62. Stajduhar KI, Davies B (2005). Variations in and factors influencing family members' decisions for palliative home care. *Palliative Medicine*, **19**(1): 21–32.

63. Gott M, Seymour J, Bellamy G, Clark D, Ahmedzai S (2004). Older people's views about home as a place of care at the end of life. *Palliative Medicine*, **18**: 460–7.

64. Folkman S, Lazarus RS, Pimley S, Novacek J (1987). Age differences in stress and coping processes. *Psychology and Ageing*, **2**: 171–84.

65. McLaughlin R, Ritchie J (1994). Legacies of caring the experiences and circumstances of ex-carers. *Health and Social Care*, **2**: 241–57.

66. Grande GE, Ewing G (2009). Informal carer bereavement outcome: relation to quality of end of life support and achievement of preferred place of death. *Palliative Medicine*, **23**(3): 248–56.

67. Payne S, Hudson P (2008). Assessing the family and caregivers. In D Walsh, AT Caraceni, R Fainsinger, KM Foley, P Glare, C Goh, et al. (eds) *Palliative medicine*, pp. 320–5. New York: Elsevier.

68. Thomas C, Morris S, Harman J (2002). Companions through cancer: the care given by informal carers in cancer contexts. *Social Science and Medicine*, **54**(4): 529–44.

69. Help the Hospices (2009). *Identifying carers' needs in the palliative setting. Report of the Carer Assessment Working Group* [Internet]. London: Help the Hospices. Available at: http://www.helpthehospices.org.uk/our-services/developing-practice/carers/publications/identifying-carers-needs/(Accessed 23 March 2010.)

70. Wenger GC (1994). Support networks and dementia. *International Journal of Geriatric Psychiatry*, **9**: 181–94.

71. Nolan MR, Keady J, Grant G (1995). Developing and typology of family care: implications for nurse and other service providers. *Journal of Advanced Nursing*, **21**: 256–65.

72. Lorenz KA, Lynn J, Dy SM, Shugarman LR, Wilkinson A, Mularski RA, et al. (2008). Evidence for improving palliative care at the end of life: a systematic review. *Annals of Internal Medicine*, **148**: 147–59.

73. Stroebe M, Schut H, Stroebe W (2007). Health outcomes of bereavement. *Lancet*, **370**(9603): 1960–73.

Chapter 14

Family carers, palliative care, and the end of life

Mike Nolan and Tony Ryan

Introduction

Although most deaths occur in hospitals the majority of people would prefer to die in their own homes (1), where the bulk of care for frail and elderly people is provided by family carers. If the aspiration of a good death at home is to be realized, our understanding of family carers' needs and the current levels of support provided to them will need to increase significantly. Family carers may also need support after the death of their relative in order to deal with the feelings of loss and grief that they experience. However the importance of supporting family carers at the end of life is not confined to the immediate home environment. A large proportion of older people die in care homes (2) and in such circumstances family carers still have an important part to play, throughout the transition into care and up until the time of death (3). This chapter explores the nature and type of support that family carers may need during the 'end of life' period and it is underpinned by the following beliefs, namely that:

- Family and professional carers need to work together as partners and that it is essential that they build a relationship based on trust.
- Family caring is best understood as a temporal experience, during which carers' needs change over time. Therefore an appreciation of the nature of prior caring experiences and relationships is central to providing good palliative and end of life care.
- A palliative care approach can be applied from an early stage, and in some instances from the point of diagnosis, as losses of differing types occur throughout a disease trajectory.
- Preparation for the death of a loved one can help in the longer-term adjustment of the family carer.
- Whilst the death of a loved one is inevitably a time of sadness and grief, it can also provide opportunities for personal growth and satisfaction, and enhancing such opportunities can be highly beneficial.
- Certain key concepts in the literature such as 'suffering' and 'grief' need to be developed more fully and applied more widely than they are at present.
- If staff are to work proactively with family carers at the end of life then they too require appropriate help and support.

Building on the above we believe that an approach to working with family carers called the PREP (PReparedness, Enrichment, and Predictability) model (4) can be adapted for use in palliative and end of life settings, whether care is being provided in the community, care homes, or more acute environments.

We begin with a brief consideration of the central role played by family carers in realizing current policies to support frail, vulnerable people.

Family carers: the lynchpin of community care

Welfare systems throughout the world promote a policy of community care in which people, despite their disabilities, are enabled to live in the environment of their choice, usually their own home or that of a relative in the community. For such a policy to be successful, the input of family carers is essential. Family carers typically provide 80% of all the care older people need (5), and in the UK their input saves the state approximately £87 billion pounds per year (6). The importance of family care was reflected in the recent Carers National Strategy in the UK, which noted that carers lie 'at the heart of 21st century families and communities' (6). Not surprisingly, policy-makers have placed growing emphasis on the need to support family carers so that they are able to continue to care, should they so wish, without detriment to their own health and well-being. Reflecting this, recent policy statements on palliative care and the end of life state that support for carers is particularly important prior to and following the death of a loved one (6–8).

In addition to such policy developments there has been considerable academic interest in the experiences and needs of family carers over the last 40 years (see reference 9 for an overview), and interventions to support family carers have become a major area of research and practice.

At the same time our understanding of palliative and end of life care has been expanding so that such concepts are no longer confined primarily to people dying of cancer in a hospice setting but are increasingly recognized as being appropriate to a much wider range of conditions and over a much longer period of time (10). For example, there are calls to recognize conditions such as dementia (11) and chronic obstructive pulmonary disease (COPD) (12), amongst others, as being terminal conditions and in such circumstances a palliative care approach is relevant from the time of diagnosis until death (8, 13). Indeed some argue that in care home settings a philosophy of palliative care provides the most appropriate model of care for all residents (14).

Staff in all care settings therefore need the relevant skills and knowledge to support family carers, and these are now recognized as being core competencies for such groups (15). Yet despite such developments there have been relatively few studies on supporting carers towards the end of life, and intervention studies in this area have been noticeably absent (13, 16, 17) and the more widespread application of palliative care principles beyond cancer and hospice settings has been slow to develop (18). Moreover, there are lessons from the wider literature on family care that can be applied to the end of life, and we elaborate upon some of these below in order to outline a framework for intervention and support for family carers at the end of life.

Palliative care and family carers: lessons from the wider literature

An important early paper exploring the relationships between family and formal systems was that of Twigg and Atkin (19). These authors suggested that professionals could work with family carers in a spirit of collaboration, as co-workers or co-clients, or in a more exploitative or disempowering way by viewing them primarily as a resource. In yet other circumstances professional support might supersede that provided by the family.

However, it is now widely recognized that one of the keys to effective support is for professionals and others to work in partnership with family carers. Such arguments are based on the belief that family carers and professionals have differing but complementary forms of expertise, both of which are needed if a complete picture is to emerge. So, for example, Harvath et al. (20) contended that professionals tend to have 'cosmopolitan' knowledge, relating to a specific disease(s) and its treatment, such as stroke, whereas carers have 'local knowledge' of what it is like to live with a stroke. Both types of 'knowing' are equally important. Somewhat later, Nolan et al. (21) proposed the 'carers as experts' model as a way of working with families which views both family carers and professionals as 'co-experts'. Here the professional role evolves from being mainly a provider of care to that of facilitator whose primary concern is to help carers to develop the skills and knowledge they need to care most effectively.

Since then partnership working has been widely promoted, with carers being described as 'expert care providers' in the recent National Carers Strategy (6). Such ideas are also prevalent in the literature on family care at the end of life, and the difficulties that arise when good relationships between carers and professionals cannot be maintained are well documented. Several authors talk about creating partnerships based on equality and interdependence (22, 23) and Fleming et al. (24) suggest that carers are 'critical partners' in the care team and that the active participation of the dying person, the family carer(s) and professionals results in an 'enriched team' effort (25). This notion of 'enrichment' is one we will consider in more detail later.

However, despite actively promoting partnerships based on the principles of user participation, Black (26) notes several potential barriers due to the reluctance of both family carers and professionals to talk openly about death, with carers often feeling guilty about focusing attention on their needs when their relative is very ill. For example in the context of end of life care for people with dementia, where the dying person may not be able to express his or her needs, some have noted a reluctance for professionals to share and acknowledge imminent death resulting in poor preparation for decision-making (27). Consequently, both carers and professionals need to be proactive in seeking to develop and maintain positive relationships. Schoot et al. (22) suggest that professionals need to demonstrate both 'attentiveness', that is a willingness to 'get to know' family carers and 'responsiveness' to their needs and wishes if critical partnerships are to flourish.

'Trust' is perhaps the most important characteristic of such relationships, and carers can lose trust in professionals more rapidly than do their relatives (24), and once lost such trust is very difficult to regain. Trusting relationships appear to be particularly important in a care home setting (14, 28), and such relationships need to be established from the outset. For example, Caron et al. (28) explored the quality of relationships between carers and staff in care homes and considered their influence on end of life decisions in people with dementia. They found that in most instances families wanted a personal relationship with staff and the opportunity to explore respective values and beliefs about a range of end of life issues. A minority of carers demonstrated 'pre-existing trust', based on the implicit belief that staff 'knew best'. However, in the majority of cases trust had to be earned based on carers' direct experience and observation of staff's knowledge and skills. Caron et al. (28) argue that the building and maintenance of relationships is an ongoing process and that both family and staff need to be more proactive than they often are in this regard.

Similarly, Munn et al. (14) highlight the importance of good relationships between residents, families, and staff to the quality of dying in care homes. In particular they noted the multifaceted, complex, and often ambiguous nature of the relationships between families and staff, which could at times be 'adversarial' with each group believing that they played the major role. They argue that such relationships require 'careful attention' and that the 'closeness' of their relationships is the primary factor promoting a good death from the perspectives of families and staff.

It has already been noted that one model of working between professionals (nurses in this instance) and family carers that we believe has wider application in the field of palliative care is the PREP model (14). PREP is based on a partnership model and is an acronym standing for:

◆ PRepardness
◆ Enrichment
◆ Predictability.

Based on their work, Archbold and colleagues argued that the goal of nursing interventions should be to 'prepare' the carer as fully as they can for their role by providing them with the information, advice, and skills they need in order to 'do caring well' (29). Secondly, staff should work actively with carers and the cared-for-person to 'enrich' their lives and to improve their relationship (30) and, thirdly, staff should try and make the future as 'predictable' as possible in order that carers can prepare for what lies ahead.

There is growing evidence to suggest that such considerations apply equally at the end of life. Predictability is, of course, more difficult in these circumstances, as specifying the likelihood of death is problematic, particularly in conditions such as dementia and COPD (12, 31), reinforcing the need to adopt the principles of palliative care as early as possible.

However, despite the unpredictability of death, the use of palliative care principles from the outset allows as much time as possible for the carer to prepare for both their caring role and the eventual death of their loved one. Preparing carers with the knowledge, skills, and understanding they need to care effectively lies at the heart of both the Carers Strategy (6) and the End of life Care Strategy in the UK (7). It is also one of the core skills identified for all groups of staff, irrespective of the care setting (15).

In addition to equipping carers with the skills and resources needed to care, preparing them for the eventual death of their loved one can be particularly beneficial. Studies show that both carers and professionals can be reluctant to discuss the death of the terminally ill person (32) and that, despite caring for a long time for a person with a progressively deteriorating condition, a substantial minority of carers do not expect the death when it occurs (33). This is unfortunate as there is growing evidence to indicate that carers who have anticipated and prepared for the death:

♦ Are more likely to report the potential of personal growth and transformation (34). This is something we will discuss more fully when we consider the satisfaction of caring at the end of life.

♦ Are less likely to experience complicated grief reactions (13).

Conversely, those carers who have not prepared for the death are more likely to experience depression, anxiety, and complicated grief (33). In this regard encouraging anticipatory grief may reduce the incidence of complicated grief at a later date (35); this is something we will discuss in more detail shortly.

However, we know relatively little about the best ways to prepare carers for the death of their loved one (33). Hebert et al. (33) suggest that preparation is a multifaceted concept comprising several elements including medical, practical, psychological, and spiritual aspects that often involve both the dying person and the carer/wider family. This is certainly an area in which more research is needed.

Enrichment, or enhancing the quality of relationships and the satisfactions and rewards of caring, is a key component of the PREP model and is one where there is considerable, but largely overlooked, potential for more widespread use with family carers in general, and those caring at the end of life in particular. The vast majority of research into family care, and subsequent interventions, has been based on a stress/coping model. The basic premise is that caregiving is a stressful situation and that efforts should be made to either reduce the stress that carers experience or to enhance their coping abilities, or both. Although the model has become increasingly sophisticated over the years the tendency is still to view caregiving as a primarily negative experience (36). However, a small minority of researchers have promoted an alternative view which is based on the belief that caring also presents opportunities for reward, satisfaction, and growth. An early pioneer was Hirschfield (37), who suggested the concept of 'mutuality', which is the extent to which carers can find gratification and meaning in their role. She argued that the higher the mutuality, the lower the stress/burden that the carer experienced and the better the caring relationship. The idea of enrichment (4, 30) is underpinned by the concept of mutuality and more recently the belief that caring is not a uniformally negative experience has gained increasing acceptance.

One of the most comprehensive attempts to gauge the type and extent of carer satisfactions led to the development of the Carers Assessment of Index (CASI) (21). Nolan and colleagues demonstrated that carers can get satisfaction and meaning from their role from a number of sources and have shown, in a range of studies in several countries, that caregiving satisfactions are more prevalent than the difficulties of caring (see, for example, references 38–40).

This is of more than academic interest as some time ago it was suggested that simultaneously reducing carer burden whilst raising satisfactions was potentially more helpful than focusing on burden alone, and that promoting satisfaction at the end of caring could be very beneficial (41). Recently there has been growing support for such beliefs.

Loboprabhu (35) argues that carers who receive affirmation of the successes and joys of caring are far more likely to feel a sense of mastery, with others concluding that if carers feel that they have 'done a good job' and experience a sense of satisfaction with their efforts, then this can also reduce their feelings of guilt and sadness (31). Such feelings of mastery and of 'doing a good job' can enhance carers' resilience in the face of difficult circumstances, and promoting resilience has a beneficial effect on carers' health and adjustment (36). The concept of resilience is something we will consider in more detail shortly.

Reflecting on the potential satisfactions/rewards of caring, and the opportunities it provides for personal growth, can help carers to find meaning in their role, which itself has beneficial outcomes on their emotional health (23, 42). Understanding how carers construct 'meaning' is seen by some to be the key to designing appropriate support (23).

Based on the above a number of authors have suggested that far greater emphasis on the positive aspects of caring should be the primary rationale underpinning future interventions (43–45). Sorensen et al. (45) term this 'accentuating the positive' and argue that we need to develop a more sophisticated understanding of caring which recognizes that burden and positive outcomes often 'coexist', and that if we only focus on reducing the negative then we are missing important opportunities to devise new and creative ways of working with carers. This is something that we would endorse and suggest that instruments such as CASI (21) can be readily adapted for application in a palliative care context.

Much of our understanding of the experience of family carers has been influenced by the application of a stress/burden model, and the above focus on satisfactions provides a more holistic view. However, even within the stress/burden paradigm authors contend that key concepts are either missing or have been neglected. Two concepts of particular relevance here are those of grief/loss and suffering.

Whilst grief and loss are an inevitable part of end of life care, many argue that losses in dementia are unique (46) due to both the extended nature of the condition and the multiple losses that occur at differing points. Consequently, grief and loss are not experienced only during the stages immediately preceding or following death, as all carers experience multiple losses, such as a loss of role, of relationships, and, in the case of dementia, loss of the person themselves. Entry of their relative to a care home is, of course, itself a major loss for many carers.

However, relatively little attention is given to the grief/bereavement experience of carers (11, 13), yet it is recognized that suitable interventions before death, and the facilitation of anticipatory grieving, can do much to enhance adjustment after significant loss (13, 35, 47). As about 20% of carers will experience complicated grief and are likely to have negative health outcomes as a consequence (48), such anticipatory work has many potential benefits.

It is also important to recognize that carers experience grief/loss differently depending on their personal characteristics and relationships. For example, spouses often report different sources and types of grief than do adult children (48), and men react differently to women (49). Men, for example, appear more reluctant to express their feelings and are less likely to see an outpouring of emotions as an appropriate response to loss. Consequently, they may need to be actively encouraged to acknowledge their emotions and begin to address these (49).

Ott et al. (44) point out that grief and depression are related but distinct concepts and that support tends to focus on the latter whilst relatively ignoring the former. As we argued above these authors stress the benefits of looking for the positive aspects of caring in order to reduce grief reactions.

The concept of anticipatory grief is promoted by Holley and Mast (46) who argue that we need to extend current interventions beyond burden and depression and to help carers to mourn for the losses they have already experienced, whilst preparing them for the ones they have yet to face. In this way carers are more likely to feel validated and supported in their role. Others take a similar view (50).

The idea of focusing on both the negative experience of loss and the potentially positive outcomes of caring is consistent with the 'dual process' model of grief (51) that highlights the need for individuals to consider both loss and restoration. The belief is that people who can achieve the appropriate balance between the two are likely to have better outcomes. Similar arguments are made in Machin's range of responses to grief model which is promoted by Relf et al. (52), as being useful in identifying those carers at 'risk' of complicated grief and so more in need of support. Assessment of risk is important as offering bereavement support when it is not needed may be harmful rather than beneficial (52). Factors that help to determine the degree of risk of complicated grief include:

- Events leading up to the death
- The meaning of the relationship for the carer
- Carers' personal vulnerability
- Their social and emotional support (see reference 52 for a more detailed discussion).

According to Machin's (53) model there are three broad types of grief reaction. People may be either:

- Overwhelmed by the experience
- Too controlled and try to deny the significance of their loss
- Resilient and strike an appropriate balance between the two above reactions.

People who are either overwhelmed or too controlling are potentially at risk of a complicated grief reaction and may need support and Relf et al. (52) provide a comprehensive and informative account of the range of factors that can be used to assess such risk (Table 14.1). Others also provide insightful accounts of how a 'grief' profile can be constructed in order both to identify carers potentially at risk, and to decide on appropriate types of support (see reference 11). These authors suggest the use of the Marwit and Meuser (54) Caregiver Grief Inventory and this would seem to have considerable potential for practical application.

Once 'at-risk' carers have been identified Relf et al. (52) suggest that they need the opportunity to engage in a range of therapeutic activities, at the heart of which lie three types of 'conversation':

- External conversations—in which people are helped to explore the events surrounding their loss—what happened and why?
- Internal conversations—which consider the impact of the loss on those involved
- Reflexive conversations—that allow people to better understand how they are coping and making sense of their situation.

Table 14.1 Assessing family carer risk at the end of life (specific indicators)

Overwhelmed response	Controlled response
• Demonstrates frequent intrusion of thoughts about the patient, illness, and outcome • Displays a sense that current issue will persist • Displays a sense that everything has changed	• Values courage and fortitude • Believes that feelings should be controlled as a demonstration of strength. • Believes that they should avoid burdening other people with their feelings. • Managing a loss is best undertaken by getting on with life
Resilient response	**Vulnerable response**
• Can face the issues of impending loss resulting from the illness • Demonstrates coping strategies that make use of inner resources and external sources of support • Demonstrates coping strategies that make use of inner resources and external sources of support	• Avoids facing the issues of impending loss resulting from the illness • Does not demonstrate coping strategies that make use of inner resources and external sources of support • Cannot acknowledge the current emotional and social impact of the illness. Does not feel hopeful that strength or meaning may come from the experience

Adapted from Relf et al. (52).

Although facilitating such conversations may at times require specialist skills and training, nurses and other practitioners are often in a position to initiate such discussions.

Another key concept that has hitherto been relatively overlooked is that of 'suffering' (55–57). Carers who are not happy with the quality of care their relative receives and believe that they 'suffer' unnecessarily, report higher distress and depression post-death (24, 58), and Schulz et al. (57) argue that this applies particularly in dementia, where the person themselves often cannot verbalize their suffering. In this context suffering is not synonymous with pain but relates to a wider concept with physical, emotional, psychological, and spiritual dimensions. Schulz et al. (57) believe that we need research that leads to a better understanding of:

• What constitutes 'suffering' in dementia

• How such suffering can be reduced

• How to support carers when suffering cannot be addressed.

Hebert et al. (55) argue that 'suffering' may be the primary, but largely overlooked, source of stress during death and dying and suggest that 'suffering' needs to be identified and relieved, which is likely to be of benefit both to the person who is dying and their carer.

Conclusion

This chapter has considered the needs of family carers at the end of life. We have explicitly promoted the application of a palliative care model from an early stage and highlighted the importance of establishing partnerships between family carers and paid staff. We have argued that using a model such as PREP enhances collaborative working so that family carers are better able to maximize their preparedness for the future, to both mitigate the risk of complex bereavement and to enhance their involvement in decision-making. Drawing upon a range of concepts from the literature it has been demonstrated that a promotion of 'trust' is an essential skill for the professional when working with family carers in an end of life context. A significant theme here, however, is the need to shift attention away from a burden model towards a perspective which recognizes that even at the end of life family carers can, and indeed should, be provided with opportunities to gain satisfaction from their caring. Such an approach has been shown to help 'protect' family carers from extended grief and a prolonged sense of guilt. Furthermore, there exist a range of theories/ models and resources to help practitioners to assess family carer risk in this context and to assist in the identification of those who may well be in a position to experience long-term emotional difficulties following the death of a loved one, and therefore need help and support. The challenge for the future is to further refine, develop, and test these concepts and tools in order to work more effectively with family carers at this difficult time.

More fundamentally, however, if staff are to work proactively with family carers at the end of life they need both the skills to do so (15) and appropriate support themselves to deal with the emotional impact of such work (3). We have already noted the importance of the relationship between family carers and professionals and it has been argued that the use of a relationship-centred approach to end of life care has much to commend it (59). This recognizes the interde-pendencies that exist between all those involved and promotes the creation of a 'enriched' environment in which all parties experience six 'senses' (60). In the present context we would see these 'senses' as being applied in the following ways:

- Security: for both carers and staff to feel safe to raise difficult and sensitive issues in a support-ive and facilitative environment.

- Belonging: for both carers and staff to feel part of a valued group who share similar values and beliefs.

- Continuity: to be able to establish relationships over time and to be able to relate the current situation to both the past and the future.

- Purpose: to recognize the complexity of end of life care for family carers and to work actively with them to prepare them for their role and their loss, now and in the future, to enrich their remaining time with their loved one, to reduce the latter's suffering and to enhance the posi-tive aspects of caring.

- Achievement: for the above to be seen as important and valued outcomes of care.

- Significance: for end of life care with family carers to be seen as valued and important, some-thing that really 'matters'.

The above represents a framework to be used with the person themselves, the family carer, and staff teams. Furthermore, the first three senses (security, belonging, and continuity) are viewed as important building blocks to enable the final three (purpose, achievement, and significance) to be achieved. We believe that using such an approach will assist all stakeholders in realizing improved outcomes in the short, medium, and longer term.

References

1. National Audit Office (2008). *End of Life Care*. London: The Stationery Office.
2. Seymour J, Witherspoon R, Gott M, Ross H, Payne S, Owen T (2005). *End-of-life Care: promoting comfort, choice and well-being for older people*. London: Policy Press.
3. Nicholson L (2006). End-of-life care. In T Owen, National Care Homes Research and Development Forum (eds) *My Home Life: Quality of Life in Care Homes*, pp. 118–28. London: Help the Aged.

4. Archbold PG, Stewart BJ, Miller LL (1995). The PREP system of nursing interventions. *Research in Nursing and Health*, **18**(1): 1–16.

5. Walker A (1995). Integrating the family in the mixed economy of care. In I Allen, E Perkins (eds) *The Future of Family Care for Older People*, pp. 201–20. London: HMSO.

6. Department of Health (2008). *Carers at the heart of 21st century families and communities*. London: Department of Health.

7. Department of Health (2008). *End of Life Care Strategy – promoting high quality care for all adults at the end of life*. London: Department of Health. Available at: http://www.dh.gov.uk/en/Publicationsandstatistics/Publications/PublicationsPolicyAndGuidance/DH_086277

8. NICE (2006). *Dementia: Supporting people with dementia and their carers in health and social care, clinical justice 42*. London: NICE/SCIE.

9. Nolan MR, Lundh U, Grant G, Keady J (eds) (2003). *Partnerships in Family Care: understanding the caregiving career*. Maidenhead: Open University Press.

10. Payne S, Seymour J, Ingleton C (2008). Introduction. In S Payne, J Seymour, C Ingleton (eds) *Palliative Care Nursing*, 2nd edn. Maidenhead: Open University Press.

11. Sanders S, Marwit SJ, Meuser TM, Harrington P (2007). Caregiver grief in end-stage dementia: Using the Marwit and Meuser Caregiver Grief Inventory for Assessment and Intervention in Social Work Practice. *Social Work in Health Care*, **46**(1): 47–65.

12. Yohannes AM (2007). Palliative care provision for patients with chronic obstructive pulmonary disease. *Health and Quality of Life Outcomes*, **5**: 17.

13. Gallagher-Thompson D (2006). Caregiving issues: Covering the spectrum from detection to end of life. *American Journal of Geriatric Psychiatry*, **14**(8): 635–41.

14. Munn JC, Dobbs D, Meier A, Williams CS, Biola H, Zimmerman S (2008). The end-of-life experience in long-term care: Five themes identified from focus groups with residents, family members and staff. *The Gerontologist*, **48**(4): 485–94.

15. St Christopher's Hospice (2009). End-of-life care competencies for nurses and health and social care staff working in the community, care homes and hospitals. *End of Life Care*, **3**(3): 63–4.

16. Herbert RS, Schulz R (2006). Caregiving at the end of life. *Journal of Palliative Medicine*, **9**(5): 1174–87.

17. McMillan SC (2005). Interventions to facilitate family caregiving at the end of life. *Journal of Palliative Medicine*, **8**(1): S132–S139.

18. Ghiotti C (2009). The Dementia End of Life Care Project (DeLCaP): Supporting families caring for people with late stage dementia at home. *Dementia: The International Journal of Social Research and Practice*, **8**(3): 349–62.

19. Twigg J, Atkin K (1994). *Carers Perceived: Policy and Practice in Informal Care*. Buckingham: Open University Press.

20. Harvath TA, Archbold PG, Stewart BJ, Gadow S, Kirschling JM, Miller L, et al. (1994). Establishing partnerships with family caregivers: local and cosmopolitan knowledge. *Journal of Gerontological Nursing*, **20**(2): 29–35.

21. Nolan M, Grant G, Keady J (1996). *Understanding Family Care: A Multidimensional Model of Caring and Coping*. Buckingham: Open University Press.

22. Schoot T, Proot I, Meulen R, Witte L (2005). Recognition of client value as a basis for tailored care: the view of Dutch expert patients and family caregivers. *Scandinavian Journal of Caring Sciences*, **19**(2): 169–76.

23. Stoltz P, Willman A, Valen G (2006). The meaning of support as narrated by family carers who are for a senior relative at home. *Qualitative Health Research*, **16**: 594–610.

24. Fleming DA, Sheppard VB, Mangan PA, Taylor KL, Tallarico M, Adams I, et al. (2006). Caregiving at the end of life: Perceptions of health care quality and quality of life among patients and caregivers. *Journal of Pain and Symptom Management*, **31**(5): 407–20.

25. Elman LB, Houghton DJ, Wu GF, Hurtig HI, Markowitz CE, McCluskey L (2007). Palliative Care in amyotrophic lateral sclerosis, Parkinson's disease and multiple sclerosis. *Journal of Palliative Medicine*, **10**(2): 433–57.

26. Black J (2008). User involvement in EoLC: how involved can patients/carers be? *End of Life Care*, **2**(4): 64–9.

27. Ryan T (2009). End-of-life care for people with dementia: A thematic review of familial involvement, practices and beliefs. *International Journal of Disability and Human Development*, **8**(1): 15–20.

28. Caron CD, Griffith J, Arcand M (2005). Decision making at the end of life in dementia: how family caregivers perceive their interactions with health care providers in long-term-care settings. *Journal of Applied Gerontology*, **24**(3): 231–47.

29. Schumacher KL, Stewart BJ, Archbold PG, Dodd MJ, Dibble SL (1998). Family caregiving skill: Development of the concept. *Image: Journal of Nursing Scholarship*, **30**(1): 63–70.

30. Cartwright JC, Archbold PG, Stewart BJ, Limandri B (1994). Enrichment processes in family caregiving to frail elders. *Advances in Nursing Sciences*, **17**(1): 31–43.

31. Ashcroft-Simpson S, Kehoe P, Butterworth L, Keady J (2008). End-of-life care and people with dementia: Admiral nurses. *End of Life Care*, **2**(4): 16–25.

32. Powers AB, Watson NM (2008). Meaning and practice of palliative care for nursing home residents with dementia at end of life. *American Journal of Alzheimer's Disease and Other Dementias*, **23**(4): 319–25.

33. Herbert RS, Dang Q, Schulz R (2006). Preparedness for the death of a loved one and mental health in bereaved caregivers of patients with dementia: Findings from the REACH study. *Journal of Palliative Medicine*, **9**(3): 683–93.

34. Caserta M, Lund D, Utz R, de Vries B (2009). Stress-related growth among the recently bereaved. *Ageing and Mental Health*, **13**(3): 463–76.

35. Loboprabhu SM (2006). The affective interpersonal bond in caregiving. In SM Loboprabhu, VA Molinari, JW Lomax (eds) *Supporting the Caregiver in Dementia: A Guide for Health Care Professionals*, pp. 85–103. Baltimore, MD: The John Hopkins University Press.

36. Gaugler JE, Kane RL, Newcomer R (2007). Resilience and transitions from dementia caregiving. *Journal of Gerontology*, **62B**(1): 38–44.

37. Hirschfield MJ (1983). Home care versus institutionalization: family caregiving and senile brain disease. *International Journal of Nursing Studies*, **20**(1): 23–32.

38. Lundh U, Nolan MR (2003). 'I wasn't aware of that': creating dialogue between family and professional carers. In MR Nolan, U Lundh, G Grant, J Keady (eds) *Partnerships in Family Care: understanding the caregiving career*, pp. 108–27. Maidenhead: Open University Press.

39. McKee K, Spazzafumo L, Nolan M, Wojszel B, Lamura G, Bien B (2009). Components of the difficulties, satisfactions and management strategies of carers of older people: A principle component analysis of CADI-CASI-CAMI. *Ageing and Mental Health*, **13**(2): 255–64.

40. Nolan MR, Keady J, Grant G, Lundh U (2003b). Introduction: why another book on family care? In MR Nolan, U Lundh, G Grant, J Keady (eds) *Partnerships in Family Care: understanding the caregiving career*, pp. 1–12. Maidenhead: Open University Press.

41. Nolan MR, Grant G, Keady J (1998). *Assessing Carer's Needs: A Practitioner's Guide*. Brighton: Pavilion Publications.

42. Riberio O, Paul C (2008). Older male carers and the positive aspects of care. *Ageing and Society*, **28**(2): 165–84.

43. Hilegman M, Allen R, DeCoster J, Burgio L (2007). Positive aspects of caregiving as a moderator of treatment outcome over 12 months. *Psychology and Ageing*, **22**(2): 361–71.

44. Ott CH, Sanders S, Kelber ST (2007). Grief and personal growth experience of spouses and adult-child caregivers of individuals with Alzheimer's disease and related dementias. *The Gerontologist*, **47**(6): 798–809.

45. Sörensen S, King D, Pinquart (2006). Care of the Caregiver: Individual and Family Interventions. In SM Loboprabhu, VA Molinari, JW Lomax (eds) *Supporting the Caregiver in Dementia: A Guide for Health Care Professionals*, pp. 168–191. Baltimore, MA: The John Hopkins University Press.

46. Holley CK, Mast BT (2009). The impact of anticipatory grief on caregiver burden in dementia caregivers. *The Gerontologist*, **49**(3): 388–96.

47. Kissane DW, McKenzie M, Bloch S, Moskowitz C, McKenzie DP, O'Neill I (2006). Family focused grief therapy: a randomized, controlled trial in palliative care and bereavement. *American Journal of Psychiatry*, **163**: 1208–18.

48. Schulz R, Boerner K, Shear K, Zhang S, Gitlin LN (2006). Predictors of complicated grief among dementia caregivers: a prospective study of bereavement. *American Journal of Geriatric Psychiatry*, **14**(8): 650–8.

49. Fromme EK, Drach LL, Tolle SW, Ebert P, Miller P, Perrin N, et al. (2005). Men as caregivers at the end of life. *Journal of Palliative Medicine*, **8**(6): 1167–75.

50. Sanders S, Swails P (2009). Caring for individuals with end-stage dementia at the end of life: A specific focus on hospice social workers. *Dementia: The International Journal of Social Research and Practice*, **8**(1): 117–38.

51. Lund DA, Caserta MS, Utz R, de Vries B (2008). 'Participants' experiences in a dual process model (DPM) intervention for bereaved spouses/partners.' Presentation at the annual meetings of the Gerontological Society of America, National Harbor, Maryland, November 2008.

52. Relf M, Machin L, Archer N (2008). *Guidance for bereavement needs assessment in palliative care*. Help the Hospices, London. Available at: www.helpthehospices.org.uk/our-services/developing-practice/bereavement/assessing-bereavement-needs/. (Accessed 3 February 2010.)

53. Machin L (2001). Exploring a framework for understanding the range of responses to loss: a study of clients receiving bereavement counselling. PhD Thesis, Keele University.

54. Marwit SJ, Meuser TM (2005). Development of a short form inventory to assess grief in caregivers of dementia patients. *Death Studies*, **29**: 191–205.

55. Herbert RS, Arnold RM, Schulz R (2007). Improving well-being in caregivers of terminally ill patients. Making the case for patient suffering as a focus for intervention research. *Journal of Pain and Symptom Management*, **34**(5): 539–46.

56. Sampson EL, Robinson L (2009). End of life care in dementia: Building bridges for effective multidisciplinary care. *Dementia: The International Journal of Social Research and Practice*, **8**(3): 331–34.

57. Schulz R, Herbert RS, Dew MA, Brown SL, Scheier MR (2007). Patient suffering and caregiver compassion: new opportunities for research, practice and policy. *The Gerontologist*, **47**(1): 4–13.

58. Dumont S, Turgeon J, Allard P, Gagnon P, Charbonneau C, Vezina L (2006). Caring for a loved one with advanced cancer: Determinants of psychological distress in family caregivers. *Journal of Palliative Medicine*, **9**(4): 912–21.

59. Nolan M, Hudson R (2008). Family and palliative care in care homes for older people. In P Hudson, S Payne (eds) *Family Carers and Palliative Care: A Guide for Health and Social Care Professionals*, pp. 169–90. Oxford: Oxford University Press.

60. Nolan M, Davies S, Brown J, Nolan J, Keady J, (2006). The Senses Framework, *Improving the Care of Older People Through a Relationship Centred Approach*, GRIP report Number 2, University of Sheffield.

Chapter 15

Cost of family caregiving

Barbara Hanratty

Introduction

Caring for another person—acting with kindness or tenderness when they are ill or dying—is arguably a defining feature of humanity. Descriptions of palliative care provided by relatives or friends can be found throughout history. And whilst health and social services may be more widely available than ever before, individuals and communities continue to provide day-to-day care at home, even in the most comprehensive welfare systems. Improvements in living conditions and disease management, have given us longer, more active lives. Few of us anticipate caring for a sick or dying relative when we are older. But as the number of people dying in frail old age and the proportion of older adults living alone increases, input from relatives and friends is likely to be an essential part of end of life experiences for many people. Care provided at little or no direct cost to organized services is attractive to governments with competing financial demands. With financial savings comes a responsibility to ensure that such care can be sustained over the course of an illness and across communities. This chapter considers the costs of end of life care from a relatively neglected perspective—that of the individual and their family. An overview of what is known about how family caregiving influences finances at the end of life is followed by discussion of the measurement challenges involved, and identification of the areas where we need to know more.

Family care

Increasing numbers of people look after an ill, frail, or disabled family member, friend, or partner, without expecting or receiving any payment (1). Although the time, and intensity of care required will vary greatly depending on the needs of the recipient, the terms carer or caregiver are used to encompass a wide range of voluntarily provided unpaid care. In the legislation relating to carers in the UK, a carer is defined as someone 'who provides, or intends to provide, a substantial amount of care on a regular basis' (2). The important distinction from care workers is that the responsibility for the physical and/or mental well-being of a person with illness or disability is unpaid. Carers are often described as 'informal', which implies that they do not have a formal contract of employment and receive no financial reward for their services. The exact nature and definition of an informal or family carer is contested, and carers have been variously described by the hours and intensity of work and the sociodemographic characteristics of the carer or recipient, particularly living arrangements (3). It is important to acknowledge that many people who are described as 'informal carers' do not embrace the term, considering that it implies a casual arrangement, which is far from the case for most people involved in caring for someone who is unwell.

The importance of family care

Populations are ageing across the developed world. Increasing life expectancy is producing a rise in the median age of populations in Europe, Japan, and North America. In 55 countries, more than 20% of the population will be aged over 65 years by 2030 (4). Soon, some of the countries of Eastern Europe where populations are shrinking will be amongst the oldest in the world (5). Declining fertility in the countries where people are living longer, add up to produce burgeoning elderly populations supported by fewer people of working age. The old age dependency ratio—which relates the number of elderly people to those at economically active ages—is predicted to almost double between 2010 and 2050 in the EU25 countries (4, 6). Not only does this reduce the pool of younger adults who could become carers, it has the potential to increase the financial burden on the working population whose taxes or insurance contributions support most welfare systems.

Another consequence of population ageing is that more people are dying at older ages. Over two-thirds of the population of England and Wales can now expect to be over 75 years old when they die (7). By 2030, over 40% of people in the UK will die when they are over 85 years old (8) a trend that is mirrored across high-income countries. A high proportion of people are admitted to hospital in their last year of life and this rises with age. For example, in a longitudinal study from a German sickness fund, over 80% of people between the ages of 55 and 84 were admitted to hospital in the 12 months before they died (9). Over the age of 85 years, people are less likely to be admitted to hospital in their last year, but when they do, they stay for longer periods than younger adults (10). Recent decades have seen reductions in morbidity and functional decline amongst older adults, so that increasing survival has not invariably led to more years of sickness and disability (11, 12) and the total time spent in hospital at older ages has not increased (13, 14). Predictions of rapid increases in the costs of end of life care may be premature, but the sheer number of older decedents will mean that the costs of providing health care for them are considerable. Attempts to quantify these costs in relation to time from death, have not produced consistent results across different health systems. Generally, approaching death is associated with increased health service expenditures, and the costs of care for decedents are greater than for comparable survivors (15–18). The overall effect of our increased survival appears to be to delay the years of high spending on health care to the end of life, with some shift away from acute hospital costs. In other words, the last months or year of life are a time when the costs of health care services are high, even if death occurs in old age. This is relevant to family care, because if friends and relatives are able to substitute for even a proportion of costly services at the end of life, they could have a significant impact on welfare expenditure. Conversely, if the existing level of family care falls, for whatever reason, the costs of providing services are likely to rise. The availability of unpaid carers is already seen as one of the most crucial determinants of long-term care costs (19) and has been described as the 'least expensive way of delivering care to elderly people' (4). In 2006, a review of long-term care for the UK King's Fund predicted an increasing role for family care in the future, with a resulting need for greater support for carers (20). Caregiving in palliative and terminal care is often more intensive, of shorter duration, and requiring greater specialist input, compared to much long-term care. Yet, even in this setting, family care is likely to substitute for some services, thereby reducing costs for the service providers.

Who are the caregivers?

The population of carers is also ageing. In the 2001 census, there were more than one million elderly unpaid carers in England and Wales. In the US, almost half of primary caregivers of frail elderly people are thought to be over 65 years of age themselves, and a similar proportion of spousal carers are older than 75 years (21). Carers of retirement age are more likely than those in other age groups to have their own medical conditions, and to find that their mental or physical health is affected by caregiving (22–25). In Australia, Abernethy and colleagues put aside assumptions about who provides care at the end of life, and decided to look at carers by the intensity of care provided (26). They analysed data from the Health Omnibus survey, an annual face-to-face survey in South Australia, which collects health-related data from a representative sample of households. More than 5000 of the 18,224 respondents had been bereaved in the previous 5 years; one in 10 had provided daily care. A picture emerged that was similar to other countries, with the most intensive carers being older, widowed females. People who were better educated, in paid work, and wealthier were more likely to provide care on an intermittent basis.

Older people who are providing care for others are drawn from a population where many live on low incomes. In retirement, it is certainly true that most people survive on a pension income that is considerably smaller than their previous earnings. Two million of the retired population in the UK has an income that would put them below the poverty line (or 60% of median equivalized income after housing costs) and a third live in fuel poverty (27, 28). There are wide inequalities in the income and wealth of retired people, and the relationship between low income and material disadvantage is complex at older ages (29). Nevertheless, increasing age and living alone do appear to be associated with increasing hardship. Across England and Wales, there are geographical differences in family caregiving, with positive associations between the intensive provision of family care and material disadvantage, whether measured by poverty, occupational groups, or area-based deprivation (30–34).

Financial consequences of caregiving

Providing care to a close friend or relative is never an easy task, and the impact on finances and material well-being is often one of the most immediate consequences for anyone who becomes a carer. The concept of carers being weighed down by their responsibilities was first discussed in the 1950s, though the term caregiver 'burden' was not defined until a little later. Initial interest focused on the strain on people who combined caring for elderly people with work outside the home—changes in employment were an important component of this. The objective pressures on the daily lives of carers, along with the more subjective psychological and emotional distress continued to interest researchers in gerontology, and most measures of carer burden attempted to measure both of these (35–37). Development of tools specific to carer burden in palliative care came much later (38) Worries about money are encompassed by the theoretical frameworks that have been proposed to understand how caregiving is converted into a burden for some people (39). One of the most influential has been the Stress Process Model, which considers caregiver burden to be linked to a negative reaction to caregiving. It adopts a broad approach to identifying stressors, including the financial along with the physical, psychological, emotional, and social challenges that may accompany caregiving (40). Although there is little consensus on which stressors have the greatest influence on the caregiver's quality of life, or the pathways involved, it is agreed that income and financial position do play a role (41).

Financial consequences of ill health

It is still the case today that illness is one of the most potent causes of poverty. Although the situation is more marked in low-income countries, the link between health care costs and financial strain is seen in most places without comprehensive welfare coverage (42). Health care costs can have catastrophic consequences for patients and carers, pushing households into bankruptcy and even homelessness. In less extreme cases, the cost of health care may discourage people from accessing care until late into an illness, with adverse effects on prognosis or increasing the help needed from unpaid carers at home. People of working age who take on caring may have to leave a job, or they may reduce or change the hours that they work. In some industries, this can have implications for their career progression, particularly if they have had career breaks to bring up children (39, 43). In most discussions of catastrophic health care costs, the USA is presented as an example of a high-income country where falling ill may have devastating effects on family finances. A lack of health insurance is one of the most important barriers to health service use, affecting some of the poorest households. Elderly people are eligible for government supported health care, and should be immune from the most severe financial consequences of health care costs. However, even if services are covered under insurance, user fees (cost-sharing) may also deter people from accessing care. Some of the most vulnerable caregivers are working people on low incomes. When people in this situation give up work to become carers, the amount of money coming into the household will reduce, but they may also sacrifice their own health care coverage if it is linked with employment. It is important to note that most of the adverse consequences of caregiving have been studied in the context of care for people with chronic illness. Whilst the likelihood of financial problems becoming serious increases with the length of caring, it also gives time for the carer to adapt to new, reduced circumstances. If the period of illness before death is short, carers may be left dealing with financial challenges at a time of practical and emotional turmoil.

Evidence for financial strain

Most of the research on financial strain at the end of life concerns people with cancer, and the largest studies were conducted in the USA. Perceptions of being under financial strain were reported more commonly than the objective measures of high spending, which suggests that paying for care was a concern even for people who could afford to do so. In analyses ranging in size from just under 1000 to more than 3000 respondents, at least one in four reported some financial hardship associated with terminal care for people with cancer and a limited number of other life-limiting conditions (44–47). In order to obtain the money to pay for care, 17–38% of households reported using most or all of the family savings to pay for care, whilst 10–40% of people had given up a job to care for someone with cancer. Selling a house, or taking on a mortgage or loan was less common. Researchers from countries with comprehensive welfare coverage have more often reported on the perception of financial hardship, and the need for more support, rather than catastrophic costs. There are no reliable data on the uptake of welfare benefits available to people with a terminal illness or their caregivers. In the UK, charitable organisations such as Macmillan Cancer Support, are working to increase the uptake of benefits, as there is a widespread feeling that some people may be missing out (48).

There is also a relative dearth of qualitative research into the effect and consequences of financial strain, and much of it relates to cancer. However, in countries as diverse as Japan and Italy, studies suggest that terminal illness and death are causing financial hardship. In Australia, Parker and colleagues (49) interviewed bereaved carers of people with cancer and found that funeral costs were a particular source of concern to carers. In northern England a qualitative study of end of life experiences of 20 patients with life-limiting illness focused on financial issues (50). Illness created increases in basic living costs, but for the most part, these costs were not linked by the interviewees to their condition, despite being more substantial than health service associated costs. For example, increased spending on food was rarely volunteered as an illness-related cost, but on reflection, all interviewees on lower incomes spoke of the burden of increased food bills, as a result of illness. The cost of fuel, telephone calls, and travel were other sources of increased expenditure. Differences between older and younger people were apparent in how financial challenges were interpreted and managed. The diagnosis of a terminal illness had profound and rapid implications for the financial well-being of younger interviewees. The initial stages of illness were characterized by financial hardship—awaiting welfare benefits, whilst income from employment disappeared. In contrast, people who developed a terminal illness after retirement, experienced fewer consequences of the financial impact of illness. Material expectations were generally lower, with an emphasis on simple pleasures that cost little. As a result, financial problems were perceived by elderly people as constraints to be managed, rather than active worries. Concern for the financial provision of others who may outlive the interviewee was common across the ages and social groups, and this is clearly a key way in which financial issues may create distress towards the end of life.

Measuring the costs of care

Both general and specialist palliative care services aim to enhance the quality of life of patients nearing the end of their lives. Compare this to surgery for osteoarthritis of the hip, for example, which aims to reduce pain and increase mobility, and it is obvious that the outcomes of palliative care may be more difficult to measure. Maintaining quality of life as death approaches and helping a family to cope with their impending loss may be short-lived benefits, but of great value to the family. Health economists are grappling with the conceptual and methodological challenges of evaluation in palliative care (51, 52), and recent work suggests that palliative care has the potential to reduce health system costs overall (53). In Spain, a Catalan demonstration project described annual savings of up to eight million Euros in a population with an estimated 60,000 deaths. (54). The picture is similar in the USA (55), where hospital palliative care teams have demonstrated savings, providing support for the inclusion of hospice care in managed care programmes (56). The effects on costs may be mediated through forward planning and open discussion of treatment preferences. In an analysis of 603 deaths in North America, Zhang found that health care costs in the last week of life were lower for people who had end of life conversations early in the course of the illness (57). People who had these conversations also had a higher home death rate than their peers. Use of primary care in the last year of life has also been linked with less costly care in the last 6 months, possibly for similar reasons (58). What is missing in most of these analyses is any consideration of the contribution of unpaid or 'family' carers. For example, in a novel analysis, Fassbender and colleagues in Canada described how costs varied with different dying trajectories. But the burden of illness approach they adopted did not encompass informal care (59). It follows that data to suggest that certain groups of the population are more costly to treat should be viewed critically, if they fail to include family care (60). Help-seeking behaviour is known to be socioculturally patterned, and will be influenced by the family care available. Family care provided to older adults by intergenerational carers in the USA appears to influence use of home care services and admission to residential care. Modelling data from the 1998 Health and Retirement Survey and the Asset and Health Dynamics Amongst the Oldest Old Panel Survey, Van Houtven and Norton (61) suggest that family care may also substitute for some hospital care and physician visits.

Much of the interest in unpaid care lies in the concern that the state will have to take over some of this in the years to come. Smaller families, greater geographical mobility, and change in social attitudes have led to more and more older people living alone in many countries around the world. Replacing the day-to-day supervision and care that families and friends provide with services or residential places would pose manpower and financial challenges for most countries.

Calculating exactly what family care does cost, requires information on time spent caregiving, and the value of that time. Neither of these is straightforward to measure.

There are three broad approaches to valuing time, and all have limitations, particularly for older carers. The 'opportunity cost' is a standard approach employed in health economics that is often used to place a value on family care. It requires caregivers to identify the next best possible use of their time that is spent on care. A value can then be placed on this time, depending on the nature of any opportunities forgone. In practice, how the time is usually spent is assumed to be the next best use. Then, a wage rate could be used to estimate the cost of a family carer of working age for example, or if someone gave up what would have been leisure time, a rate for that could be used. Although this approach appears to be conceptually straightforward, it requires a range of assumptions when put into practice.

When older people who are not undertaking paid work become carers, they often give up time that might have been spent on domestic or leisure activities such as gardening, visiting family, or shopping. The value placed on leisure by individuals may vary considerably from person to person. It is likely to depend on who they are caring for, and whether it is an activity that affords them any pleasure or benefit. If the caring responsibilities consist of supervision of an elderly person, then it is possible that the carer may continue some of their own activities. They might be able to read, watch television, or knit, for example, whilst they are watching over their charge. It could be argued that this time should be valued at a lower level than time that has to be devoted exclusively to caregiving. If, on the other hand, the carer is giving up time that could be spent in paid work, the time spent on family care may be valued using a wage rate that an employed person would receive for providing a similar service.

The opportunity cost approach attempts to value the resource (in this case time) that is put into family caregiving. In contrast, the market price method estimates the market value of the caregiving work, or output. The equivalent cost of employing a professional carer to do the same work is used to value the family caregivers time. However, this may be inaccurate if people who are untrained, and older are considered to work at different rates to younger, paid care workers. Contingent valuation, the third broad approach to valuing family care, has been used less often. Caregivers or members of the public are asked to estimate how much they are willing to pay to provide care themselves, or to pay someone else to provide the services. A number of useful critical reviews of the approaches to valuing caregiver time have been produced (62–64). An understanding of these methods is helpful, as the cost of family care does seem to vary with the method used for the calculation (65).

What does family care cost?

When the total cost of family care to a country is calculated, it will include care provided to people at the end of their lives, along with much longer episodes of caregiving. Such estimates are crude, but invariably point to substantial sums of money. Annual costs for England and Wales have been estimated at anywhere from 50–160% of gross expenditure on personal social services for all age groups. In the USA, figures for family care may be double the cost of nursing home care, and more than six times that of formal home care (66). Hayman and colleagues (67) used a population-based survey to estimate the cost of family care for elderly people with cancer. Treatment for cancer was associated with additional hours of family care each year, which at the time of the study, would have cost an extra US $1 billion to provide. Family care costs have been shown to be higher in the USA when hospice is used (68). In the palliative phase, Canadian data suggest that family care costs rank third behind hospital stays and home care, with the family contributing one-quarter of the total costs of care (38).

Conclusion

The costs of family care are worthy of attention at two levels. For welfare systems, however, the nature, duration, and value of the care are estimated; the costs of providing equivalent services would be substantial. Meeting the care needs of changing societies requires forward planning, and that will inevitably include caring for the growing population of elderly people without family carers. For people receiving and providing care towards the end of life, illness may have significant implications for financial well-being and health. Such consequences at the household level merit greater scrutiny, if any inequities are to be addressed. We know relatively little about how the hardship that results from family caregiving varies with social position, or the relationship with uptake of available support, such as welfare benefits. A greater understanding of these issues, and the influence of financial strain on quality of life and health status, would allow services to target those in greatest need and prevent deterioration in the health of the caregivers. Care at the end of life is provided, in one form or another, for most of the population. Ensuring that family care can be financially supported in our ageing societies should be given priority.

References

1. The Princess Royal Trust for Carers. *Who is a carer?* Available at: http://www.carers.org/what-carer (Accessed 4 January 2010).
2. Department of Health (1995). *The Carers (Recognition and Services) Act 1995.* London: HMSO.
3. Arber S, Ginn J (1990). The meaning of informal care: gender and the contribution of elderly people. *Ageing & Society*, **10**(4): 429–54.
4. Giannakouris K (2008). Ageing characterises the demographic perspectives of the European societies. *Eurostat Statistics in Focus*, **72**: 1–12.
5. Chawla M, Betcherman G, Banerji A, Bakilana AM, Feher C, Mertaugh M et al. (2007). *From Red to Gray: The 'Third Transition' of Ageing Populations in Eastern Europe and the former Soviet Union.* Washington, DC: The World Bank.
6. Carone G Costello D, Diez Guardia N, Mourre G, Przywara B, Salomäki A. (2005). *The economic impact of ageing populations in the EU25 Member States.* Report No. 236. Brussels: European Commission Directorate General for Economic and Financial Affairs Publications.
7. Office for National Statistics (2002). *Mortality statistics general 2000.* Series DH1. London: The Stationery Office.
8. Gomes B, Higginson IJ (2008). Where people die (1974—2030): past trends, future projections and implications for care. *Palliative Medicine*, **22**(1): 33–41.
9. Busse R, Krauth C (2002). Use of acute hospital beds does not increase as the population ages: Results from a seven year cohort study in Germany. *Journal of Epidemiology and Community Health*, **56**(4): 289–93.
10. Henderson J, Goldacre M, Griffith M (1990). Hospital care for the elderly in the final year of life: a population based study. *British Medical Journal*, **301**(6742): 17.
11. Fries J (2005). The compression of morbidity. *Milbank Quarterly*, **83**(4): 801–23.
12. Mor V (2005). The compression of morbidity hypothesis: A review of research and prospects for the future. *Journal of the American Geriatrics Society*, **53**: S308–S309.
13. Himsworth RL Goldacre M (1999). Does time spent in hospital in the final 15 years of life increase with age at death? A population based study. *British Medical Journal*, **319**(7221): 1338–9.
14. Dixon T, Shaw M, Frankel S, Ebrahim S (2004). Hospital admissions, age, and death: retrospective cohort study. *British Medical Journal*, **328**(7451): 1288.
15. Roos NP, Montgomery P, Roos LL (1987). Health care utilization in the years prior to death. *Milbank Quarterly*, **65**(2): 231–54.

16. Werblow A, Felder S, Zweifel P (2007). Population ageing and health care expenditure: a school of 'red herrings'? *Health Economics*, **16**(10): 1109–26.

17. Seshamani M, Gray AM (2004). A longitudinal study of the effects of age and time to death on hospital costs. *Journal of Health Economics*, **23**(2): 217–35.

18. Breyer F, Felder S (2006). Life expectancy and health care expenditures: a new calculation for Germany using the costs of dying. *Health Policy*, **5**(2): 178–86.

19. Pickard L (2008). *Informal Care for Older People Provided by Their Adult Children: Projections of Supply and Demand to 2041 in England. Report to the Strategy Unit (Cabinet Office) and the Department of Health. PSSRU Discussion Paper 2515*. London: PSSRU.

20. Wanless D (2006). *Securing Good Care for Older People - taking a long term view*. London: The Kings Fund.

21. Wolff JL, Kasper JD (2006). Caregivers of frail elders: updating a national profile. *Gerontologist*, **46**(3): 344–56.

22. Hirst M (2005). Carer distress: a prospective, population-based study. *Social Science & Medicine*, **61**(3): 697–708.

23. Pinquart M, Sorensen S (2003). Associations of stressors and uplifts of caregiving with caregiver burden and depressive mood: a meta-analysis. *Journals of Gerontology Series B-Psychological Sciences & Social Sciences*, **58**(2): P112–28.

24. Hanratty B, Drever F, Jacoby A, Whitehead M (2007). Retirement age caregivers and deprivation of area of residence. *European Journal of Ageing*, **4**(1): 35–43.

25. Schulz R, Sherwood PR (2008). Physical and mental health effects of family caregiving. *American Journal of Nursing*, **108**(9 Suppl): 23–7.

26. Abernethy A, Burns C, Wheeler J, Currow D (2009). Defining distinct caregiver subpopulations by intensity of end-of-life care provided. *Palliative Medicine*, **23**(1): 66–79.

27. Anon (2008). *Automatic payment of benefits and improving the basic state pension. Help the Aged Policy Statement*. London: Help the Aged.

28. Office for National Statistics (2010). *Inequalities and poverty in retirement*. London: The Stationery Office.

29. Berthoud R, Blekesaune M, Hancock R (2006). *Are 'poor' pensioners 'deprived'? Department for Work and Pensions Research Report 364*. London: Corporate Document Services for DWP.

30. Hutton S (1998). *Poverty over time for those recorded as informal carers in the British Household Panel Survey*. York: University of York.

31. Arber S, Ginn J (1999). Class, caring and the life course. In S Arber, M Evandrou (eds) *Ageing, Independence and the life course*, pp. 149–68. London: Jessica Kingsley.

32. Glaser K, Grundy E (2002). Class, caring and disability: evidence from the British Retirement Survey. *Ageing & Society*, **22**: 325–42.

33. Leontardi R, Bell D (2002). *Informal care of the elderly in Scotland and the UK*. Edinburgh: Scottish Executive Central Research Unit.

34. Hanratty B, Holland P, Jacoby A, Whitehead M (2007). Financial stress and strain associated with terminal cancer—a review of the evidence. *Palliative Medicine*, **21**(7): 595–607.

35. Townsend P (1957). *The family life of old people: An Enquiry in East London*. London: Routledge and Kegan Paul.

36. Hoffmann RL, Mitchell AM (1998). Caregiver burden: historical development. *Nursing Forum*, **33**(4): 5–11.

37. Gilbar O (2004). The elderly cancer patient and his spouse: two perceptions of the burden of caregiving. *Journal of Gerontological Social Work*, **21**(3-4): 149–58.

38. Dumont S, Fillion L, Gagnon P, Bernier N (2008). A new tool to assess family caregivers' burden during end-of-life care. *Journal of Palliative Care*, **24**(3): 151–61.

39. Carretero S, Garces J, Rodenas F, Sanjose V (2009). The informal caregiver's burden of dependent people: theory and empirical review. *Archives of Gerontology & Geriatrics*, **49**(1): 74–9.

40. Pearlin LI, Mullan JT, Semple SJ, Skaff MM (1990). Caregiving and the stress process: an overview of concepts and their measures. *Gerontologist*, **30**(5): 583–94.

41. Lim JW, Zebrack B (2004). Caring for family members with chronic physical illness: a critical review of caregiver literature. *Health & Quality of Life Outcomes*, **2**: 50.

42. Xu K, Evans B, Kawabata K, Zeramdini R, Klavus J, Murray CJL (2003). Household catastrophic health expenditure: a multi-country analysis. *Lancet*, **362**: 111–17.

43. Jenson J, Jacobzone, S (2000). *Care Allowances for the Frail Elderly and their Impact on Women Care-Givers*. Paris: Directorate for Education, Employment, Labour and Social Affairs; Employment, Labour and Social Affairs Committee (OECD).

44. Emanuel EJ, Fairclough DL, Slutsman J, Emanuel LL (2000). Understanding economic and other burdens of terminal illness: the experience of patients and their caregivers. *Annals of Internal Medicine*, **132**(6): 451–9.

45. Emanuel EJ, Fairclough DL, Slutsman J, Alpert H, Baldwin D, Emanuel LL (1999). Assistance from family members, friends, paid care givers, and volunteers in the care of terminally ill patients. *New England Journal of Medicine*, **341**(13): 956–63.

46. McCarthy EP, Phillips RS, Zhong Z, Drews RE, Lynn J (2000). Dying with cancer: patients' function, symptoms, and care preferences as death approaches. *Journal of the American Geriatrics Society*, **48**(5 Suppl):S110–21.

47. Covinsky KE, Landefeld CS, Teno J, Connors AF, Jr., Dawson N, Youngner S, et al. (1996). Is economic hardship on the families of the seriously ill associated with patient and surrogate care preferences? SUPPORT Investigators. *Archives of Internal Medicine*, **156**(15): 1737–41.

48. Tunnage B, Tudor-Edwards R, Linck P. (2004). *Estimation of the extent of unclaimed Disability Living Allowance and Attendance Allowance for people with a terminal diagnosis of cancer*: Centre for the Economics of Health, University of Wales.

49. Parker D, Grbch C, Maddocks I (2001). Financial issues in caring for someone with terminal cancer at home. *Australian Journal of Primary Health*, **7**(2): 37–42.

50. Hanratty B Jacoby A, Whitehead MM (2006). *The financial consequences of terminal illness - a qualitative study*: Liverpool: University of Liverpool.

51. Normand C (2009). Measuring Outcomes in Palliative Care: Limitations of QALYs and the Road to PalYs. *Journal of Pain and Symptom Management*, **38**(1): 27–31.

52. Haycox A (2009). Optimizing decision making and resource allocation in palliative care. *Journal of Pain and Symptom Management*, **38**(1): 45–53.

53. Murray E (2009). How advocates use health economic data and projections: The Irish experience. *Journal of Pain and Symptom Management*, **38**(1): 97–104.

54. Paz-Ruiz S, Gomez-Batiste X, Espinosa J, Porta-Sales J, Esperalba J (2009). The costs and savings of a regional public palliative care program: The Catalan experience at 18 years. *Journal of Pain and Symptom Management*, **38**(1): 87–96.

55. Morrison RS, Penrod JD, Cassel JB, Caust-Ellenbogen M, Litke A, Spragens L, et al. (2008). Cost savings associated with US hospital palliative care consultation programs. *Archives of Internal Medicine*, **168**(16): 1783–90.

56. Smith TJ, Cassel JB (2009). Cost and non-clinical outcomes of palliative care. *Journal of Pain and Symptom Management*, **38**(1): 32–44.

57. Zhang B, Wright AA, Huskamp HA, Nilsson ME, Maciejewski ML, Earle CC, et al. (2009). Health care costs in the last week of life: associations with end-of-life conversations. *Archives of Internal Medicine*, **169**(5): 480–8.

58. Kronman AC, Ash AS, Freund KM, Hanchate A, Emanuel EJ (2008). Can primary care visits reduce hospital utilization among Medicare beneficiaries at the end of life? *Journal of General Internal Medicine*, **23**(9): 1330–5.

59. Fassbender K, Fainsinger RL, Carson M, Finegan BA (2009). Cost trajectories at the end of life: the Canadian experience. *Journal of Pain & Symptom Management*, **38**(1): 75–80.

60. Hanchate A, Kronman AC, Young-Xu Y, Ash AS, Emanuel E (2009). Racial and ethnic differences in end-of-life costs: why do minorities cost more than whites? *Archives of Internal Medicine,* **169**(5): 493–501.

61. Van Houtven CH, Norton EC (2008). Informal care and Medicare expenditures: testing for heterogeneous treatment effects. *Journal of Health Economics,* **27**(1): 134–56.

62. Tranmer JE, Guerriere DN, Ungar WJ, Coyte PC (2005). Valuing patient and caregiver time: a review of the literature. *Pharmacoeconomics,* **23**(5): 449–59.

63. McDaid D (2001). Estimating the costs of informal care for people with Alzheimer's disease: methodological and practical challenges. *International Journal of Geriatric Psychiatry,* **16**(4): 400–5.

64. Wright K (1987). *The Economics of Informal Care of the Elderly.* York: Centre for Health Economics, University of York.

65. Andersson A, Levin L-A, Emtinger BG (2002). The economic burden of informal care. *International Journal of Technology Assessment in Health Care,* **18**(1): 46–54.

66. Arno PS, Levine C, Memmott MM (1999). The economic value of informal caregiving. *Health Affairs,* **18**(2): 182–8.

67. Hayman JA Langa KM, Kabeto MU, Katz SJ, De Monner SM, Chernew ME, et al. (2001). Estimating the cost of informal caregiving for elderly patients with cancer. *Journal of Clinical Oncology,* **19**: 3219–25.

68. Taylor DH, Jr. (2009). The effect of hospice on Medicare and informal care costs: the U.S. Experience. *Journal of Pain & Symptom Management,* **38**(1): 110–4.

Chapter 16

Workforce development: an international perspective on who will provide care

Philip Larkin and Meg Hegarty

Introduction

Defining workforce development is challenging and fundamental differences exist in its interpretation and meaning. The term can refer to occupational preparation, but also the ongoing education needed to sustain an individual in a specific role. One definition defines workforce development as a coordinated activity which assists both individuals and organizations to develop their work potential and to reach the highest organizational goals respectively (1, 2). In the context of this chapter, a recent description of palliative care service planning offers an important backdrop to understanding workforce development for older person palliative care (3). The first challenge is the ad hoc manner in which UK hospice and palliative care services have developed. The second is its continued reliance on the voluntary sector for funding services and capital developments. Inequity in service provision is mirrored in the history and experience of many hospice and palliative care services internationally (4–5). Clearly, engagement with statutory health services must be a key objective if palliative care hopes to transform end of life care of the wider community. From a workforce planning perspective, the revision of the World Health Organization definition of palliative care (6) from 'speciality' to 'approach', has been a mixed blessing. On the one hand, it expands the capacity of hospice and palliative care to reach the wider domains of chronic and life-limiting illness beyond the cancer arena. On the other, the breadth of what now constitutes specialist palliative care practice within chronic life-limiting illness has raised legitimate concerns that when people refer to 'palliative' care, it is no longer clear what position they hold in relation to end of life care (7). Hence, who provides care remains a grey area with marked diversity in terms of its definition and description (8).

The complexity of older person palliative care

For older people in need of optimal end of life care, the rationale for integrated palliative care into elder health care provision is well documented (9–14). Multiple comorbidities and fluctuating patterns of health including functional impairment and frailty evidence why many older people would clearly benefit from a palliative care intervention (13, 15, 16). Slow decline, interspersed by crisis interventions, emphasizes dying in old age as an ill-defined process (17–19). This demands a palliative approach with meticulous assessment, advance care planning, and the continuing balancing of benefit over burden regarding interventions (20). The significance of symptoms in older people is often unrecognized due to their difficulty in articulating what is happening. Advanced dementia provides particular challenges in this respect. Prognostication, both of the dementia itself and of accompanying medical conditions, is difficult. The physiological response of the very old to polypharmacy which may affect legal competence must also be considered (12, 21–23).

The challenge of integrating palliative and older person care

Given this complex picture, the challenge of providing integrated appropriate palliative care involvement to the ever-increasing residential care sector remains contentious. The proliferation of and complex classification of place of residence for older people is equally fraught. In one study, at least seven different statutory and voluntary providers of older person care were identified, with different funding streams and access to palliative care services (24). This, coupled with the reality of the changing social demography of the family and increasing reliance on professional and non-professional carers, both inside the home and in institutional care settings, means that the 21st century is going to bring a particular set of challenges and demands for practitioners (25).

Integration may be further compromised where institutionalized care of the dying older person is limited in addressing its spiritual and emotional brief (26). 'Social' death' often occurs for older people long before physical death (26–28). They may adapt to multiple losses of ageing, gaining wisdom which will serve them in dealing with the final losses of dying (29). Palliative care cannot simply be imposed on aged care without adapting it to incorporate these factors and prepare the workforce appropriately (14). Recognizing this enables clinicians to acknowledge the ways palliative care can and should be managed differently in this context.

In this chapter, we propose to address current and future perspectives on who will care for older people at the end of life. More particularly, we will explore workforce development and the barriers which challenge the provision of good end of life care. Since most recent innovative work in this area is framed within nursing, we will use this as the basis for discussion, notwithstanding our call for greater multidisciplinary approaches. We will reflect on education and training in developing a skilled and caring workforce and why that should remain as a priority in terms of service development and sustainability. Finally, given the reality that professional care options are in rapid decline, we will reflect on the reality of family as carers, solicited or otherwise, in supporting older family members at end of life. We begin by outlining the context that determines the international picture of contemporary caregiving for older people.

The changing demography of professional caring: barriers and challenges

We write this chapter at a time of global economic recession, rising unemployment, migration, and burgeoning health care systems, often unable to adequately address fully the needs of their populations. Changing family structures and work patterns (for example, women as the traditional family carers now working outside the home) and the reality of limited choice regarding place of death for older people, are real issues that will impact on workforce development now and in the decades ahead (16, 30). An interesting perspective proposed is that we have inadvertently obscured the reality of older peoples' dying by over-emphasizing a healthy ageing agenda (31, 32). Ultimately, all these perspectives influence the way in which care for older people is offered. International generic health policy frameworks envisage an innovative, creative, and sustainable workforce that can attend to the complex needs of service users and achieve optimal standards in quality of life based on a principle of integrated teamwork (33). Such policies have strong messages for those involved in the delivery of end of life care in terms of choice on final place of care, defining team and preparing that team to meet the complexity of older person care.

Current statutory funding priorities and policy constraints limit the energy and vision needed for workforce development in end of life care for older people. Quite simply, innovation requires flexibility in resource allocation, increasingly less evident in health care structures.

There is clearly a demand for trained, skilled health care workers across both older person residential and community care settings. Assuming the importance of professional nursing to end of life care (we define that as someone registered to practise as a nurse in accordance with State law), the shift in the perception of 'nursing' work and self-identity is a relevant considera- tion (34, 35). The administration demands on professional nursing practice have resulted in a perceived division of labour between nurses and non-professional caregivers (such as health care assistants or social carers), increasingly the bedside provider of care, usually, though not always, under supervision. The rise of the non-professional health care worker is evidenced by the indi- cated shortfall of 275,000 nurses in the USA in 2010. In order to balance the ageing population of nurses rapidly approaching retirement age, there is a need to educate a further 1.1 million nurses, almost half of the existing US workforce (36). This reality, albeit in smaller numbers, can be rep- licated across many countries. Add to this the issue of economic migration. Ireland is frequently cited as a country which achieved its strong economic growth in the 'Celtic Tiger' years because of well-managed immigration policies for foreign labour (37). To fill gaps in the workforce, first employment for many overseas nurses and non-professional carers has largely been in the public and private long-stay and residential care settings. In terms of end of life care, this has led to the concomitant problems of limited cultural awareness around issues of death and dying, language barriers which inhibit communication and social support to the family, and misunderstanding over ritual and practice at life closure (24, 38). The success of recruitment and retention of overseas nurses and carers is based on the quality of the adaptation programme provided by the host country, which sadly has been, at best, variable (39). Now that Ireland is in economic decline, migrant health care workers seek opportunity elsewhere, since a reversal to restrictive immigra- tion policies now fail to offer health care workers permanent residence or the possibility to bring their families to the country. The gaps once filled are now again vacant. Preparing the future workforce will require a reconfiguration of the way in which care is delivered, a clearer delineation in work role between the professional and non-professional carer, and a stronger sense of how recruitment may be managed and sustained.

Education and training provision: reflections on preparing the workforce

As noted earlier, workforce development requires acknowledgement of the specific issues and care needs of this population at the end of their lives. Barriers in education include the limited number of available courses and training opportunities for learning the skills and knowledge required for this work and, commonly, a poor understanding of what is needed to train and provide ongoing education for this workforce. The lack of higher academic training in this area compounds the problem as shown in two main areas: 1) the content of such training, and 2) the most effective ways of learning and teaching such content. These will be explored later in this chapter.

Palliative care education in the older care setting draws on three inter-related, but discrete bodies of knowledge: gerontology, geriatric care, and palliative care. This symbiotic relationship is defined not only in terms of its complementary nature but also in its ability to drive health and social policy. Incorporating work by Ryan et al., (40), it is argued that:

> All three deal with issues society tends to ignore – ageing, living with life-limiting illness and dying. Each has challenged acute, highly technological medicine and health care models and because of this stance, have operated at the margins of health care. (13)

Each discipline brings a wealth of discreet, evidence-based knowledge. Examples from gerontology include the psychology of ageing, social gerontology, and demographic implications for care planning; from geriatric care, the impact of 'the geriatric giants' in causing morbidity; and from palliative care, the physical, psychosocial, and spiritual issues in end of life care. Each discipline challenges how we respond to the most vulnerable in society and each holds a body of knowledge and skills which has potential to inform current palliative care practice. Synthesizing this knowledge effectively requires a balancing of the prescribed philosophy of healthy ageing with the realities of chronic disease and the losses associated with dying. Equally, it warrants learning to better maintain function and comfort during disease progression (13, 16).

Palliative care education: a European perspective

Globally a key challenge for workforce development has been the overemphasis on specialist education for specialist practice. In the European context, this has largely been driven by national policy agenda to embed palliative care into health systems (5, 41). European palliative care curricula and recommendations for education espouse a three-level approach with specialist practice at the pinnacle (42–44). At the non-specialist level, emphasis on the palliative care 'approach' (6) is made but with limited attention to its detail and integration into generalist health care. This said, the recommendations of the EAPC Nurse Education taskforce (42) do reflect the disparate knowledge needed to apply palliative care outside the specialist setting, through a series of 'statements for practice' which offer advice as to nursing competency following a specific programme of education and training. This can offer real benefit in older person care settings and has been used as a basis for the development of some innovative programmes of education linking palliative and gerontological care (45).

Education: motivational and inhibitory factors in workforce learning

Overall, the structured implementation of palliative care education within older person care settings remains largely unfocused and under-resourced. This can only impact negatively on who will provide palliative care for older people in the future. Much end of life care education of residential aged care staff has been conducted, formally and informally, through visiting community palliative care nurse consultation. Failing to acknowledge fully the need to rigorously adapt specialist palliative care learning to older people's needs as different from the general palliative care population, reinforces an ageist agenda (46). Further, the motivation for palliative care education must be considered. For example, in Ireland, a review of older person care provision following an inquiry into neglect in one nursing home led to the development of national standards, of which *Standard 16* relates directly to end of life care (47, 48). The need for residential care settings to meet the standard resulted in an exponential increase in demand for palliative care education. How far this relates to a desire to optimize care or to meet legal inspection requirement, remains unclear. This has led to the rise of private colleges offering vocational training for those working in older person residential care settings around 'palliative care' but with wide variance in terms of links to palliative care professional teams for clinical guidance and educational materials. A similar situation appears evident in Australia, with short courses in aged care varying from 6 weeks to 18 months, offered by the Vocational Education and Training (VET) sector. Though some clearly offer a specific elective module in end of life care, it remains peripheral to core competency for non-professional health care workers. Nor is it entirely clear who is responsible for its delivery. Since formal training in end of life care for non-professional health care workers is not mandatory and given low wage levels, particularly in the private sector, incentives to undertake such courses are also low. In Australia, teaching methods and resources in accredited courses for this group presume a literacy level equivalent to a high school Year 10 level. As noted earlier, a higher than average percentage of health care workers in residential aged care facilities with English as a second language, limited fluency and lower educational qualifications compounds the problem (24, 37).

Addressing the challenges of training and education for older person palliative care

There have been initiatives to mitigate these problems. It is noted that the translation of palliative care knowledge into the clinical arena is of equal if not greater importance to what is taught in the classroom (49). Working directly in a residential care setting can demonstrate increased skills and competencies in the provision of palliative care (9, 50–52). The work of Hockley in particular demonstrates that working directly with older person care staff using an action research approach will improve end of life care outcomes (52). Developing staff capacity through skill augmentation and empowerment in clinical decision-making is clearly a sound model for integrative working.

The link nurse model: an example of innovation

A further positive development has been the link nurse/link worker model in Australia. Based on earlier work in the UK (including that of Hockley), projects have aimed at developing and strengthening Link Nurses (sometimes referred to as Resource Nurses) within residential aged care facilities (RACFs) (53). Nominated by their RACF, these nurses act as palliative care champions within their institutions. Specialist palliative care services provide initial and ongoing training for the Link Nurses and support the network of Link Nurses, which meets on a regular basis to discuss difficult cases and liaise with palliative care specialist nurses. This peer networking is a pivotal strategy in this model of supportive training. In later years, development has included sustainability measures through selecting Link Nurses who have the aptitude for, and interest in effecting attitudinal and clinical change within their institutions. The mutually respectful, collaborative relationship between the RACF and the specialist palliative care service is crucial in its success (personal communication, Peter Jenkin, project manager, CEBPARAC project, 20 January 2010). At the time of writing, a similar national pilot sustainability project has been evaluated and developed in the UK and Ireland, underpinned by the Gold Standards Framework for Care Homes (see http://www.goldstandardsframework.nhs.uk/GSFCareHomes).

Self-directed learning

While self-directed learning can be an excellent model for professional health care providers confident in accessing programmes and learning/online resources, most health care workers and non-professional carers in aged care learn more effectively with greater face-to-face support.

Personal support for these students is very important in reducing attrition rates and establishing best practice in the care setting. One Australian self-directed learning package in palliative care for community caregivers working with older people (*Establishing the careworker role in palliative care project 2003–2006*) demonstrated a need for face-to-face personal communication and support from the educator. A similar finding was demonstrated in a pilot project in Ireland (45). Inadequate dialogue and collaboration between palliative care and aged care hinder workforce development by limiting understanding of the wealth of knowledge and skills in each field and the value of synthesizing these in the development of a new body of knowledge—palliative aged care. Therefore, self-directed learning alone may not meet the needs of this group.

Workforce development: an academic perspective

Developing the workforce for palliative care for older people occurs in the context of 'the drive to develop an evidence based practice' in end of life care (54). The skills needed to assimilate this knowledge are taught most usually in formal learning environments. However, educating the older person workforce also requires teaching the skills of life-long learning. This enables practitioners to access and evaluate new evidence and to incorporate it appropriately into their clinical work, thus maintaining currency of practice. There is evidence that those working in the older person care setting are less likely to have engaged with formal academic studies (24). Being able to translate theory to practice is therefore essential for such staff.

Palliative aged care and the undergraduate curriculum

Limited attention to palliative care education in the undergraduate programme is well documented (5). What is available tends towards medicine and nursing and in most academic centres undergraduate education develops as a discreet discipline, with little or no application to shared learning or multidisciplinary education included. Aged Care and Palliative Care content are often treated separately and taught to varying degrees across health care undergraduate courses. A positive development is the *Palliative Care for Undergraduate Curricula (PCC4U)* project, funded by the Australian Government Department of Health and Ageing. This has developed educational resources, with uptake in 33% of Australian health care undergraduate courses. This includes 30 of the 36 nursing schools, 13 of the 20 medical schools, and several allied health schools, incorporating the PCC4U resources in a variety of teaching methods, adapted to course needs. The template developed by the PCC4U project has the potential to base palliative care within core curricula which can then be utilized across a variety of disciplines and care settings. Further information on this development can be downloaded at http://www.caresearch.com.au/Caresearch/Default.aspx?alias=www.caresearch.com.au/Caresearch/pcc4u and http://www.caresearch.com.au/Caresearch/Portals/4/Documents/AgedCare_FINAL_Principlesforinclusion.pdf.

Palliative aged care and the postgraduate curriculum

At the postgraduate level, the synergy between palliative care and older person care is often dependent on personal contacts between educators who see the value in reciprocal learning. As with the undergraduate curriculum, there is evidence of change. In 2004, a decision was taken by the Australian Government to fund the development of the first ever suite of postgraduate courses in palliative aged care. These courses were developed jointly through a partnership of the Centre for Ageing Studies (CAS) and the Department of Palliative and Supportive Services (DPSS), Flinders University, Adelaide, in a clear acknowledgement of the need to incorporate the knowledge-base of gerontology, geriatrics and palliative care. The resultant multidisciplinary *Palliative Care in Aged Care* courses (from Graduate Diploma to PhD) are undertaken by clinicians, managers, and policy planners from a range of disciplines within aged care and palliative care. Online teaching is by a combined faculty of academics, clinicians, and researchers from health care and social science. During the development of the courses, collaborative partnership between these fields enabled shared understanding between faculty members from the different specialties regarding the philosophies and policies of each paradigm. These philosophical debates are crucial in informing the development of palliative aged care. Learning to work effectively in multidisciplinary and interdisciplinary care teams became an important priority in the planning of responsive curricula. Such sensitive collaborations are rarely easy (55).

The language and perspectives of differing paradigms must be learnt and respected. Shared dialogue between academics has fed this multidisciplinary curriculum, to engage students' thinking and gain knowledge and skills for wise, evidence-based clinical practice. Student feedback shows that supported study with an online network of multidisciplinary peers strengthens ongoing leadership in palliative aged care, at all levels of service planning and provision.

The challenges for education are great. We have focused here on those who provide immediate and personal care but there are other resources specifically designed to support and inform the wider health care community, including general practitioners and the multidisciplinary team who play a crucial role in older person care (see, for example, http://www.scdgp.org.au/page/Programs/Palliative_Care_/Palliative_Care_General_Practice_Support).

In summary, workforce development requires an understanding of the most effective education approaches for different groups within the workforce, including professional and non-professional health care workers. There is a dearth of evidence in the literature about training needs of non-professional health workers caregivers on end of life. As the context of service delivery changes with older people entering residential aged care facilities later in life, with higher levels of dependency and shorter stays before death ensues, the implications for workforce training are that care which is increasingly complex, requires staff to have a broader skills base drawn from a range of disciplines (56, 57).

Beyond formal care: family as workforce

The discussion so far has focused really on the formal care of older people at end of life in a variety of care settings. However, as is increasingly recognized in the literature, the real workforce in end of life is usually the family with variable levels of support through statutory and voluntary services (58). In the UK, it is estimated that approximately 500,000 unpaid carers (as family members may be termed) undertake this role (59). This estimate should be paralleled with the falling numbers in nurse recruitment and retention cited earlier in the chapter.

Comprehensive reviews of the evidence regarding family as carer conclude that their substantial contribution in economic terms to the State is often overlooked, as is the burden to their own health from the demands of caring placed upon them (58, 60, 61). Family as carer is a global phenomenon (62, 63). The immensity of burden to the unpaid carer cannot be underestimated in terms of lack of access to support mechanisms and resources, prolonged ill health, and poor long-term bereavement outcomes (25, 64, 65). There is also evidence that these experiences are determined and greatly exacerbated by the relative age and gender of the carer, with predictably worse outcomes noted as age increases (66–68). Carers have become an important topic for research, although there are clearly gaps in the types of research undertaken and a need to improve empirical evidence, tools for assessment and evaluation methods in relation to life quality (69). The benefit of respite care to family carers has been highlighted, albeit critical of the inflexible terms of short-stay inpatient care (70). The lack of available respite care in many centres, attributable to increasing inability to offer beds for 'social admission' is worthy of note.

Adequate preparation and supporting family carers in their role is key to success. Group psycho-educational initiatives have been reported as beneficial to sustaining relatives in their caring role (71). Similarly, family meetings, often seen as core practice in palliative care, have been shown to be effective in meeting the needs of family carers (72). However, evidence from the field of palliative aged care is lacking. Clinical practice guidelines are needed to make the care planning for family carers understandable and achievable. The *Guidelines for a Palliative Approach in Residential*

Aged Care (2006) and *Guidelines for a Palliative Approach for Aged Care in the Community Setting* (currently being prepared for publication) have, for the first time, provided evidence-based guidelines for practice in end of life care for older people across care settings. The community guidelines specifically incorporate a document written in lay language for family and non-professional carers. Translating guidelines into practice requires targeted educational approaches.

Conclusions

Key to addressing the question 'Who will provide care?' is an appreciation of how to embed palliative care principles into the language and practice of older person caring.

Sustainability measures must be built into any project providing education or training. Continuing access to education resources and peer-support networks beyond the life of a project is essential. Use of a highly credible, evidence-based, and freely accessible online hub such as Caresearch, an active, palliative care networking repository for linked resources, sites and updated information (http://www.caresearch.com.au), enables this to happen. The changing dynamic of older person care means that practitioners need to 'roll with the punches'—prepare for change where we can and adapt to change when we need to. There is an imperative on health systems and government agencies to embrace the realities which will face an older dying population in future years. Preparing for a motivated, knowledgeable, innovative, and cohesive multidisciplinary health care workforce is the greatest challenge for palliative aged care at this time.

References

1. Jacobs RL (2002). 'Understanding workforce development: definition, conceptual boundaries and future perspectives.' Paper presented at the International Conference on Technical and Vocational Education and Training, Canadian Vocational Association and UNEVOC-Canada, Winnipeg, Manitoba.
2. Gray K, Herr E (1997). *Workforce education: The basics.* Boston, MA: Allyn-Bacon.
3. Finlay IG (2009). Developing a template to plan palliative care services: The Welsh experience. *Palliative Medicine*, **38**: 81–6.
4. Gwyther L, Brennan F, Harding R (2009). Advancing palliative care as a human right. *Journal of Pain and Symptom Management*, **38**: 767–74.
5. Stjernswärd, J, Foley KM, Ferris FD (2007). Integrating palliative care into national policies. *Journal of Pain and Symptom Management*, **33**: 514–20.
6. Centeno C, Clark D, Lynch T, Rocafort J, Praill D, De Lima L, et al. (2007). Facts and indicators on palliative care development in 52 countries of the WHO European region: results of an EAPC taskforce. *Palliative Medicine*, **21**: 463–71.
7. World Health Organization (2002). *WHO Definition of palliative care.* Available at: http://www.who.int/cancer/palliative/definition/en/. (Accessed 3 February 2010.)
8. Illhardt FJ (2001). Scope and demarcation of palliative care. In H Ten Have, R Janssens (eds) *Palliative care in Europe concepts and policies*, pp. 109–16. Amsterdam: IOS Press.
9. Block S, Portenoy RK (2008). Workforce and Leadership. *Journal of Palliative Medicine*, **11**: 955–6.
10. Badger F, Clifford C, Hewison A, Thomas K (2009). An evaluation of the implementation of a programme to improve end-of-life care in nursing homes. *Palliative Medicine*, **23**: 502–11.
11. Morrison RS (2009). Suffering in silence: addressing the needs of nursing home residents. *Journal of Pain and Symptom Management*, **12**: 671–2.
12. Lloyd-Williams M, Kennedy V, Sixsmith A, Sixsmith J (2007). The end of life: a qualitative study of the perceptions of people over the age of 80 on issues surrounding death and dying *Journal of Pain and Symptom Management*, **34**: 60–6.

13. Shega JW, Hougham GW, Stocking CB, Sachs GA (2008). Patients dying with dementia: experience at the end of life and impact of hospice care. *Journal of Pain and Symptom Management*, **35**: 499–507.

14. Hegarty M, Currow D (2007). Palliative aged care: collaborative partnerships between gerontology, geriatrics and palliative care. *International Journal of Gerontology*, **1**: 112–17.

15. Froggatt K. Palliative care and nursing homes: where next? *Palliative Medicine* 2001; **15**: 42–8.

16. Higginson IJ, Foley KM (2009). Palliative care : no longer a luxury but a necessity? *Journal of Pain and Symptom Management*, **38**: 1–3.

17. Currow DC, Hegarty M (2006). Residential aged care facility palliative care guidelines. *International Journal of Palliative Nursing*, **12**: 231–3.

18. Davies E, Higginson IJ (eds) (2004). *Better palliative care for older people*. Geneva: World Health Organization.

19. Evers MM, Meier DE, Morrison RS (2002). Assessing differences in care needs and service utilization in geriatric palliative care patients. *Journal of Pain and Symptom Management*, **23**: 424–32.

20. Seale C (1989). What happens in hospices: a review of research evidence. *Social Science & Medicine*, **28**: 551–9.

21. Lunney J, Lynn J, Foley D, Lipson S, Guralnik JM (2003). Patterns of functional decline at the end of life. *Journal of the American Medical Association*, **289**: 2837–392.

22. Amella E (2003). Geriatrics and palliative care: Collaboration for quality of life until death. *Journal of Hospice and Palliative Nursing*, **5**: 40–8.

23. Evans B (2002). Improving palliative care in the nursing home: from a dementia perspective. *Journal of Hospice and Palliative Nursing*, **4**: 91–102.

24. Herr K (2002). Chronic pain in the older patient: management strategies. *Journal of Gerontological Nursing*, **28**: 28–34.

25. O'Shea E, Murphy K, Larkin P, Payne S, Froggatt K, Casey D, et al. (2008). *End-of-Life Care for Older People in Acute and Long-Stay Care Settings in Ireland*. Dublin: National Council for Ageing and Older People and The Irish Hospice Foundation.

26. Grande GE, Farquhar MC, Barclay SIG, Todd CJ (2006). The influence of patient and carer age in access to palliative care. *Age & Ageing*, **35**: 267–73.

27. Costello J (2001). Nursing older dying patients: findings from an ethnographic study of death and dying in elderly care wards. *Journal of Advanced Nursing*, **35**: 59–68.

28. Johnson G (2004). Social death: The impact of protracted dying. In S Payne, J Seymour, C Ingleton (eds) *Palliative care nursing: Principles and evidence for practice*, pp. 257–91. Maidenhead: Open University Press.

29. Chicin ER, Burak OR, Olson E, Likourezos A (2000). *An end-of-life ethics and the nursing assistant*. New York: Springer.

30. Baltes PB (1997). On the incomplete architecture of human ontology: Selection, optimization and compensation as foundation of developmental theory. *American Psychologist*, **52**: 366–80.

31. Drennan V, Levenson R, Goodman C, Evans C (2004). The workforce in health and social care services to older people: developing an education and training strategy. *Nurse Education Today*, **24**: 402–8.

32. Miller EA, Mor V (2008). Balancing regulatory controls and incentives: towards smarter and more transparent oversight in long-term care. *Journal of Health Politics, Policy and Law*, **33**: 249–79.

33. Abbey J, Abbey B, Bridges P, Elder R, Lemcke P, Liddle J, et al. (2006). Clinical placements in residential aged care facilities: the impact on nursing students: perception of aged care and the effect on cancer plans. *Australian Journal of Advanced Nursing*, **23**: 14–19.

34. Page S, Willey K (2007). Workforce development: planning what you need starts with knowing what you have. *Australian Health Review*, **31**: s98.

35. Buchan J, Aiken L (2008). Solving nursing shortages: a common priority. *Journal of Clinical Nursing*, 2008; **17**: 3262–8.

36. Murray MA (2007). Crossing over: transforming palliative care nursing services for the 21st Century. *International Journal of Palliative Nursing*, **13**: 366–76.

37. The Center for Nursing Advocacy. Available at: http://www.nursingadvocacy.org. (Accessed 8 February 2010).

38. Humphries N, Brugha R, McGee H (2008). *Overseas nurse recruitment: Ireland as an illustration of the dynamic nature of nurse migration. Epidemiology and Public Health Medicine Articles*. Dublin: Royal College of Surgeons in Ireland.

39. Payne S, Froggatt K, O'Shea E, Murphy K, Larkin P, Casey D, et al. (2009). Improving palliative end of life care for older people in Ireland: a new model and framework for institutional care. *Journal of Palliative Care*, **25**: 218–26.

40. Gerrish K, Griffith V (2003). Integration of overseas Registered Nurses: evaluation of an adaptation programme. *Journal of Advanced Nursing*, **45**: 579–87.

41. Ryan DP, Carson MG, Zorzitto ML (1989). The first international conference on palliative care of the elderly: an overview. *Journal of Palliative Care*, **5**: 40–2.

42. Centeno C, Noguera A, Lynch T, Clark D (2007). Official certification of doctors working in palliative medicine in Europe: data from an EAPC study in 52 European countries. *Palliative Medicine*, **21**: 683–7.

43. De Vlieger M, Gorchs N, Larkin P, Porchet F (2004). Palliative nurse education: towards a common language. *Palliative Medicine*, **18**: 401–3.

44. European Association for Palliative Care (2007). *Curriculum in palliative care for undergraduate medical education. Recommendations of the European Association for Palliative Care*. Available at: http://www.eapcnet.org.

45. European Association for Palliative Care (2009). *Recommendation of the European Association for Palliative Care for the Development of postgraduate Curricula leading to Certification in Palliative Medicine*. Available at: http://www.eapcnet.org.

46. Cooley MC, Keegan O, Larkin P (2010). *Evaluation of the Pilot Introductory End of Life Education Programme for Staff Working in Residential Care Settings for Older People*. Dublin: Irish Hospice Foundation.

47. Reed J, Cook M, Cook G, Inglis P, Clarke C (2006). Specialist services for older people: issues of negative and positive ageism. *Ageing & Society*, **26**: 849–65.

48. Department of Health and Children. *The commission of investigation (Leas Cross Nursing Home) Final Report* 2009. Dublin: DOHC.

49. An bord Altranais (2009). *Professional Guidance for Nurses working with older people*. Dublin: An bord Altranais.

50. Ferris FD, Gunten CF, Emanuel LL (2001). Knowledge: insufficient for change. *Journal of Palliative Medicine*, **4**: 145–7.

51. Miller SC, Han B (2008). End-of-life care in U.S. nursing homes: nursing homes with special programs and trained staff for hospice or palliative/end-of-life care. *Journal of Pain and Symptom Management*, **11**: 865–77.

52. Froggatt K (2007). The 'regulated death': a documentary analysis of the regulation and inspection of dying and death in English care homes for older people. *Ageing & Society*, **27**: 233–47.

53. Hockley J, Froggatt K (2006). The development of palliative care knowledge in care homes for older people: the place of action research. *Palliative Medicine*, **20**: 835–43.

54. Maddocks I, Abbey J, Pickhaver A, Parker D, Beck K, DeBellis A (1996). *Palliative care in nursing homes. Report to the Commonwealth. Department of Health and Family Services*. Adelaide: Flinders University.

55. Hegarty M, Currow D (2009). Postgraduate education in palliative care. In G Hanks, NI Cherny, NA Christakis, M Fallon, S Kaasa, R Portenoy (eds) *Oxford Textbook of Palliative Medicine*, 4th edn, pp. 00-00. Oxford: Oxford University Press.

56. Seymour J, Clark D, Philp I (2001). Palliative care and geriatric medicine: shared concerns, shared challenges. Editorial. *Palliative Medicine*, **15**: 269–70.

57. Fox J (2008). Shaping education for tomorrow's workforce. [comment] *British Journal of Nursing*, **17**: 218–19.

58. Kelly D (2003). Regulation of the social care workforce. *Nursing & Residential Care*, **5**: 178–9.

59. Grande G, Stajduhar K, Aoun S, Toye C, Funk L, Addlington Hall J, et al. (2009). Supporting lay carers in end of life care: current gaps and future priorities. *Palliative Medicine*, **23**: 339–44.

60. Payne, S, Hudson, P (2009). Assessing the family and caregivers. In D Walsh, AT Caraceni, R Fainsinger, FM Foley, P Glare, C Goh, et al. (eds) *Textbook of Palliative Medicine*, pp. 320–5. New York: Elsevier.

61. Kennedy S, Seymour J, Almack K, Cox K (2009). Key stakeholders' experiences and views of the NHS End of Life Care Programme: findings from a national evaluation. *Palliative Medicine*, **29**: 283–94.

62. Aoun SM, Kristjanson LJ, Currow DC, Hudson PL (2005). Caregiving for the terminally ill: at what cost. *Palliative Medicine*, **19**: 551–5.

63. Australian Institute of Health and Welfare (2003). *Australia's welfare 2003*. (AIHW, Cat No. AUS-41.) Canberra: Australian Institute of Health and Welfare.

64. Greaves L, Hankivsky O, Kivadiotakis G, Cormier R, Saunders L, Galvin L, et al. (2002). *Final payments: Socioeconomic costs of palliative home caregiving in the last months of life*. Vancouver, BC: British Columbia Centre of Excellence for Women's Health, Canada.

65. Buckner L, Yeandle S (2007). *Valuing carers–calculating the value of unpaid care*. London: Carers UK. Available at: http://www.carersuk.org/Policyandpractice/Research/Profileofcaring/1201108437/ ValuingcarersFINAL.pdf. (Accessed 11 February 2010.)

66. Seymour JE, Witherspoon R, Gott M, Ross H, Payne, S (2005). *End of Life Care: promoting comfort, choice and well-being among older people facing death*. Bristol: Policy Press.

67. Fromme EK, Drach LL, Tolle SW, Ebert P, Miller P, Perrin N, et al. (2005). Men as caregivers at the end of life. *Journal of Palliative Medicine*, **8**: 1167–75.

68. Thomas C, Morris SM, Harman JC (2002). Companions through cancer: the care given by informal carers in cancer contexts. *Social Science & Medicine* **54**: 529–44.

69. Ringdal GI, Jordhoy MS., Ringdal K, Kaasa S (2001). Factors affecting grief reactions in close family members to individuals who have died of cancer. *Journal of Pain and Symptom Management*, **22**: 1016–26.

70. Cohen R, Leis AM, Kuhl D, Charbonneau C, Ritvo P, Ashbury FD (2006). QOLLTI-F: measuring family carer quality of life. *Palliative Medicine*, **20**: 755–67.

71. Skilbeck JK, Payne S, Ingleton MC, Nolan M, Carey I (2005). An exploration of family carers' experience of respite services in one specialist palliative care unit. *Palliative Medicine*, **19**: 610–18.

72. Hudson P, Thomas T, Quinn K, Cockayne M, Braithwaite M (2009). Teaching family carers about home-based palliative care: final results from a group education program. *Journal of Pain and Symptom Management*, **38**: 299–308.

73. Hudson P, Thomas T, Quinn K, Aranda S (2009). Family meetings in palliative care: are they effective? *Palliative Medicine*, **23**: 150–7.

The significance of place at the end of life
Introduction

Merryn Gott and Christine Ingleton

Whilst place of care at the end of life has long been a topic of importance within palliative care research and policy, the views and preferences of older people have received little specific attention. Moreover, the complexities of these preferences are rarely articulated; home may be a preferred place to die for many, but what does 'home' actually mean? In Chapter 17, Habib Chaudhury and colleagues consider this key issue, framing their discussions around the question: 'what are the physical, environmental characteristics responsive to end of life care?' They consider how the (built) hospice environment can be optimally designed to support people and their families at the end of life, recognizing that the same design principles apply to both residential and acute care facilities. Having critiqued the widely accepted view that home is always preferred as a location of end of life care by older people, they consider the ways in which 'home-like' environments can be recreated in institutional settings. The authors conclude by arguing for the recognition of two basic issues in creating such environments: firstly that physical environmental concerns need to be balanced by considerations of the social and organizational milieu; and secondly that notions of 'home' are determined by the cultural understandings of patients and their families. More research is required to understand the optimum means of balancing these considerations to best achieve an end of life environment that supports 'a positive living and dying experience'.

The numbers of older people living out the end of their lives in nursing and residential care facilities is set to rise in coming years within all developed countries. In Chapter 18, Katherine Froggatt and colleagues argue that a whole systems approach is required to achieve optimum care in these environments. Key challenges in delivering palliative care in nursing and residential care facilities are outlined, including responding to the diversity of needs amongst older residents and their families, workforce issues, the care culture, and wider organizational constraints. Three examples of innovative practice in palliative care provision are presented from Canada, the UK, and Austria. The authors use these as a springboard for considering how change in palliative care provision within care home settings can be achieved for and by individuals, teams, organizations, and the wider system. They conclude that 'there is no one optimal way of implementing palliative care in long-term care settings for frail older people' and that, as ever, more research is needed. Moreover, they argue that it is policy and practice decision-makers who need to take the lead in implementing 'a comprehensive, multilevel approach towards improving care'. Otherwise attempts to improve care of the dying in long-term care facilities, however well intentioned, are doomed to failure.

In Chapter 19, Deborah Parker continues the theme of how to effect change in the provision of palliative care within residential care homes. She outlines the development and implementation of evidence-based palliative care guidelines for these settings in Australia, the only evidence-based guidelines of this type to have been developed internationally. Through her discussions she provides a framework which could guide the development of similar work in other countries and provides examples of specific projects in different regions. The lessons she draws are salutary for others charged with the difficult task of ensuring high-quality palliative care provision in care home settings. The chapter concludes by identifying that more evidence regarding the effectiveness of the guidelines in improving 'resident and family outcomes' is needed and that it is this which will 'be the best driver for change'. Indeed, all chapters in this section prioritize change if end of life environments are to be optimized and older people are to have a real choice about where they die.

Clare Gardiner and Sarah Barnes take up the themes of physical environment and design in Chapter 20. They turn their attention to the setting in which most people will die, but the least research attention has been paid—acute hospitals. The significant impact of the hospital environment upon patient, carer, and staff well-being is identified and the authors consider strategies to optimize this impact for all groups concerned. They conclude by stating that 'hospital environments are not always optimal for older people reaching the end of life' and call for lessons to be learnt from the design of other end of life care environments, such as children's hospitals, hospices, and residential care homes. The importance of soliciting user views to inform the design of new hospitals or wards is identified. However, in light of previous discussions throughout this book, it is perhaps unsurprising that they identify that older people are rarely consulted in this capacity, despite being the major users of acute hospitals internationally.

Chapter 17

Place matters: an exploration of the role of physical environment in end of life care

Habib Chaudhury, Gloria Puurveen, and Jennifer Lyle

Introduction

There is a growing acknowledgement and understanding of the interrelationship between the physical environment of health care institutions and the quality of life of care recipients and those involved in care giving (1). The physical characteristics of a setting influence the quality of care and its delivery, the ability to modulate the intensity of service, and the likelihood that a person will need to be transferred to another care location (2, 3). While research has uncovered preferences for place of death as well as where people die, there is little scholarship related to the questions of 'What are the physical environmental characteristics responsive to end of life care?' There is recognition that the physical environment is an important therapeutic element in end of life care. A well-designed environment responsive to physical, psychosocial, and spiritual needs can minimize suffering of older people and their families at the end of life, and maximize independence, encouraging social interaction and enabling self-expression (4). However, empirical research and design guidelines for responsive environments for death and dying have not kept pace with the advances observed in other settings.

This chapter focuses on the place of dying and death for older adults. The aims of this chapter are as follows. First, we will examine the relative benefits and challenges of 'home' as the place of end of life care. Second, we will review the literature on environmental design in hospice and residential care, and synthesize the design considerations for end of life care setting. The final aim is to present brief conceptual reflections on the interrelationship between place and end of life care.

Home as a place for end of life care

There is a presumption that a home death is ideal (5). The desire to die at home is related to a myriad of reasons such as maintaining close connections with family, a sense of continuity, being in a familiar environment, and maintenance of control over daily routine (3, 6). Dying at home also allows the older person to dictate the conditions for social interactions and can provide the opportunity for family caregivers to remain intimately connected with their loved one (3, 7, 8). However, dying at home may pose substantial challenges due to complex interrelationships between individual, social, environmental, and systems factors.

First, older people may not have caregivers to support them at home. If family caregivers are available, they may be unable, unwilling, or overwhelmed by the intensity of care required. They may become financially and emotionally bankrupt in the face of increasing care demands (2, 6, 7). Moreover, fulfilling the role of a caregiver in the home may reshape the meaning of home for the family member (9, 10). These challenges for the family may be compounded if professional resources are inadequate (3) and if the living-dying trajectory is prolonged (11). In addition, the older person needing care may not want to encumber her/his family members with personal care needs (12) or the emotional burden of bearing witness to their suffering (13).

Second, although care recipients who receive hospice services within the home are able to stay at home significantly longer than those who do not (14), the older person may be unable to access appropriate services due to finances, geographical location, or lack of availability of home hospice programmes within their community (3). Moreover, the decision to intensify services is largely determined by the older person and/or their family, and when the care needs are higher and complex, there is incongruence between what the older person wishes and the practicalities of home-based care provisions (3). Further, the physical environment of the home may not support the persons' changing functional needs (3, 8, 15, 16). While environmental modifications may enable a person to remain at home, there may come a point when the home is more a burden than a support and relocation is necessary.

Finally, as the face of home changes to support terminal care, are the positive meanings of home sustained for the older person? Are the associations of 'home' obscured or changed by the increasing medicalization of the home environment during the dying process (7, 10)? Arras and Neveloff-Dubler (7) raise the concern about how a person can be at 'home' if the home is transformed into a mini intensive care unit with the import of medical equipment and personnel. Receiving home care can change the face of the family home in such a way that values associated with meaning of home, such as privacy, social relations, dignity, and control, become compromised (17, 18).

The next section examines the design principles of hospice architecture. Many of these principles are also found in the residential care literature. As such, while the hospice literature is the framework for the discussion on design principles, it is as relevant to residential care and acute care.

Physical environment of hospice: an overview

The Canadian Hospice and Palliative Care Association (CHPCA) defines hospice palliative care as 'whole-person health care that aims to relieve suffering and improve the quality of living and dying' (19) Central to this definition is the term 'whole-person'. It is commonly understood that the ethos of end of life care is to address the individual's needs, expectations, hopes, and fears with respects to their physical, social, emotional, and spiritual well-being. Moreover, hospice care is based on the concept that death is a natural event, and that the dying and their loved ones have the right to a peaceful and empowering end of life experience (20–23). There are several models for hospice design—each based on different principles regarding the relationship between the hospice and the recipients of care (22).

First, hotel-type models are based on the concept that hospice facility users are guests, and they are there to rent and use the space temporarily. These models feature a high degree of patient autonomy and privacy; however, there is also a higher chance of isolation and little emphasis on building community. Second, co-housing models provide persons with private rooms and shared spaces to promote a sense of community and support. Third, monastic models emphasize the idea that the dying process is a time for quiet reflection and meditation, borrowing from the medieval concept of cloister to design their building plans. Finally, residential models incorporate architectural characteristics common in private homes, such as kitchens, family rooms, private bedrooms, and easy access to the outdoors into a facility building plan to create an environment that is reminiscent of a typical family home. Overall, hospice units are not only modern health care facilities; they are also a home to a wide variety of people with differing needs. Providing optimal clinical care needs to be balanced with the provision of a calm, tranquil environment that enables a person to truly live until they die.

Private spaces: the bedroom

Within a hospice, the bedroom is the primary unit of the physical environment. As a person enters into the final days of life, his or her world progressively shrinks from the community to a bed (8). Throughout this progression, the person's bedroom becomes the central locus for all activity (8, 24, 25). Socialization, retreat, palliative care, reminiscence, grieving, and finally death all occur within this room. As such, the bedroom significantly impacts an older person's end of life experience (25). Sensitive design of the bedroom can help support a number of therapeutic goals. Apart from supporting a person's clinical needs, the bedroom can support continuity of the self and of relationship through personalization of the room and accommodating spaces for visitors. It also enables control, independence and dignity through adaptive design and choice. A particular challenge in the design of bedrooms is to ensure that the environment does not become overly clinical. That is, it must balance the emerging clinical needs with psychosocial needs.

Personalization and enabling a sense of identity

Studies have shown that familiar and cherished objects are symbolic representations of an individual's connection to home that offer a sense of comfort, familiarity, and continuity of self (10, 13, 26). As such, opportunities for personalization enable older people to retain a sense of connection with their personal history and allow them to develop a connection and sense of control over their current environment (8). Shelving units, dresser tables, and generous window ledges provide space for the display of personal items such as photographs and mementos (4, 8, 20, 23, 25, 27). Storage space should be provided to accommodate other personal items that a person may wish to bring with him or her (20, 25). Flexible furniture arrangements enable the person or families to move furniture into a configuration that suits them, and space can be provided for the addition of some personal furniture items, such as a favourite chair. The incorporation of familiar objects enhances the individualization of a room.

Socialization and enabling relationships

While dying is a time for quiet reflection, it is also a time for human connection. Connecting with loved ones and other residents enables people to feel supported during a period of life that is physically and emotionally challenging (24, 28). However, a commonly cited fear around dying and death is that of dying alone or in isolation from others (6, 29). This is especially true as the person spends more time in the bedroom and opportunities to connect with others become less frequent. Therefore, design of the bedroom must support socialization. Personalization of the space can serve as the basis of personal narratives and provides a platform for meaningful activity; for sharing stories and life review. In addition, the space needs to support family vigils as well as moments of celebration. Thus, bedrooms must be designed to accommodate visitors. There should be adequate seating for several guests, and options for visitors who wish to stay the night in the older person's room, either in the form of a recliner, or space for a cot or roll-out bed (4, 8, 20, 27, 30, 31).

Privacy and preserving dignity

It is observed that older people exhibit an increased desire for privacy as their condition worsens (28). Thus, bedrooms should also provide visual and acoustic privacy as needed particularly when the space is shared between two or more people (8, 31, 32). Single-bed rooms offer their occupants more privacy than multiple bedrooms; however, multiple-bed rooms enable peer support during their end of life experiences (28, 33, 34). Generally, two persons per room should be avoided, as the negative emotional impact on the surviving roommate when his or her companion dies is significantly greater in this situation versus a four-bed configuration (20).

The location of the rooms is an important consideration in the design of a hospice facility. The bedroom is the inner sanctum of the hospice environment. The location of this private space should allow easy access to other areas of the hospice, while maintaining separation from the higher traffic areas to create a sense of protection and privacy. To accomplish this, hospices can incorporate the principles of cloistering, whereby open public spaces gradually feed into smaller, more private spaces until one finally reaches the bedroom area (20, 22, 25). This creates a sense of privacy and provides staff, visitors, and residents with a gradient between public and private spaces (22).

Maintaining independence

As a person progresses through the final stages of life, his or her functional abilities decrease. As a result, the environment has an increased impact on the person's ability to function independently (8, 20, 35). Therefore, the hospice environment should support a range of abilities to enable the person to function independently for as long as possible. For example, bedrooms should be able to accommodate a wheelchair, a wheeled bed, or other mobility aides (8, 20, 22, 25). Older people should be provided with options to vary the intensity of the light to meet their needs. Adjustable features can include blinds and curtains, dimmer switches, and table lamps (25). Independent temperature and ventilation controls enable the individual to change the climate of their rooms (8, 20, 25, 35). Remote controls can allow low-functioning older people to control their room's temperature and lighting levels (8).

Each private room should have access to its own washroom to support the functional abilities of the person receiving care and provide them with a measure of privacy (7, 8, 25). Elements such as handrails, elevated toilet seats, non-slip flooring, a place to sit, ample lighting, and adequate space to accommodate a variety of mobility aids support a range of functional abilities and prolong independence (20, 25, 34). Moreover, space for personal items such as toiletries and towels can help create a place that is more homelike (34).

Creating a community: design of public spaces

Public spaces within a hospice facility give its users the option of different social settings outside of the bedroom and support a diverse group of functions. The design features in these spaces communicate the function and atmosphere of the room, but also provide a commentary as to the overall atmosphere of the facility itself.

Socialization and maintaining relationship

Public spaces are important for supporting social interactions and fostering relationships. Due to various concerns regarding the older person's comfort or care regime, visitors may also wish to have overnight accommodations outside of the individual's bedroom. These accommodations should be located near the older person's room, and can vary from dormitory-style sleeping arrangements to separate apartments depending on space availability (20, 24, 25). Having these options enables family members to remain in close contact to provide support and comfort their loved ones.

From a cultural standpoint, the sharing of meals is an important component of daily social life. Food is strongly associated with major celebrations and time spent with family and friends, and is a vehicle for displays of affection across different cultures (8, 20, 21, 22). As such, dining options in hospice facilities should support this association of food with care and good company. Dining spaces within the hospice facility can incorporate home-like elements such as smaller table sizes (e.g. groups of four or six), placemats, home-like furniture pieces, and decorations (e.g. a china hutch, paintings, wooden tables and chairs) (25, 34). The space should promote a sense of intimacy among diners. This does not necessarily imply a small room; a larger room may be necessary due to space and staffing constraints, but can be subdivided using screens or furniture to create the impression of multiple, smaller social spaces (34).

Finally, each public space on the facility grounds can be regarded as an opportunity for memorialization of people who have had a prior stay at the hospice. Providing families the opportunity to preserve the memory of their loved ones on site enables them to honour their loved one and show appreciation for the hospice staff and facility. As the majority of hospice facilities rely on donations to fund their operations, providing opportunities for donations from prior users is important (25, 36). Options include naming wings in honour of people who are no longer at the hospice, having inscriptions along outdoor walkways or interior walls, and dedicating benches or exterior architectural pieces like fountains or gazebos.

Purpose-specific areas

Facilities should also have a few purpose-specific areas. An important goal of hospice care is to support the grieving and bereavement process. Thus, older people and their families need to be provided with a private, quiet space outside of the bedroom. Such spaces provide the opportunity for meditation and spiritual reflection, for grieving, and retreat (25, 32). A multidenominational space such as a chapel, a meditation room, a small private nook that is located near bedrooms, or an outdoor area can provide users with an isolated space for quiet contemplation. A designated bereavement room can provide the privacy in which family members can view the body of the deceased and say their goodbyes. This space is particularly important in facilities where the bedrooms are shared or where it is not otherwise possible to use the bedroom as a private viewing space after death has occurred (25, 28). Other spaces may also be designed to provide the older person with the opportunity to engage in self-expression and sensory exploration. Art rooms create a space to communicate feelings through a medium other than speech, in addition to providing sensory stimulation. Multisensory rooms can be used to provide multifaceted sensory experiences, and can be designed to suit a range of functional and cognitive abilities (25).

The sensory environment

Since an individual's ability to function within a given environment differs with age and disease progression, the sensory environment must be carefully considered in the context of user populations, the function of a space, and the therapeutic goals of that space (4, 8, 30, 37, 38). This section explores design principles along the visual, aural, and olfactory domains.

The visual environment

The visual sensory environment can be divided into two categories: ambience and functional support. Ambience refers to how physical aspects of the environment can evoke a set of emotions regarding that space. In modern hospice design, emphasis is on creating spaces with residential appeal. Visual elements such as pictures, home-like flooring (e.g. laminate, carpet, wood), fabric window coverings, and residential-style furnishings can be used to create the impression of a welcoming, home-like environment (25, 39). Moreover, distractive elements such as paintings and interesting ceiling patterns can help an older person to transition their focus from themselves to the external environment, helping to reduce anxiety and pain (27, 30).

The visual environment also plays a large role in enabling persons in hospice and their families to function independently. Objects within a space can be used to provide visual cues with respect to that space's function (34, 37). For example, the presence of residential dining table(s) can be used to identify the room used for eating. The advantages of this approach are threefold: it minimizes the amount of signage required to identify each room, thereby increasing the overall residential ambience; it increases the level of redundancy with respect to the information provided for room identification; and it enables users to navigate the facility based on landmarks with minimal outside assistance (34, 37).

Adequate illumination is also a prerequisite for supporting independent functioning. A room that requires high visual acuity, such as a space for reading or for food preparation, will have a higher minimum lighting level needed than a space that does not have similar functions to serve (20, 22, 37, 38). Transition spaces between outdoor and indoor areas will require a higher level of lighting than interior spaces in order to minimize glare and facilitate light-dark adaptation as a person moves from outside to inside or vice versa (20, 37). Areas that have changes in depth, such as stairways, also require a higher level of lighting than spaces with level flooring, to better highlight the changes in depth (34, 37). The characteristics of the user population also impact the level of lighting required. Disease progression and ageing impact the visual system, decreasing sensitivity to contrast and colour, and increasing the minimum amount of light required for a given task (37, 38). Moreover, as a person nears death, his or her lighting preferences change from bright to dark (25). In order to address the needs of a diverse population, lighting levels must be modifiable and designed to meet the needs of its most visually impaired users. For example, table lamps can be placed near reading areas, overhead task lighting can be employed in food preparation areas to augment existing levels, and hallways should be brightly lit to meet the needs of all age groups (e.g. see reference 37).

The auditory environment

In addition to the visual environment, the auditory environment has an important impact on how facility users view the hospice. Facilities where alarms, noisy television sets, and shouting staff are clearly audible have higher levels of anxiety among the people who reside there (30). Moreover, environment-related noise is related to sleep fragmentation and consequently with depressive symptoms (40), as well as agitated behaviours (41). Consequently, efforts should be made to ensure a quiet environment by controlling excess noise through the use of sound absorbing materials, or isolating/containing the sound sources by using partitions or doors. Research also shows that creating a calm pleasant environment is related to increased well-being (41). Acoustic privacy is also important, as sounds from other people can distress those in proximity to them (8).

The olfactory environment

Smell can have a powerful impact on how a space is perceived. Home-like odours such as fresh coffee can evoke pleasant memories of home, allowing older people to connect with previous experiences and life roles (34). Facility policy should support the general use of kitchen areas and encourage on-site as opposed to off-site meal preparation. Conversely, smells of bodily odours and harsh chemicals create the impression of an institutional environment (34) and are associated with a lower level of care (30). Ventilation should be of high standard and if possible, use natural ventilation.

The tactile environment

Finally, the tactile environment impacts the atmosphere of a space. An overabundance of hard surfaces results in a high ambient noise load and creates a cold, institutional space, while soft surfaces increase the perception of warmth and absorb noise within a space (34). Varied tactile surfaces can provide a source of positive stimulation as well, which is particularly important for older people who may otherwise experience sensory deprivation, leading to increased agitation and higher self-reported pain levels (34).

Natural spaces

Being in natural spaces has a powerful, positive effect on a person's psyche and overall well-being. Providing a secure outdoor space offers a choice for the person to leave the confines of the building into a natural setting that promotes sensory stimulation, reminiscences, and supports quality of life (42). Persons residing in hospice report an increased sense of calmness and fewer symptoms when provided with the opportunity to connect with nature, either through outdoor access or views, or even paintings of natural scenes (28, 32). The benefits of the natural environment extend to staff and visitors as well (30). The outdoor areas of a hospice facility can incorporate a variety of design features. For example, facilities can have gardens with level, paved paths to allow non-ambulatory older people to move through the area, along with handrails for those who are ambulatory but have difficulty with gait and balance. Paths can be designed to loop back to the facility to enable those with cognitive impairments to more easily navigate the space (25, 34, 39). Sheltered seating areas can provide a comfortable space to rest and passively enjoy the outdoor scenery for those with low energy levels, and can be located in quiet areas to provide a private space outside or can be situated near high-traffic areas to encourage social interaction (25, 38, 39).

Concluding thoughts: the complexity of 'home' in designing for end of life care

As the concept of 'home' holds powerful social and symbolic meaning and is connected to maintenance and support of self-identity in older people, it is important that the design concepts associated with 'home-like' environment should be incorporated in the design of end of life care settings. Within long-term care environments, there is an increasing recognition that person-centred models of care are essential for providing optimal care. Indeed, promoting an institutional environment as 'home' or 'home-like' is equated with best practice in design of institutions and is a method for evaluating quality of life. In this respect, it is not surprising that most hospices are domestic in nature—both in terms of scale and ambience, giving the 'visual reassurance which enables people to enter unafraid and to find within them a sense of calm, light, space, peace and supportive order' (39). Design of residential care facilities are increasingly becoming domestic in nature or at the very least, being designed as homes as opposed to places where one accesses health care (43).

Notwithstanding the relevance and richness of 'home' as a benchmark for creating a supportive end of life care environment, the meaning of 'homelike' environment remains open-ended and subjective. Two basic issues need to be acknowledged and addressed in this regard. The physical environmental aspects of a homelike setting do not work in isolation of the social and organizational milieu. The full potential of a homelike physical environment can afford positive experiences when the social interactions and relationships are supportive of the end of life experience. For example, a view of the garden from one's bedroom can be effected by the design of the room, window, and landscaping. However, at another level, the garden could be better experienced for some individuals if they are able to actually go outside with the assistance of staff members. What is the value of an outdoor space if access to it is restricted due to facility policy or lack of appropriate staffing? Care approaches and a physical environment that compete with each other only add to confusion and incongruence (44). Thus, organizations need to be flexible and willing to tailor the environment to reflect the lived experiences of the older people who reside there. Organizational structures, care approaches, and the physical environment must be aligned to create a therapeutic environment (45). Without these integrating components, the benefits of a supportive physical environment can be undermined. A place gains meaning when the physical and social aspects of the experience are aligned and supportive of each other.

A second aspect concerning the 'home-like' physical environment supportive of a person-centred dying experience is related to the cultural background of the individuals. 'Homelike' and family-oriented healing environments are experienced in the context of cultural notions of privacy, social interaction, independence, etc. Design decisions based on normative expectations of how environment can support behaviour need to be sensitive of cultural variations in activities and beliefs. The process of a desired dying process is individually, socially, and culturally shaped necessitating a need to take a multifaceted approach and associated care-planning strategies. Culture itself needs to be situated in the religious or faith based context of the individual. What might be the religious or spiritual practices and beliefs that are part of one's frame of mind and need to be supported by the environment? There could be individual and social dimensions as well.

Much research needs to happen in expanding theoretical understanding, empirical evidence and strategies for implementation in practice. There needs to be a conceptual exploration of person-environment interaction in the last phase of life in terms of how it might be different or nuanced from our current understanding. The environmental scale, sensory properties, mobility, familiarity, etc. represent a few of the relevant environmental issues that could be taken into account as we consider the possible nature of this relationship. Given the dearth of empirical studies on the role of physical environment at the end of life phase, it is critical that multiple studies undertake well-grounded approach in examining the impact of micro- and macroscale environmental issues, private and public spaces, interrelationships of sensory characteristics, elements of nature, etc. on objective and subjective aspects of the dying phase of older people. It is important to design studies that are based on population-based contexts as well as qualitative approaches that will lead to a rich and deeper understanding of the environmental experience. Finally, intervention studies with environmental modifications in the private and public spaces could explore the feasibility and efficacy of renovation in existing hospice or long-term care facility environments. Most importantly, it would be critical not to lose sight of the important role of physical environment at the end of life for older people and the positive role it can play in supporting a positive living and dying experience.

References

1. Ulrich R (2006). Evidence-based health care architecture. *Lancet*, **368**: S38–S39.
2. Lynn J (2002). A commentary: Where to live while dying. *The Gerontologist*, **42**: 68–70.
3. Mezey M, Dubler N, Mitty E, Brody A (2002). What impact do setting and transitions have on the quality of life at the end of life and the quality of the dying process? *The Gerontologist*, **3**: 54–67.
4. Davis S, Byers S, Nay R, Koch S (2009). Guiding design of dementia-friendly environments in residential care settings: Considering the living experiences. *Dementia*, **8**(2): 185–203.
5. Bowling A (1983). The hospitalization of death: Should more people die at home. *Journal of Medical Ethics*, **9**: 158–61.
6. Fisher R, Ross MM, MacLean MJ (2000). *End of life care for Canadian seniors*. Toronto: University of Toronto.
7. Arras J, Neveloff DN (1994). Bringing the hospital home: Ethical and social implications of high-tech home care. *Hastings Center Report*, **24**(Special Supplement 5): S19–S28.

8. Tofle R (2009). Creating a place for dying: Gerontopia. *Journal of Housing for the Elderly*, **23**(1): 66–91.

9. Noddings N (1994). Moral obligation or moral support for high-tech home care. *Hastings Centre Report*, **24**: S6–13.

10. Rubinstein RL (1990). Culture and disorder in the home care experience: The home as sickroom. In J Gubrium, A Sankar (eds) *The home care experience*, pp. 37–57. Newbury Park, CA: Sage.

11. Lynn J, Adamson DM (2003). *Living well at the end of life: Adapting health care to serious chronic illness in old age*. Rand White Paper. Available at: http://www.rand.org. (Accessed 3 March 2009.)

12. Yamasaki M, Ebihara S, Freeman S, Ebihara T, Asada M, Yamanda S, et al. (2008). Sex differences in the preference for place of death in community-dwelling elderly people in Japan. *Journal of the American Geriatrics Society*, **56**: 376.

13. Gott M, Seymour J, Bellamy G, Clark D, Ahmedzai, S (2004). Older people's views about home as a place of care at the end of life. *Palliative Medicine*, **18**: 460–7.

14. Volicer L, Hurley A, Blasi Z (2003). Characteristics of dementia and end-of-life care across care settings. *American Journal of Hospice and Palliative Care*, **20**(3): 191–200.

15. Angus J, Kontos P, Dyck I, McKeever P, Poland B (2005). The personal significance of home: Habitus and the experience of receiving long-term home care. *Sociology of Health and Illness*, **27**(2): 161–87.

16. Dyck I, Kontos P, Angus J, McKeever P (2005). The home as a site for long term care: Meanings and management of bodies and spaces. *Health and Place*, **11**(2): 173–85.

17. Mahmood A, Martin-Matthews A (2009). Dynamics of carework: Boundary management and relationship issues for home support workers and elderly clients. In A Martin-Matthews, JE Phillips (eds) *Ageing and caring at the intersection of work and home life: Blurring the boundaries*. New York: Lawrence Erlbaum Associates.

18. Tamm M (1999). What does a home mean and when does it cease to be a home? Home as a setting for rehabilitation and care. *Disability and Rehabilitation*, **21**: 49–55.

19. Canadian Hospice and Palliative Care Association. Available at: http://www.chpca.net/general_information.html. (Accessed 22 March 2010.)

20. Becher MM (1999). *Hospice: A place for the dying*. Calgary: University of Calgary.

21. Kayser-Jones J, Chan J, Kris A (2005). Model long-term care hospice unit: care, community, and compassion. *Geriatric Nursing*, **26**(1): 16–25.

22. Wagner JDC (1999). *Hospice affirming life: a sanctuary for palliative care and bereavement (British Columbia)*. Calgary: University of Calgary.

23. Zweig S, Oliver D (2009). Returning from the total institution to a home environment: A journey for birthing and dying. *Journal of Housing for the Elderly*, **23**(1): 116–29.

24. Movahed A (1994). *Physical and environmental features that contribute to satisfaction with hospice facilities*. Portland, OR: Portland State University.

25. Verderber S, Refuerzo B (2006). *Innovations in hospice architecture*. New York: Taylor & Francis.

26. Sherman E, Dacher, J (2005). Cherished objects and the home: Their meaning and roles in late life. In G Rowles, H Chaudhury (eds) *Home and identity in later life*, pp. 63–80. New York: Springer.

27. Renzi J (2008). Life and afterlife. *Interior design*, **79** (2): 104–7.

28. Rowlands J, Noble S (2008). How does the environment impact on the quality of life of advanced cancer patients? A qualitative study with implications for ward design. *Palliative Medicine*, **22**: 768–75.

29. Kaufman SR (2005). *And a time to die: How American hospitals shape the end of life*. Chicago, IL: University of Chicago Press.

30. Edvardsson D (2008). Therapeutic environments for older adults: Constituents and meanings. *Journal of Gerontological Nursing*, **34**(6): 32–40.

31. Russell C, Middleton H, Shanley C (2008). Dying with dementia: The views of family caregivers about quality of life. *Australasian Journal on Ageing*, **27**(2): 89–98.

32. Kayser-Jones J, Schell E, Lyons W, Kris A, Chan J, Beard R (2003). Factors that influence end-of-life care in nursing homes: the physical environment, inadequate staffing, and lack of supervision. *The Gerontologist*, **43**(Special Issue 2): 76–84.

33. Chaudhury H, Mahmood A, Valente M (2005). Advantages and disadvantages of single vs. double occupancy patient rooms in acute care environments: A review and analysis of the literature. *Environment and Behavior*, **37**(6): 760–86.

34. Brawley E (2006). *Design innovations for ageing and Alzheimer's: Creating caring environments.* Hoboken, NJ: Wiley.

35. Vohra J, Brazil K, Szala-Meneok K (2006). The last word: family members' descriptions of end-of-life care in long-term care facilities. *Journal of Palliative Care*, **22**(1): 33–9.

36. Ryder J (1999). Design Centre—Petaluma Hospice. *Nursing Homes/Long Term Care Management*, **48**(4): Centerfold (6).

37. Jones G, van der Eerden W (2008). Designing care environments for persons with Alzheimer's disease: visuoperceptual considerations. *Reviews in Clinical Gerontology*, **18**: 13–37.

38. Tyson M (1998). *Healing landscape: therapeutic outdoor environments*, 2nd edn. Madison, WI: University of Wisconsin-Madison.

39. Worpole K (2009). *Modern hospice design: The architecture of palliative care.* New York: Routledge.

40. Gentilli A, Weiner DK, Kuchibhatil M, Edinger, JD (1997). Factors that disturb sleep in nursing home residents. *Ageing*, **9**: 207–13.

41. Cohen-Mansfield J, Werner P (1995). Environmental influences on agitation: An integrative summary of an observational study. *American Journal of Alzheimer's Care and Related Disorders*, **10**: 32–9.

42. Kwack H, Relf PD, Rudolph J (2005). Adapting garden activities for overcoming fifficulties of individuals with dementia and physical limitations. *Activities, Adaptation & Ageing*, **29**(1): 1–13.

43. Commission for Architecture and the Built Environment (CABE: 2009). Homes for our old age. Available at: http://www.cabe.org.uk/files/homes-for-our-old-age.pdf. (Accessed 30 October 2009.)

44. Keane WL, Shoesmith JAM (2005). Creating the ideal person-centred program and environment for residential dementia care: 10 steps and 10 challenges toward a new culture. *Alzheimer's Care Quarterly*, **6**: 316–24.

45. Cohen U, Moore KD (1999). Integrating cultural heritage into assisted living environments. In B Schwarz, R Brent (eds) *Ageing, Autonomy, and Architecture: Advances in Assisted Living*, pp. 90–109. Baltimore, MA: Johns Hopkins Press.

Chapter 18

Improving care for older people living and dying in long-term care settings: a whole system approach

Katherine Froggatt, Kevin Brazil, Jo Hockley, and Elisabeth Reitinger

Introduction

Better palliative care for older people is, as has been described, a worldwide priority (1). The long-term care context has been identified as a setting where palliative care is provided for older people towards the end of life, internationally (1) and nationally; for example, in the UK (2), Austria (3), and Canada (4). A significant proportion of older people die in these settings with figures ranging from 13% in Austria (5), 20% in England (6), to 39% in Canada (4). In this chapter we will use the term long-term care settings to describe the range of institutions and organizations that provide health and social care for older people in a collective environment that is not a domestic home, hospital or hospice. We draw specifically upon examples from the UK, Canada, and Austria to illustrate our discussions.

In this chapter we will outline the current knowledge about the provision of palliative care in long-term care settings. The challenges that exist in supporting older people to die well in long-term care settings across the whole health and social care system are also outlined. In response to these challenges, examples of interventions that have been implemented across the different levels in the system are presented as ways to raise the quality of care provision in this setting for older people. In this chapter we do not aim to describe how to provide palliative care for older people living and dying in long-term care settings; rather we wish to critically consider, using a whole system perspective, the ways in which palliative care provision has been developed in, for, and with, this setting and indicate the importance of a whole system perspective for this work. In this chapter a whole system perspective means a consideration of all the elements of the health and social care system that shape the care an individual receives, from the staff that care for him or her, through to the organizational culture and wider agencies that work together to support people towards the end of life.

Long-term care settings: context and cultures

Many countries worldwide are addressing similar questions about how to provide appropriate care and support for older people as they live with ongoing disabilities, adverse health events, or increasing frailty (7). Whilst many countries would seek to find ways to enable people to live in their own homes, for some individuals because of their specific health needs and their particular social circumstances, a move into an institutional setting is required.

The complexity of the long-term care context can be captured across a number of dimensions that encompass the whole health and social care system (Table 18.1): the types of long-term care settings, the status of long-term care providers, how long-term care is funded, and the place and form of regulation of the sector. Whilst there are similarities between different developed countries, differences also exist. Under a generic term of long-term care settings there appear to exist different types of support and care, dependent upon the nature of the needs an older person is assessed to have. A differentiation is often made between personal and health care needs, with some settings providing personal and nursing care as in nursing homes (Austria), and care homes (nursing) (UK). Other settings only provide personal care in retirement homes (Austria) and care homes (personal care) (UK). Nursing and medical care is provided from primary care services for long-term care settings that provide only personal care, but nursing care is available on-site in nursing homes. In the three countries considered here the funding status of long-term care providers sits across the private, public, and not-for profit sector. Interestingly Austria has the highest proportion of public sector providers (53%), in contrast to the UK (12%) and Canada (18%). The UK has a high proportion of private providers (74%) which encompass large global international businesses to small individual owner manager homes. Not-for-profit providers are present in all three countries, often meeting the needs of specific faith and ethnic cultural groups. Funding for care in long-term care settings again draws upon a range of sources in these three countries indicating the challenge it is to finance long-term care for older people. Whilst state/public funding is available for elements of care this is often means tested or provided on the basis of a needs assessment. In Austria, diverse levels of reliance on universal public health care systems, health insurance, and social insurance systems can be observed which reflects an ongoing debate about the scope and coverage of public funding.

Regulation of the long-term care sector is present in different forms: some countries have more national legislation (England, Scotland), others have fewer regulations at a national level and more on a provincial level (Canada, Austria). National standards for care in these settings are also present and are then used as a basis for regular inspections. These processes of regulation are one way in which provision of high-quality care is ensured and maintained in the sector, but for specific areas of care, e.g. palliative care, other more targeted drivers for change exist: these include national strategies within palliative care (England) and more general policy initiatives that indirectly influence the use of long-term care settings (Austria, Canada, England).

It is possible to identify developments that have been undertaken to support the provision of palliative care in long-term care settings working at different levels in many countries. These include interventions that seek to promote care for individuals classified as either as: decision-making interventions; care pathways for the last days of life; and specific support for individuals at the point of and following death (11). At a service provision level interventions have been classified as follows: the provision of hospice services; the establishment of specialist palliative care units; and use of consultation services (12). However, the evidence of their effectiveness and impact remains generally descriptive and small scale (11, 13), reflecting that only recently has palliative care provision in long-term care settings been considered seriously. Research in the area has also only recently begun alongside the clinical developments. Evidence derived from the research to date that has initially arisen from local needs and issues has therefore remained less predictive and generalizable (11).

Key challenges to the delivery of high-quality care towards the end of life

A number of key challenges shape the nature and extent of palliative care developments within these settings. These concern the varying needs of the older people resident in these settings and their family, the different concerns of family and friends, issues of staffing and team working, the

Table 18.1 Long-tern care settings

Country	Terminology and types	Status of long-term care providers	Funding for long-term care	Regulation	Key drivers for change
Austria (8–11)	*Nursing homes*: provide personal and nursing care (domestic help and basic care), 24 hours a day, 7 days a week. Medical care (medical treatment) is provided by primary care service providers	Three types of provider: 1) Public provision, especially community supply (53%)	Federal funding for long-term care (received by person in need, care levels from 1 to 7) Provincial funding for long-term care (received by person in need)	On national level: Nursing home residency statutes ('Heiaufenthalts-gesetz'); nursing home contract statutes ('Heimvertragsgesetz').	Federal and National concepts that include Palliative Care for nursing homes
	Retirement homes: provide a place of residence and personal care if necessary. Focus on social activities and social care	2) NPOs (non-profit organizations), many of them established by confessional providers (26%)	For all: medical treatment covered by statutory health insurance. Private contributions towards care: pensions, private care insurance, personal assets, assets of relatives[a]	On provincial level: Provincial legislation regulates care standards and structural frames	Regional projects integrating Hospice and Palliative Care into long-term care settings
	Geriatric centres: provide personal, nursing, and medical care 24 hours a day, 7 day a week. Focus is on medical and interdisciplinary health care	3) Private providers (21%)		No legal regulations concerning Palliative Care Guidelines for the implementation and development of Hospice and Palliative Care in nursing homes.	Efforts to improve quality of care and life within nursing homes: 'National certificate of Quality' (NQZ)[b]
Canada (Ontario)	Long-term care homes (nursing homes or homes for the aged) are designed for people who require 24-hour nursing care and supervision within a secure setting. Medical care is provided by primary care services, and other health professionals	Approximately 600 LTC homes in Ontario. Three types of LTC home ownership: 1) Private corporation (57% of LTC homes)	The Ontario Ministry of Health and Long-term Care provides funding for LTC homes which will cover nursing and personal care; programming and support services; food; and other accommodations. The amount paid by residents for their accommodation is called a 'co-payment'. The amount depends on the	Three pieces of provincial legislation govern long-term care homes. 1) Homes for the Aged and Rest Homes Act	Public policy to minimize the use of hospitals and mental instructions'
		2) Non-profit corporations such as faith, community, ethnic, or cultural groups (25% of LTC homes)	type of accommodation (private, semi-private, and ward). If resident income is not sufficient to pay for basic accommodation, there is a subsidy available to reduce accommodation rates. Subsidies are only available for basic accommodation Nursing, personal care,	2) Nursing Home Act 3) Charitable Institutions Act The Ontario Ministry of Health and Long-Term Care set standards for care and inspect long-term care homes annually. The Ministry also encourages homes to get accredited by	
		3) Municipally-run facilities (18% of LTC homes)	medical care, and other therapies to assist optimal level of functioning are publicly funded Residents have the option of privately purchasing further personal care	Accreditation Canada by providing a funding incentive to accredited homes. The Ministry also conducts annual compliance reviews and homes are required to post this report to make it available to residents, families and prospective residents	

(Continued)

Table 18.1 (Continued)

Country	Terminology and types	Status of long-term care providers	Funding for long-term care	Regulation	Key drivers for change
UK (England)	Care homes (nursing) provide personal and nursing care 24 hours a day, 7 days a week. Medical care provided by primary care services Care homes (personal care) provide only personal care. Nursing and medical care provided by primary care services	In the UK: 15,700 care homes (OFT 2005) Mixed provider status: 1) Private provision (74%): corporate organizations; small business chains; owner managed enterprises 2) Not for profit organizations (14%): large chains to small groups 3) Public sector provision (12%) in some places	Mixed Individual is means tested provision Needs assessed for nursing care provision in nursing homes, but nursing care provided free to residents in care homes (personal care) by primary care nurses Medical care free to all, although some care homes may pay GPs a retainer for extra services such as regular visits to the care home.	National Minimum Standards exist against which care homes are inspected by an inspectorate now located in a health care body (Care Quality Commission)	End of Life Strategy (2) Strong emphasis upon improvement of care in care homes. The National Dementia Strategy (Department of Health, 2009) identifies needs of people with dementia towards the end of life needing to be met, many of whom are living in care homes

aDifferent regulations exist in the nine provinces of Austria.

bhttp://www.e-qalin.net (Accessed 3 August 2009.)

culture of care, and wider organizational constraints (14). Alongside these challenges, inherent to the system of care provision, lie factors associated with the processes by which change is brought about within the long-term care sector with respect to palliative care provision. Of particular concern here are the issues of transferability and sustainability (15).

The resident population is changing with an increasingly frail population living with multiple morbidities, a higher incidence of dementia, and a range of complex physical, psychological, social, and spiritual needs to be met (16). Family members too, are not a unified group and the specific dynamics within any family group require specific attention (14). Gender aspects also have to be taken into account: residents, professionals, relatives, informal care givers, and volunteers are primarily women (17).

Quality care is of paramount importance to long-term care settings and the ability to provide such care depends on its employees. There are a number of issues and challenges that staff in these settings face in relation to end of life care (18–21). Staff turnover is an important issue (22). Factors found to be associated with turnover specifically in nursing homes include working hours, advancement opportunities, communication, role clarity, autonomy, participation in decision-making, supervision, and keeping employees informed (22, 23). Addressing staffing issues in these settings is complex. Decision-makers are required to consider a range of issues related not only to sufficient staffing levels, but also to such factors as, training, service delivery models, and the use of team approaches to care as well as staff skill mix and experience (24).

Within long-term care settings, organizational research has shown that, alongside professional values, management and leadership play an essential role for giving care in a needs-oriented way. Values that influence perceptions, communication, and decision processes are crucial in understanding the logic of the dominant cultures within an institution. Therefore management can be seen as an important factor influencing the practice of palliative care in nursing homes (3, 25) Leadership influences the culture of care in long-term care settings. There has been an emphasis in many long-term care settings on a rehabilitative philosophy of enablement in order for an older person's potential to be maximized (18, 26). This has led to staff isolation with respect to training in palliative care/end of life care (21, 27) as this approach to care has not been recognized within the focus on rehabilitation.

Wider societal attitudes also make the development of palliative care in long-term care settings a challenge (14). The marginalization of older people and the care settings where they reside has not facilitated innovative developments to care. Attitudes about death and dying in today's modern society, mean that dying as a 'natural, final event' in old age has been usurped by technologies now available to maintain life at any cost (28). A 'striving to keep alive' mentality can then be present within the staff encouraging a closed communication culture that limits learning and expertise in death and dying (21, 29).

Process issues regarding change management also shape the development of palliative care in long-term care settings. The transferability of palliative care as an approach to care in long-term care settings has to address the issues of attitudes and beliefs just outlined, alongside the underlying investment of such initiatives (15). Too often, short-term funding initiates developments, but this is not always sustained, leaving staff frustrated and isolated again.

Framing good practice

Although challenges exist and shape the nature of palliative care provided for, and experienced by, older people in long-term care settings, they are not insurmountable. In this section we describe three initiatives which have been undertaken to support the development of palliative care in long-term care settings in Canada (Enhanced Care Project), the UK (collaborative learning groups), and Austria (transdisciplinary organizational development).

The Enhanced Care Project

This quality initiative was focused upon individuals as it sought to improve care by educating the staff working in one institution: St Joseph's Villa, a long-term care facility in Hamilton, Ontario, Canada.

Increasing resident complexity in care needs requires staff expertise that is often not available. Recognizing the need to strengthen staff capacity and competency to deliver better care, St Joseph's Villa, a 378-bed long-term care home, launched the Enhanced Care Project. Funded by the Ontario Government, as a 19-month demonstration project, the leadership in the facility identified the importance of developing educational support for frontline staff to improve the quality of their work life and improve resident care. The initiative was designed to optimize the role for health care aides and personal support workers. Although these workers had some clinical skills training, the skills were rarely used in their daily practice. The main objective of the programme was to both enhance and support the use of clinical skills as well as foster greater ability to contribute in a team approach to care.

Initially, a learning needs assessment was completed to determine educational needs in the facility. The gaps identified contributed to the development of training sessions that included both class room instruction combined with e-learning modules. Four modules were developed by facility staff, with input from experts and the literature. The completed modules included clinical and leadership content alongside clinical content regarding: 1) respiration and hydration; 2) vital signs, 3) pain management, 4) dementia.

A total of 140 staff participated in a programme that consisted of four half-day training sessions. Throughout the demonstration period efforts were made to share key messages generated by the project with all staff in the facility, via posters and newsletter. Participants who took part in the training sessions reported an increase in their level of knowledge and confidence in regards to the training material. Clinical observers responsible for documenting the transfer of clinical training from the classroom to the bedside reported most participants were effective in applying trained skills into practice. Participants who participated in post-programme focus groups reported the programme meeting their expectations and had increased their confidence in providing care.

Collaborative learning groups

Experienced-based learning as a way of improving knowledge about end of life care for staff in long-term care settings would appear to be a useful tool in light of some of the issues highlighted earlier. In order to create a greater learning culture amongst staff, collaborative learning groups (CLGs) (experienced-based learning groups) were set up on two nursing care homes in Scotland in the UK (21). The groups met 5–7 days following the death of a resident in the home. The groups comprised of staff from the both morning and afternoon shifts; some staff while on a 'day-off' attended if they had been particularly involved with the resident prior to the death. Domestic and kitchen staff also attended on occasions alongside some night staff. The groups were scheduled to last no longer than 45 minutes.

The CLGs followed a clear format (Table 18.2).

This format gave the group a degree of structure but also allowed flexibility for staff to participate within the CLGs as they felt able. At the beginning of each session, one of the staff present gave a brief résumé of the resident's life, their time in the nursing home, and their family. Group members

Table 18.2 Stages of CLG session

---

1. Brief résumé of resident/family whose death was being discussed.

2. What happened?

- Description of own and other peoples' actions/involvement

- Different times, shifts, experiences

3. How did the participants feel?

- Exploration of personal and interpersonal feelings

- Anticipation of unexpected expressions of emotion

- What was 'good' . . . what was 'bad'?

4. What does it mean?

What can we learn . . . how does practice need changing?

---

were invited to 'tell what happened' on the different shifts during the last few days of the resident's life which created a collective narrative around the death. Arising from the accounts, specific issues related to the situation were identified and could then be addressed, e.g. issues of pain control for people with dementia.

The CLGs facilitated the discussion of topics relevant to the older age context instead of formal teaching sessions being superimposed from a background in specialist palliative care. As a result, topics specific to end of life care in their setting actively engaged staff members. The CLGs enabled staff to talk openly about not only their own fears and concerns of death and dying but also how they might improve their care of the resident who was dying and the family. Three core functions have been identified for these groups (21): educational, communicative, and supportive. Education was not just from the basic premise of 'being taught' but there was evidence that staff were also gaining greater in-depth understanding as well as starting to critically think through some of the issues. The support and communication with the wider team were also very positive elements reported by those who took part in the CLGs (21).

Organizational development through transdisciplinary cooperation

A well-developed example of transdisciplinary cooperative projects between long-term care settings and the wider system exists in Austria. Here the Faculty for Interdisciplinary Research and Education (IFF) Department of Palliative Care and Organizational Ethics has worked with long-term care providers in both Austria and Germany (30–32). The first project ('Organizational Culture of Dying') using this methodology for the development of palliative care in long-term care settings was a partnership between the Diakonie (a not-for-profit provider in Düsseldorf, Germany) and the IFF Department of Palliative Care and Organizational Ethics in Vienna, Austria. Three main parameters shaped this project (30, 33):

1) Resident-focused orientation: the perspectives of those who were concerned with living and dying within nursing homes were the main drivers for change.

2) Organizational change: the project design made sure that interdisciplinary cooperation across hierarchies and homes took place. The project architecture connected the different social systems (management, homes, the project coordinator, public relations, and research) in a systematic coordinated way.

3) Participation of staff and knowledge management: the learning processes aim to include all those who were involved.

In this approach to organizational development the following elements were present at different levels, external to, and within the long-term care organizations concerned:

- *Steering committee or round tables:* leading members of the long-term care institutions and researchers formed a team that was responsible for formulating the aims, processes and decision making of the project. The executives of the parent organizations were involved as well as the individual facilities.

- *Individual homes and project groups:* within each individual home a specific palliative care project group was established. Specific issues were identified by members of the staff working in the home. Issues that were addressed included: ethical dilemmas, use of rituals, communication with relatives. One way that was used to find out more about the needs of residents and relatives was to educate the care staff in ways to communicate with their residents about their needs concerning their end of life.

- *Interactive discussions:* an important part of the change process within these projects was the establishment of spaces where open dialogue could occur between groups and people who may not have had contact before. Thus discussion rounds between different homes, between homes and parent organizations, or between different parent organizations provided participants with an opportunity to learn from the perspectives of others. Learning from differences, and learning through unexpected connections of people, professions, and social settings were important concepts that lay behind these initiatives (34).

- *Analyses and reflection within the research team:* reflective sessions within the research team were undertaken. These helped to identify assumptions and formulate assessments of the actual situation and new perspectives for further steps. Conflicts that flared up within the research team often mirrored tensions within the cooperating organization and showed where critical issues and themes existed (32, 35).

- *Feedback processes and validation:* the findings were converted into presentations, shared within the project teams and then discussed by practitioners and researchers. Findings about how end-of-life care was provided and what changes were desired led to agreements which further the development of a palliative care culture with management and staff. These presentations also reappraised and validated the findings.

- *Public relations:* in order to publicize the project and its results to the broader public, exhibitions, open house, symposia, or publications were organized.

Developing a way forward

The initiatives we have described here work at different levels across the whole health and social care system. We utilize Ferlie and Shortell's framework (36) to understand better the strengths of addressing palliative care provision in multiple levels present in and around long-term care settings. Ferlie and Shortell (36) argue that four levels of change are required to maximize the probability of success in promoting sustainable organizational change: at the level of individuals, teams, organizations, and the wider system.

Beginning at the level of the individual care workers, education and training is an important consideration (37). The different ways this education can be undertaken are illustrated within the examples described above. Most care is provided in a team-based environment; reinforcing a collaborative team-based approach to resident care can be an enabler for improving care and meeting the demands that individual providers face. The collaborative learning groups described earlier were one way to develop teams within an organization. Improving collaboration and teamwork across occupational groups can assist caregivers to work even more effectively.

There is mounting evidence that this process, described as interprofessional care, offers multiple benefits (38).

However, efforts to target individual providers or teams are little more than symbolic gestures if institutional leadership is not shown to support these initiatives. Institutional leadership is required to support systems, processes, and tools that will allow individual providers and teams to be organized and practised in a systematic way (36). The wider perspectives taken by the Austrian organizational development approach addresses this level of change. A further example of an intervention that has been developed that addresses multiple levels in the system can be seen in the Australian initiative to develop Palliative Care Guidelines for Residential Aged Care Facilities, which is described in Chapters 19 and 24, this volume. Change strategies also require larger systems reform such as the determination of adequate funding for the long-term care system or improved external oversight that hold nursing homes accountable for quality care (37). According to Heimerl (33), a palliative culture needs intervention to address values and attitudes as well as personal and organizational actions and knowledge. Thus, four fields of change can be described: palliative care attitudes; palliative care knowledge; implicit and explicit values of the organization and communication structures; and decision making.

Conclusions

In terms of the provision of palliative care for older people residing in long-term care settings we have identified that older people living in such settings often have complex needs. The location of the sector crosses different health and social care economies so making the funding and delivery of care similarly complex. We have provided examples of initiatives that have addressed one or more levels of quality improvement change as identified by Ferlie and Shortell (36). Generally the current evidence as regards the impact of these initiatives is generally descriptive and small scale and we agree with the recommendations from Shipman et al. (39) that there is a need for more rigorous evaluations of interventions and initiatives to identify their efficacy, costs, and benefits. As illustrated by these different international examples there is no one optimal way of implementing palliative care in long-term care settings for frail older people. Cultural, structural, and economical factors all influence the manner in which change processes are undertaken and organizational, professional, and personal values, competences, and backgrounds shape the palliative care approaches which seem to be appropriate within a specific setting. Current work by a recently implemented Taskforce on Palliative Care in Long-Term Care Settings for Older People, under the auspices of the European Association of Palliative Care, will seek to identify these different approaches across Europe, and internationally, and appraise their prevalence.

We therefore argue that many well-intentioned efforts to improve care of the dying in long-term care settings will fail unless policy and practice decision-makers consider and implement a comprehensive, multilevel approach towards improving care. Whether change to improve quality of care for the dying is top-down or bottom-up, whether it occurs incrementally or dramatically, change must be considered from a multilevel perspective. In order to meet the needs of individuals we recommend that best practice be shared internationally using a whole system approach to ensure that the development of quality care for older people living and dying in these organizations is attained.

Acknowledgements

The authors acknowledge the European Association of Palliative Care and their support for the Taskforce on Palliative Care in Long-Term Care Settings for Older People and Katharina Heimerl for her support regarding the Austrian perspective.

References

1. Davies E, Higginson I (2004). *Better Palliative Care for Older People*. Copenhagen: World Health Organization.

2. Department of Health (2008). *End of Life Care Strategy—promoting high quality care for all adults at the end of life*. London: Department of Health.

3. Heller A, Dinges S, Heimerl K, Reitinger E, Wegleitner K (2003). Palliative Kultur in der stationären Altenhilfe. *Zeitschrift für Gerontologie und Geriatrie*, **36**: 360–5.

4. National Advisory Committee on End-of-Life Care for Seniors, Fisher R, Ross M, Maclean M (eds) (2001). *A Guide to End-of-Life Care for Seniors*. Toronto: University of Toronto.

5. Statistics Austria (2009). *Todesursachenstatistik 1984–2008. Table of places of death*. Vienna: Statistics Austria.

6. Office for National Statistics (2008). *Mortality Statistics. Deaths registered in 2008*. London: Office for National Statistics.

7. Froggatt K, Davies S, Meyer J (2009) Research and development in care homes: setting the scene. In K Froggatt, S Davies, J Meyer (eds) *Understanding Care Homes: A Research and Development Perspective*, pp. 9–22. London: Jessica Kingsley Press.

8. Badelt C, Österle A (2001)*Grundzüge der Sozialpolitik. Sozialpolitik in Österreich*. In *Spezieller Teil, 2. Auflage*. Vienna: Manz.

9. Federal Ministry of Social Security Generations and Consumer Protection (2005). *Provision for long-term care in Austria*. Vienna: Federal Ministry of Social Security.

10. Hospiz Österreich (2008). *Umsetzung und Entwicklung von Hospiz und Palliative Care im Pflegeheim. Arbeitsgruppe Hospiz und Palliative Care im Pflegeheim*. Wern: Hospiz Österreich.

11. Froggatt K, Wilson D, Justice C (2006). End-of-life care in long-term care settings for older people: a literature review. *International Journal of Older People Nursing*, **1**: 45–50.

12. Ersek M, Wilson S (2003). The challenges and opportunities in providing end-of-life care in nursing homes. *Journal of Palliative Medicine*, **6**(1): 45–57.

13. Goodman C, Evans C, Wilcock J, Froggatt K, DrennanV, Sampson E, et al. (2010) End of life care for community dwelling older people with dementia: an integrated review. *International Journal of Geriatric Psychiatry*, **25**(4): 329–37.

14. Froggatt K (2004) *Palliative Care in Care Homes for Older People*. London: The National Council for Palliative Care.

15. Abbey J, Froggatt K, Parker D, Abbey B (2006). Palliative care in long-term care: a system in change. *International Journal of Older People Nursing*, **1**: 56–63.

16. Bowman CE, Whistler J, Ellerby M (2004). A national census of care home residents. *Age and Ageing*, **33**: 561–6.

17. Milligan C (2009). *There's No Place Like Home: Place and Care in an Ageing Society*. Farnham: Ashgate.

18. Hanson L, Henderson M, Menon M (2002). As individual as death itself: A focus group study of terminal care in nursing homes. *Journal of Palliative Medicine*, **5**(1): 117–25.

19. Forbes-Thompson S, Gessert C (2005). End of life in nursing homes: connections between structure, process and outcomes. *Journal of Palliative Medicine*, **8**(3): 545–55.

20. Kayser-Jones J, Schell E, Lyons W, Kris AE, Chan J, Beard RL (2003). Factors that influence end-of-life care in nursing homes: the physical environment, inadequate staffing, and lack of supervision. *The Gerontologist*, **43**: 76–84.

21. Hockley J (2006) *Developing high quality end-of-life care in nursing homes: an action research study. Unpublished PhD*. Edinburgh: University of Edinburgh.

22. Cohen-Mansfield J (1997) Turnover among nursing home staff. A review. *Nursing Management*, **28**(5): 59–62.

23. Parsons S, Simmons WP, Penn K, Furlough M (2003). Determinants of Satisfaction and Turnover Among Nursing Assistants. The Results of a Statewide Survey. *Journal of Gerontological Nursing*, **29**: 51–8.

24. Chou S, Boldy D, Lee A (2002). Staff satisfaction and its components in residential aged care. *International Journal for Quality in Health Care*, **14**: 207–17.

25. Reitinger E (2006) *Bedürfnismanagement in der stationären Altenhilfe*. Systemtheoretische Analyse empirischer Evidenzen. Heidelberg: Systemische Forschung im Carl-Auer Verlag.

26. RCP, RCN, BGS (2000). *The health and care of older people in care homes: a comprehensive interdisciplinary approach. A report of a joint working party*. London: Royal College of Physicians.

27. Komaromy C, Sidell M, Katz J (2000) The quality of terminal care in residential and nursing homes. *International Journal of Palliative Nursing*, **6**(4): 192–200.

28. McCue JD (1995). The naturalness of dying. *Journal of the American Medical Association*, **273**(13): 1039–45.

29. Travis S, Loving G, McClanahan L, Bernard M (2001). Hospitalisation patterns and palliation in the last year of life among residents in long-term care. *The Gerontologist*, **41**(2): 153–60.

30. Heimerl K, Heller A, Stelling C (2001) Regeln, Routinen, Rituale in den 'Leben im Alter Zentren': Organisations Kultur des Sterbens von Diakonie in Düsseldorf. In K Heimerl, A Heller (eds). *Eine grosse Vision in kleinen Schritten. Aus Modellen der Hospiz- und Palliativbetreuung lernen*, pp. 131–39. Freiburg im Breisgau: Lambertus.

31. Pleschberger S (2007). Dignity and the challenge of dying in nursing homes: the residents' view. *Age and Ageing*, **36**(2): 197–202.

32. Reitinger E (ed) (2008) *Transdisziplinäre Praxis. Forschen im Sozial-und Gesundheitswesen*. Heidelberg: Systemische Forschung im Carl Auer Verlag.

33. Heimerl K (2006) *Palliative Care in Organisationen umsetzen. Habilitationsschrift zur Erlangung der venia legendi in Palliative Care und Organisationsentwicklung*. Self published. Vienna.

34. Grossmann R, Heimerl K, Heller A, Scala K (1997). Organisierte GesellschaftIff-texte. Bd. 1. In R Grossmann (ed) *Wie wird Wissen wirksam?* pp. 43–51. Wien/New York: Springer.

35. Zepke G (2005). *Reflexionsarchitekturen. Evaluierung als Beitrag zum Organisationslernen*. Heidelberg: Systemische Forschung im Carl-Auer Verlag.

36. Ferlie E, Shortell S (2001). Improving the quality of health care in the United Kingdom and the United States: A framework for change. *The Millbank Quarterly*, **79**(2): 281–315.

37. Institute of Medicine, Wunderlich G, Kohler P (eds) (2001). *Improving the Quality of Long-Term Care*. Washington, DC: National Academy Press.

38. Lemieux-Charles, L, McGuire W (2006). What do we know about health care team effectiveness? *Medical Care Research Review*, **63**: 263–300.

39. Shipman C, Gysels M, White P, Worth A, Murray SA, Barclay S, et al. (2008). Improving generalist end of life care: national consultation with practitioners, commissioners, academics, and service user groups. *British Medical Journal*, **337**: a1720.

Chapter 19

The development and implementation of evidence-based palliative care guidelines for residential care: lessons for other countries

Deborah Parker

Guidelines are 'systematically developed statements to assist practitioner and patient decisions about appropriate health care for specific clinical circumstances' (1). In the last decade there has been worldwide interest in development and use of evidence-based guidelines. This has been driven by the imperative to limit variations in clinical practice for people with the same condition, uncertainty about the effectiveness of interventions in making a change in people's health, and making the best of limited health resources within fiscal constraints. Whilst initially the focus was on how guidelines should be developed, this is now well defined and in Australia the National Health and Medical Research Council (NHMRC) (1) provides details of this process as does the National Institute for Health and Clinical Excellence (NICE) (2) in the UK. Several countries such as Australia, the UK, the USA, and Canada have national bodies that collate, synthesize, and publish evidence.

Attention has now moved to the more difficult task of implementation. The assumption that getting evidence into practice is as straightforward as providing the evidence in a digestible format for clinicians has well and truly been debunked. While in the early days of the evidence-based movement assumptions were made that once evidence was generated this would be transferred to the clinical setting in a linear and technical process, this is not reality for those engaged in this process. Rather, system changes at both the individual and organizational level are required in addition to the evidence (3).

Language around evidence-based practice reflects the evolution of the evidence into practice movement. In the 1970s clinicians needed to be engaged in research translation; in the 1980s it was research utilization—today the task is knowledge translation or KT. Research translation and research utilization assumed the linear process and led to what has been called the 'two communities' problem. That is, one community is generating the research and the other community uses the research (4). KT aims to overcome this duality by being a dynamic and iterative process that includes synthesis, dissemination, exchange, and ethically-sound application of knowledge to improve the health, provide more effective health services and products, and strengthen the health care system (5). The extent to which KT has been successful has not been systematically evaluated as yet.

This chapter discusses the principles of guideline development and implementation using the Australian Palliative Approach in Residential Aged Care Project (APRAC) as an example. These guidelines are the only evidence-based palliative care guidelines that have been specifically developed for this setting. A review of the process of the development and dissemination of the Australian palliative care guidelines for residential aged care will be discussed as will be the current knowledge on the implementation of these guidelines into practice. Finally, some comments on the issues raised in implementing evidence into practice will be discussed with particular reference to the residential aged care sector.

The development of evidence-based guidelines

Guidelines are sometimes based on consensus amongst experts, however with the explosion of evidence-based practice it is increasingly recognized that where possible guidelines should be based on the systematic identification and synthesis of the best available evidence. In Australia, the NHMRC has principles for developing guidelines as well as strategies for dissemination (1). Table 19.1 provides a summary of these.

In Australia, the NHMRC encourages the development of different versions of the published guidelines targeted at different groups. However, the uptake of this depends on the guideline developers and funding provided. In the UK all NICE guidelines (2) have four versions published:

1. The full guideline which contains all the background details and evidence for the guideline, as well as the recommendations

2. A version which contains only the recommendations from the full guideline, without the information on methods and evidence

3. A quick reference guide which summarizes the recommendations in an easy-to-use format for healthcare professionals

4. 'Understanding NICE guidance' which summarizes the recommendations in the NICE guideline in everyday language for patients and carers.

Table 19.1 NHMRC principles for developing guidelines and strategies for dissemination

Principles for developing guidelines	Strategies for dissemination
Focus on outcomes and the use of outcome measures	Provide short summaries on the Internet
Use the best available evidence and include a statement about the strength of the recommendations	Engage potential users in development
Utilize the strongest method to synthesize the available evidence and ensure that the group developing the guidelines have sound judgment, experience, and good sense	Media to publicize development and availability
Ensure the development team is multidisciplinary and involve consumers	Professorial journals and magazines to publicize the development
Be flexible and vary to local conditions	Communication with specialist organizations
Be developed with resource constraints in mind	Engagement with clinical leaders to promote the guidelines
Be disseminated and implemented, taking into account target audiences	Provide economic incentives
Should be evaluated for their impact	Use educational processes of professional organizations including conferences and workshops
Be reviewed regularly	Incorporate into routine procedures such as quality assurance

All NICE guidelines have three support tools: a Power Point presentation, audit support, and a costing report and costing template.

The next section of the chapter discusses the development and implementation of the palliative approach in residential aged care guidelines in Australia.

Development of the guidelines for a palliative approach in residential aged care

In Australia, as part of the National Palliative Care Strategy the Australian Palliative Residential Aged Care (APRAC) project was undertaken to develop evidence-based guidelines—*Guidelines for a Palliative Approach in Residential Aged Care Facilities* (6). These guidelines are thought to be the only evidence-based guidelines addressing this issue that have been developed anywhere in the world and the process of development and subsequent implementation of these guidelines may assist other clinicians or academics embarking on this process.

The working party of APRAC consisted of 22 academic and clinical professionals in aged care and palliative care. In addition, during the project 18 project staff from a range of disciplines were employed as well as an expert reference group to provide further professional and consumer oversight. The development of the guidelines was a two-step process: firstly the systematic review of the literature and secondly guideline formulation. Each of these steps is briefly described. Fuller details are available in the guidelines document (6).

Step 1: systematic review of the literature

The literature review was conducted by a sub group of APRAC. However, all members of APRAC were involved in guideline formulation.

While guideline development is often undertaken on a systematic review based around a clinical question, the interface between palliative care and aged care is complex and identification of specific clinical questions that would satisfy different professional groups would have been difficult. Palliative care medical specialists may be more concerned with clinical questions regarding symptoms or pharmacological management while aged care nurses' focus may be more on care of people with dementia which may include symptoms and environmental or non-pharmacological management. For allied health professionals, such as speech pathologists, the priority is swallowing and communication, whereas for physiotherapists functional independence may be the focus. To accommodate these potential competing interests of different professional groups the APRAC team identified 13 domains of literature that were considered relevant to search. The domain areas were not disease limited and were chosen to reflect the multidisciplinary care that older people would require. The 13 domains were:

1. A palliative approach, including care models and practices

2. Assessment and management tools

3. Comorbidities

4. Cognitive impairment

5. Physical care

6. Psychological support

7. Spiritual support

8. Family/carer support

9. Indigenous support

10. Cultural support
11. Advance care plans
12. Dignity and quality of life
13. Rural and remote issues.

Searching the literature

Two strategies to search the literature were employed. Firstly, searches for articles relevant to the 13 domains were conducted from 1990 to Week 3 September 2002 on MEDLINE, CINAHL, EMbase, Cochrane Library and Current Contents, APAIS, DRUG, PsychINFO, and Dissertation Abstracts International. At this point, secondary references as well as government and non-government publications, standards of care, existing guidelines, and reports were also undertaken. Secondly, following a preliminary review of the evidence captured by these searches specific searches were conducted on any perceived gaps. Full details of search strategies are available in the guidelines (6).

Evaluation of the literature

As both quantitative and qualitative articles were included in the review, a separate rating of level of evidence was devised. For articles on intervention studies a level of evidence was assigned based on the NHMRC levels of evidence (1) (Table 19.2).

As the NHRMC levels of evidence did not have provision for rating qualitative studies, an evaluation tool drawing on guidelines from the Cochrane and Campbell Collaboration was developed. This tool consisted of eight questions which reviewed the theoretical and methodological rigour of the article (for further refer to the guidelines document).

Using the first search strategy, a total of 12,000 references were preliminary assessed by the review working party and of these 939 articles were formally evaluated for relevance to the project. Of these 939 articles, 446 received met these criteria and were further evaluated for assessment of quality and strength. After these ratings *206 of the 939* were included.

Using the second more targeted search strategy, another 483 articles were rated as relevant but of these only *87* met the assessment of quality and strength. The final number of articles on which the guidelines was based was therefore *293*.

Step 2: guideline formulation

The development of the guidelines then followed a two-step process. Firstly, under each domain heading relevant evidence was examined and recommendations for best practice formulated and

Table 19.2 Level of evidence categories of the NHMRC, 1999

Level of evidence	Criteria
I	Systematic review of all relevant randomized controlled trials (RCTs)
II	At least one properly designed RCT
III-1	Well-designed pseudo-RCT
III-2	Comparative studies with concurrent controls and allocation not randomized, case–control studies, or interrupted time series with a control group
III-3	Comparative studies with historical control, two or more single-arm studies, or interrupted time series without a parallel control group
IV	Case series, either post-test or pre-test and post-test

a guideline statement drafted. At this point 104 draft guidelines covering the 13 domains were developed. The second step involved a series of 10 feedback loops of relevant stakeholders. These included health professionals in both aged and palliative care, peak body groups representing aged and palliative care, and public consultation via advertising in national newspapers. A summary of the main issues raised were:

◆ Inclusion of complementary therapies

◆ Distinguishing between delirium, dementia, and depression

◆ More information about the physical symptoms of advance dementia

◆ Clarification of the difference between a palliative approach, palliative care, and terminal care.

The last point led to a separate chapter specifically on end of life care. Following this extensive feedback loop, 79 guidelines were identified, each guideline consists of a statement, a note to which reference(s) the guideline has been developed from, and the level of evidence of the guideline.

Guideline implementation and evaluation

As the guidelines were developed as part of the Australian National Palliative Care Strategy, the Department of Health and Ageing in conjunction with Palliative Care Australia and the Community Services and Health Industry assisted with their implementation. Initially, each residential aged care facility in Australia received a free copy of the guidelines and further electronic copies are available for free download from http://www.nhmrc.gov.au/publications.

In addition to the circulation of a copy of the guidelines, a series of 1-day national workshops was provided free for staff from residential aged care facilities (RACFs) to attend. At this point the Residential Aged Care Palliative Approach Network (RACPAN) was formed to coordinate the dissemination and provide workshops. RACPAN workshops were held in major cities (127), inner regional (69), outer regional (33), remote (5) and very remote areas (2) ensuring that the maximum number of RACFs could access the training. Of the 3000 RACFs in Australia, 1864 (plus 42 Multipurpose centres) sent 3361 staff to one of 236 RACPAN workshops. Thirty-five Divisions of General Practice (DGP) and local palliative care services attended 135 of the workshops. The evaluation of the workshops was very positive and participants reported developing skills that would enable them to act as resource people within their RACF. Follow-up evaluation, 6 months after the RACPAN workshop rollout, indicated that many staff who had attended the workshops were acting as resource people and champions for a palliative approach in their facility (7). This evaluation did not however extend to evaluation of how the guidelines were implemented in each facility and whether this had any impact on resident and family outcomes.

Ongoing education and training

In addition to the RACPLAN workshops a broad range of education and training was developed to target all levels of staff working in residential aged care and general practitioners (GPs). Table 19.3 provides a summary of the target groups of this education.

General practitioners

For GPs two resources were developed. As part of the initial implementation a multidisciplinary active learning module (ALM) that covered specific topic areas within the guidelines was developed. The module comes in kit form and comprises a manual and CD, a copy of the guidelines, a selection of useful brochures on palliative care, Power Point presentation, handouts, and suggestions on how to run the activity. For individual GPs wanting to complete training individually, an interactive online module has been developed and is hosted on sites that will enable free access for GPs.

Table 19.3 Summary of education and training for guideline implementation

	GP	RN	EN	AIN	Allied Health
Certificate III and IV				√	
Self-directed learning package		√	√	√	√
Workbook		√	√	√	√
Palliative care topics		√	√	√	√
Active learning module	√				
Online GP module	√				

Education for all levels of aged care home staff

Three educational resources have been designed to be used for all levels of residential aged care home staff.

1. A self-directed learning package that is designed to be incorporated as part of structured education sessions
2. A workbook of eight modules with specific learning outcomes and assessment criteria (8)
3. Self-paced palliative care topics.

Education for assistants in nursing

The Community Services and Health Industry Skills Council have developed two units of competency about a palliative approach for Certificate III and Certificate IV qualifications. In Australia, these qualifications are available for the lowest level of worker in residential aged care—the careworker or assistant in nursing.

To continue to raise awareness of the guidelines and encourage implementation the RACPAN continues. It is supported by the Department of Health and Ageing and is hosted by Palliative Care Australia. The aim of the newsletter is to provide a forum for sharing of experiences in implementing the guidelines.

Australian examples of implementation of the guidelines

As previously discussed the evaluation of the initial phase of guideline implementation focused on education and 'awareness raising' of the guidelines for staff working in residential aged care and general practitioners. However, the necessary infrastructure to evaluate the impact of the guidelines on practice including changes in resident and family outcomes was not available at the time of initial dissemination. Since then a number of research projects have been conducted that use the *Guidelines for a Palliative Approach in Residential Aged Care Facilities* (6).

The New South Wales Institute of Clinical Service and Teaching conducted a comparative study looking at the effectiveness of two different teaching methods used to improve the integration of the palliative approach into rural residential aged care facilities (9). Conducted in five residential aged care facilities in two rural areas, staff in facilities either receive education in providing palliative care using two different education models. The first was the use of in-service education and the second case conferencing. The *Guidelines for a Palliative Approach in Residential Aged Care Facilities* were used to help prepare all the education sessions. Three facilities were allocated to in-service and two to case conferencing (6).

Evaluation of the effectiveness of the different models was undertaken using a questionnaire ascertaining views about palliative care, views about death and dying, and attitudes towards palliative care. The questionnaire was administered prior to the intervention, then 6 and 12 months during the intervention. Interviews were also conducted at the end of the 12-month intervention. Rate of referrals to the specialist palliative care services for each facility was also measured. The authors conclude that the study demonstrates that case conferencing was more effective than in-servicing in relation to:

• Enabling appropriate referral to specialist palliative care services

• Increasing the understanding of the role of the specialist palliative care team

• Creating practice changes

• Increasing communication between team members.

These results should, however, be interpreted with caution as the response rate for evaluation of either model using the questionnaire was quite low (case conferencing 35.8% pre to 44.4% post, and in-service model 5.5% to 20.1%).

The Anglican Retirement Villages project, *Implementing a Palliative Care Approach in an Aged Care Organisation* (10), aimed to increase awareness and promote discussion of death and dying, improve care at the end of life, and provide appropriate grief and bereavement support for care staff, families, and volunteers. The project involved the employment of a full time Palliative Care Clinical Nurse Consultant to provide clinical support and education. Case conferences have been integrated into care, a palliative care section has been developed in the policy and procedure manual, and information on spiritual and cultural care is available with a spiritual kit in each RACF. Environmental wishes and needs are also addressed with the introduction of a palliative leisure and lifestyle questionnaire. Education was a key focus and this was delivered in a variety of formats. The project has, to date, resulted in more than 300 residents having been referred to the Palliative Care Clinical Nurse Consultant to support staff in caring for resident at the end of life. Ongoing education is available for staff and Advance Care Planning is promoted in all the facilities. End of life documentation is now available with an End of Life pathway and a comfort care plan to assist staff and GPs in delivering high-quality care. This project, similar to the previous one, did not directly evaluate the impact of the guidelines on resident and family outcomes.

Abbey and colleagues (11) conducted a study using the guidelines as a basis for a model of multidisciplinary care for residents with end-stage dementia in two residential aged care facilities in Queensland. The model of care included education for all staff and the use of palliative care case conferences and care planning. The model of care was evaluated using a pre- and post-study design. That is, care was compared for 25 residents prior to the implementation of the model with care for 17 residents who received the model of care. Outcomes were measured by chart audits, the Symptom Management at the End-of-Life in Dementia (SM-EOLD), and the Satisfaction with Care at the End-of-Life in Dementia (SWC-EOLD) (12) scales. The SM-EOLD records the occurrence of nine common symptoms in the 90 days prior to the person's death—fear, anxiety, shortness of breath, depression, agitation, resistiveness to care, pain, skin breakdown, and calm. These audits were completed by a research nurse with experience in dementia. The SWC-EOLD is a 10-question scale with questions focused on satisfaction with care, involvement in decision-making, and care planning. This scale was administered by the research nurse with the resident's closest relative. The main findings were that the use of palliative care case conferencing increased from 12% to 71% and a there was a slight increase in the use of advance health directives (8% to 12%). However, documentation of the occurrence of all symptoms using the SM-EOLD increased. This was most probably due to the focus in the education sessions on the importance of assessment and documentation rather than a decrease in care. Carer satisfaction using the SWC-EOLD increased slightly for carers whose family members received the new model of care (mean 30.68% pre and mean 31% post). However, the sample size was not large enough to calculate statistical significance. The authors concluded that providing a structured multidisciplinary approach for residents with end-stage dementia shows some promising results but more work in this area is required.

Most recently, a programme by the Australian Government Department of Health and Ageing—Encouraging Best Practice in Residential Aged Care (EBPRAC)—is providing support for residential aged care homes to translate evidence into practice. EBPRAC aims to improve the level of clinical care for residents in aged care home by supporting the uptake of existing evidence-based guidelines by funding organizations to translate the best available evidence into easy approaches for staff to use in their everyday practice. To date, there have been two rounds of EBPRAC and 13 projects have been funded. Rounds 1 and 2 have focused on key clinical areas for which there are existing bodies of knowledge to support evidence-based practice as well as existing tools and resources to support implementation. Five projects were funded under Round 1 of EBPRAC and focused on the clinical areas of nutrition and hydration, PRN ('as required') medication management, oral health care, falls management and pain management. Projects ran from November 2007 to December 2009. Eight projects were funded under Round 2 of EBPRAC, focusing on the clinical areas of palliative care (three projects), behaviour management (three projects), wound management, and infection control. Round 2 projects run from December 2008 to December 2010 (13). The three palliative care projects funded in Round 2 are briefly described although as these three projects are not due for completion in December 2010 no results are available.

The first project, *Implementing an evidence based palliative approach in residential aged care* (CEBPARAC), led by the author (http://www.caresearch.com.au/caresearch/CEBPARAC.aspx) aims to develop and implement an evidence-based model of palliative care. This will be achieved through a range of strategies including: providing education to nursing and care staff at all levels working in aged care homes using existing training materials; establishing training and supporting link nurses in each aged care home; and promoting the use of existing GP online training modules to support GPs in providing a palliative approach to residents in their care. The project will develop a tool kit comprising generic templates for policies, procedures, documentation, production of a case conferencing DVD, and self-directed learning packages (13).

The second project, *Encouraging best practice palliative care in residential aged care facilities* (http://www.mdgp.net.au/), is led by the Murrumbidgee General Practice Network. This project aims to encourage best practice in palliative care in residential aged care homes with a focus on rural communities within New South Wales, South Australia, and Victoria. Particular emphasis is placed on: a multidisciplinary, palliative approach provided in the resident's familiar surroundings; and systematic development and implementation of advance care planning involving communication between the resident, family and doctor (13).

The third project, *A good death in residential aged care* (http://www.nevdgp.org.au), is coordinated by the North East Valley Division of General Practice. This project aims to implement evidence-based use of medications, to manage symptoms in the end of life phase for residents in aged care homes. The project will result in a number of improvements including: improved assessment and monitoring of symptoms at the end of life; improved prescribing; appropriate and effective use of 'as required' (PRN) medicines for symptom management; improved collaboration between aged care home staff, GPs, specialist palliative care services, and pharmacists in ensuring timely availability of medicines for symptom management; and improved processes to support informed choice by residents and families at the time of prescribing and administration of medication and/or in advance (13).

Lessons from the development and implementation of the Australian guidelines

At the beginning of the chapter, nine principles for guideline development from the NHMRC were proposed. Reviewing the Australian experience of APRAC it appears that at least seven of these nine principles have been completed (Table 19.4). The evaluation of the impact of these guidelines in practice will be enhanced by the funding of the three palliative care EBPRAC projects. All NHMRC guidelines require revision every 5 years and for these current guidelines this is scheduled for September 2010. Revision is unlikely to change the intent of the guidelines but with a dramatic increase in publications in many of the literature domains the review will provide a stronger evidence base.

In regard to recommended dissemination and implementation tasks identified by the NHMRC as discussed earlier in the chapter (Table 19.5), the guideline dissemination and implementation strategy was closely aligned with that recommended.

The guidelines were published as a full document and in the original dissemination a shorter navigational tool booklet with a summary of guidelines and tips for implementation was produced. However, this shorter version is not widely disseminated anymore and not available electronically. Unfortunately no resources were available to develop a consumer booklet. A version suitable for consumers would have been useful for the large workforce in residential aged care who are untrained—these are the assistants in nursing or care workers. No options for including the guidelines into routine quality assurance activities were made available.

While there are issues with the complexity of the guidelines themselves, the residential aged care sector is a complex and challenging environment in which to embed evidence-based practice. Eight key factors that have been identified that will assist getting evidence into practice include (14):

1. Receptive context for change
2. Model for change (including a role for change agents)
3. Adequate resources
4. Staff with the necessary skills
5. Stakeholder engagement, participation, and commitment

Table 19.4 NHRMC principles of guideline development

Principle	APRAC guidelines
Focus on outcomes and the use of outcome measures	Yes
Best available evidence/statement about the strength of the recommendations	Yes
Strongest method to synthesize the available evidence/experienced development group	Yes
A multidisciplinary team and involve consumers	Yes
Flexible and vary to local conditions	Yes
Resource constraints in mind	Yes
Disseminated and implemented taking into account target audiences	Yes
Evaluated for their impact	In process
Reviewed regularly	Due 2010

Table 19.5 NHRMC strategies for dissemination and implementation

Dissemination and implementation	APRAC guidelines
Short summaries on the Internet	No
The involvement of potential users in development	Yes
Media to publicize development and availability	Yes
Professorial journals and magazines to publicize the development	Yes
Communication with specialist organizations	Yes
Engagement with clinical leaders to promote the guidelines	Yes
Provision of economic incentives	No
Use of educational processes of professional organizations including conferences and workshops	Yes
Incorporating into routine procedures such as quality assurance	No

6. Local adaption and interpretation to fit with current practice

7. Systems to support the use of evidence

8. Demonstrable benefits of change.

Some of these factors are more difficult to solve. Australia, like other developed countries has concerns regarding resources and staffing. Strategies for implementation must take into account that staff with limited formal training may need to be up-skilled in the use of assessment tools and management strategies to support the use of evidence-based practice.

Janes et al. (15) identified two factors that influence successful facilitation in long-term care homes—those at the level of the individual and those relating to the context of care. Those at the individual level included those of the facilitator and those receiving the facilitation. An approach where best practice knowledge was framed by the facilitators so that it was relevant to practice and the reality of care was important. Case-based learning using current residents as examples was preferred by staff and it was important to break evidence into digestible pieces. Engagement with staff not as expert but as coaches was useful as was trying to encourage staff to develop skills for continued practice improvement. A key factor for the receivers of evidence-based practice was for the individual to be motivated to learn and improve care through evidence-based practice. Contextual factors included supportive leadership and a cooperative relationship between nursing staff and administrators. An organizational culture that promotes a learning environment, partnership, person-centredness, honesty, compassion, creativity, and enquiry were key features. Workload is a common barrier to practice change and while backfill for staff to attend education may assist, new practices still require extra time for staff to become familiar with new protocols and for these to become usual care.

A final context factor was the regulations long-term care are governed by, which seemed to conflict with some best practice changes.

Conclusion

This chapter has provided an overview of the development and implementation of what is understood to be the world's first evidence-based guidelines for a palliative approach in residential aged care. Recognizing that this is a complex and difficult area to distil into specific clinical guidelines, a broad approach to collecting evidence relevant to providing a palliative approach was used.

While this provided a rich source of evidence, translating this to practical everyday clinical guidelines is a challenge. In countries such as Australia that have an accreditation standard for palliative care, linkages with guidelines may assist practice change.

While developing evidence-based guidelines is a complex and time-consuming task, implementation into clinical practice remains the real challenge. At present there are encouraging signs that the Palliative Approach in Residential Aged Care Guidelines have the potential to impact on the health outcomes for residents and family. The development and dissemination of the guidelines so far in Australia has raised the awareness of palliative care in the residential aged care sector. The extent to which they will improve resident and family outcomes is yet to be determined, but if demonstrated will be the best driver for change.

References

1. National Health and Medical Research Council (1999). *A guide to development, implementation and evaluation of clinical practice guidelines.* Canberra: National Health and Medical Research Council.
2. National Institute for Health and Clinical Excellence (2009). *The guidelines manual.* London: NICE.
3. Kitson A, Rycroft-Malone J, Harvey G, McCormack B, Seers K, Titchen A (2008). Evaluating the successful implementation of evidence into practice using the PARiHS framework: theoretical and practical challenges. *Implementation Science*, 3(1).
4. Graham B, Cheek J, Alde P (2009). The research/practice nexus: underlying assumptoms about the nature of research uptake into practice literature pertaining to the care of the older person. *International Journal of Older People Nursing*, 4: 219–26.
5. Canadian Institutes of Health Research (2008). About knowledge translation. Available at: http://www.cihr-irsc.gc.ca/e/29418.html. (Accessed 1 April 2010.)
6. Commonwealth of Australia (2006). *Guidelines for a palliative approach in residential aged care facilities—NHMRC endorsed edition.* Canberra: Commonwealth of Australia. Available at: http://www.nhmrc.gov.au/publications/synopses/ac12to14syn.htm.
7. Palliative Care Australia (2007). *Introducing the guidelines for a palliative approach in residential aged care project—evaluation report.* Canberra: Palliative Care Australia.
8. Commonwealth of Australia (2004). *Training modules for a palliative approach in residential care.* Canberra: Commonwealth of Australia.
9. Giugni C (2009). *A comparative study looking at the effectiveness of two different teaching methods used to improve the integration of the Palliative Approach into Rural Residential Aged Care Facilities.* Dubbo, Australia.
10. Lancaster C (2009). *Implementing a palliative approach.* RACPAN Newsletter, March: 2.
11. Abbey J, Sacre S, Parker D (2008). *Develop, trial and evaluate a model of multidisciplinary palliative care for residents with end-stage dementia.* Brisbane: Queensland University of Technology.
12. Volicer L, Hurley AC, Blasi ZV (2001). Scales for evaluation of End-of-Life Care in Dementia. *Alzheimer Disease & Associated Disorders*, 15(4): 194–200.
13. Department of Health and Ageing (2009). *Encourageing Best Practice in Residential Aged Care Program.* Canberra: Department of Health and Ageing. Available at: http://www.health.gov.au/internet/main/publishing.nsf/Content/ageing-bestpractice-program-second-round.htm. (Accessed 14 January 2010.)
14. Masso M, McCarthy G (2009). Literature review to identify factors that support implementation of evidence based practice in residential aged care. *International Journal of Evidence Based Healthcare*, 7: 145–56.
15. Janes N, Fox M, Lowe M, McGilton K, Shindel-Martin L (2009). Facilitating best practice in aged care: exploring influential factors through critical incident technique. *International Journal of Older People Nursing*, 4: 166–76.

Chapter 20

Improving environments for care at the end of life in hospitals

Clare Gardiner and Sarah Barnes

Where people die and how people are cared for at the end of life is a subject of recognized importance. In the industrialized world the majority of deaths now occur in institutionalized settings; 2004 data reported by the World Health Organization showed that most people in the UK, USA, Germany, Switzerland, and France die in hospitals (1). This is a marked change from previous centuries (as discussed in more detail by Kellehear, Chapter 2, this volume). In the UK, for example, in 1900 the majority of people died in their own homes, with a minority in workhouses. By the middle of the 20th century around half of people died at home, and by the early 21st century over 50% of deaths occurred in acute hospitals (2). A 20% increase in the proportion of deaths in institutionalized settings such as acute hospitals, nursing homes, and hospices is predicted over the next 20 years (3).

Across the world, and particularly in developed countries, the number of older people is increasing (4). Over the next 25 years the number of people in the UK aged over 65 years is expected to increase by over 50% (5). Long-term projections indicate that if recent trends continue, people will die at increasingly older ages, with deaths in those people aged over 85 predicated to increase by more than 10% in the next 20 years (2). Adults aged over 75 years now account for approximately two-thirds of all deaths in the UK and experience the highest proportion of hospital deaths and the lowest rates of death at home or in hospice. Whilst the proportion of people dying at home has been decreasing steadily for all age groups over the last 25 years, this trend is most marked for people aged over 65 years (3).

Meeting patients' preferences for place of care at the end of life is clearly an important priority when providing high-quality end of life care. However preferences for place of care are not always consistent and patient preferences may change with time and with the course of any illness. A study by Higginson (2000) (6) exploring preferences for place of care in advanced cancer suggested well over 50% of patients would choose to die at home, with inpatient hospice care a second preference for the majority of patients. However, although many people would prefer to be cared for and to die at home, the requirements for high-quality care and the potential burden to families and carers can impact on preferences, particularly for older people. Some older people have expressed mixed views as to whether a home death is either achievable or desirable and, for a proportion of patients, the acute hospital may be the preferred setting for end of life care (7). In particular, older people report feeling reassured by the presence of medical expertise and technologies in hospitals. Indeed, although dying at home is often considered central to the 'good death', many older people anticipate they would prefer to be cared for somewhere else when actually dying (7). Recent international policy developments and initiatives have prioritized home as a place of death (2, 8). Nevertheless, hospital remains the most common place of death across the developed world and it is therefore imperative that hospital environments for dying are prioritized. This chapter considers the need to improve hospital environments for older people at the end of life within this context. Whilst the discussion focuses primarily on the UK situation, there are many similarities between the UK experience and that of other developed countries.

Hospital environments for older people at the end of life

The environment in which older people are cared for can profoundly affect their health, well-being, independence, and quality of life, particularly at the end of life (9). Many older people in hospital are cared for on geriatric (or 'care of the elderly') wards, often typified by various common environmental characteristics. In recent years there has been considerable public concern about the suitability of these environments for the care of older people and their relatives. This section briefly outlines the nature of hospital provision for older people in the UK, before moving on to identify essential elements to consider in designing appropriate hospital environments for older people and their family carers.

Although some single room accommodation is available in UK hospitals, many older people are cared for on small public wards or larger multiple bed 'Nightingale' type wards. Multiple occupancy wards clearly necessitate some sharing of communal spaces and facilities, and older people and their families lack privacy in this setting. Despite the UK government's recent commitment to phase out mixed-sex hospital wards, a minority of hospitals still accommodate patients in this setting, a situation which today few people find acceptable and which raises questions regarding infringements of patient dignity (10). Whilst there is little consensus regarding the most effective model of care and care setting for older people in hospital (11), there are recognized differences between care settings in terms of the delivery of health care, and the coordination of comprehensive care. It is important to recognize that any ward which houses large numbers of older people will have some patients who will recover and some who will die. An ideal hospital environment should be designed to support the dignity of all older people, irrespective of diagnosis, prognosis, and place of care.

When older people move into or between care settings, new environments are encountered and some degree of adaptation to the new environment normally occurs. Whilst the ability to adapt to new environments may be relatively unproblematic in younger people, this ability can be compromised in later life by changes in vision, hearing, sense of touch, dexterity, mobility, and cognition. Changes in these senses may affect the ability to respond and adapt to new environments, and this ability may be further compromised in hospital inpatients by illness, disability, frailty, and cognitive impairment (12). Hospitals often provide care for large numbers of dementia sufferers, and these patients may have specific difficulties adapting to new environments. Adaptation to change in environment can also be particularly difficult for patients reaching the end of life; patients are highly vulnerable at this time and the impact of environment on patients' families is also significant. Recognition of these various factors is vital when considering ways in which hospital environments can be appropriately designed to meet the needs of older patients, particularly those reaching the end of life.

Elements to consider in an end of life care environment

There are a number of elements which have been highlighted by patients and relatives as important in the environments of older people (13, 14). Many are universal and can be applied to any environment, some specifically relate to hospital environments, and some relate to the dying environment. These can be divided into a number of themes:

Privacy

Research findings suggest that privacy is one of the most important aspects of the environment of older people (15–17). It is well documented that older people and their relatives have expressed a dislike of having to share wards and bathrooms with people of the opposite sex (10). However, it is the way the environment enables patients to be private or not as they wish which is of greatest importance to them. Privacy in a hospital setting can largely be defined by being in a single or multiple-occupancy room and there can be advantages and disadvantages to both environments. For example, there is evidence to suggest that satisfaction with treatments is higher in patients with single bed accommodation (13). On the other hand, patients often express a preference for multiple-bed spaces citing a wish for company and a feeling they are more likely to be given attention by staff. This conflict is equally prevalent amongst patients reaching the end of life. For practical reasons shared rooms are difficult when patients are actively dying as there is a lack of privacy as well as a potential to cause disturbance or distress to others. Conversely some seriously ill patients report feeling safer knowing there are other people close by, and patients often provide support to one another. Often, it is family members rather than patients who consider having a single room to be important (18). Older hospital inpatients often complain of loneliness or boredom. Psychologists have pointed out that social interaction in hospital is just as important a determinant of well-being as environmental factors, and spatial arrangements themselves can facilitate or inhibit such interaction (19). However, not all patients want to mix with others, and some prefer to remain in their own room. It is the provision of good privacy options that can make social interaction more welcome.

Control of the environment

The comfort of a building is mediated by light, temperature, air quality, and noise levels and hospital environments offer a low level of control over these aspects of the environment, even in relatively new buildings. Evidence shows that patients want more control over heating, lighting, windows, blinds, and noise, and an inability to control the environment is associated with reduced satisfaction among older people in care settings (13, 14). Intrusive noise is a concern that is frequently raised by patients, particularly when the noise is generated by members of staff talking or shouting to each other (20). Building design can give patients a measure of control over aspects of comfort, for example by ensuring that windows are accessible and easily opened, that heat and cooling sources can be controlled by patients, and that light fittings are localized. However, research in residential and nursing homes has shown that, in an institutional environment, a hierarchy of control needs to be acknowledged as control over communal spaces is unlikely to be afforded to patients (21).

Homeliness

There is evidence that the issue of homeliness is frequently raised by patients and their families (22). Within a hospital setting patients can reside in one place for a long period of time and can come to regard it as their home. However, equipment within a hospital, including the bed itself, can make the environment less homely. Older people spending long periods of time in hospital often attempt to make their immediate environment more homely by personalizing their bed area or room with photos, cards, religious artefacts, radio, television, etc. (23). This ability to personalize space provides them with a greater sense of territory.

Cleanliness

A desire for a clean environment with no offensive odours is also important to patients, who appreciate an environment that appears to be cared for. Untidiness and lack of cleanliness within a care setting can be seen to equate to a lack of care, attention, or love of the place by those responsible for it (19).

Views and outdoor spaces

There is evidence to suggest that patients with a view get discharged from hospital more quickly than those without, and lack of view is a common complaint amongst patients (24). It is not necessarily a view of nature that is required, just a view of everyday life in which something happens, such as children leaving school (13). Older patients nearing the end of life can enjoy contact with the natural world in the form of sunshine, gardens, indoor plants, bird boxes, and ponds. These can be viewed from a window if patients are unable to get outside. Well-conceived outdoor environments can provide older people and their relatives with spaces for privacy, activity, and stimulation, all of which contribute to quality of life (25). Easy access to outdoor spaces with visual and sensory stimulation is particularly beneficial for patients with dementia but it is often the case that outdoor spaces can only be accessed with the help of staff, so are not used frequently.

Provision for visitors

Being able to receive visitors is of paramount importance to older people who are staying in hospital for long periods of time. These visitors are often family members who are older people themselves and, as such, prioritize ease of access and navigation around the hospital building which, ideally, would be in close proximity to their home. If they are required to make a journey to visit their friend or family member, access to public transport and availability of parking are also important issues. When patients are nearing the end of life, their relatives often like to stay with them overnight and some hospitals do provide a dedicated space elsewhere in the hospital for visitors to stay. However, many relatives prefer to stay near the patient and sleep on the floor next to the bed, in some cases for companionship and in other cases to perform religious rituals. Whilst families welcome the provision of a chapel or faith room as well as access to gardens for spiritual expression, it is often the space within the patient's own room which is of most value. There is no reason why both cannot be made available.

Environment requirements of hospital staff

Whilst the needs and preferences of patients and families are clearly a priority when considering improvements to hospital environments, the requirements of the staff working within this setting are also of key importance. Health and allied professionals, auxiliary staff, and support staff all have specific environmental requirements in order that patients are afforded the highest quality care whilst staff are provided with an appropriate working environment. Legal requirements dictate certain standards of health and safety, e.g. regarding hygiene and infection control. Medical equipment must be robust and fit for purpose, and patient areas need to provide the flexibility required to support the needs of all patients. By and large the architectural and design principles informing the design of hospitals remains largely functional, with the efficient delivery of medical and technical services being given priority over patient preferences (26). Finding the balance between an appropriate environment for staff and a preferred environment for patients forms one of the key dilemmas for hospital design teams.

In buildings which are poorly adapted, staff often complain of a lack of space to carry out appropriate care. Some single patient rooms barely reach minimum space standards and staff can face difficulties in carrying out their role effectively. Privacy options favoured by staff include being able to maintain patient confidentiality and privacy for patients actively dying. Staff also express concerns about the layout of buildings which do not allow privacy for bereaved relatives (22). While there is some consensus on issues such as privacy, dignity, and spirituality, there is a clear potential for conflicting views. These include stringent health and safety requirements versus patient choice and control; conversing with patients and other members of staff versus a quiet ambience preferred by patients; and the homely environment favoured by patients versus the need for institutional and often cumbersome medical equipment.

Potential impact of environments on patients at end of life

The impact of an environment will almost certainly have a direct effect on the patient experience in hospital. There is evidence to suggest that some design elements impact positively on quality of life and even health outcomes. Generous, appropriately orientated windows which allow sunlight, have provision for shading and a view of the outside world, improve both the quality of life of patients and the morale of the carers (27). Environments which facilitate spatial orientation and navigation can contribute positively to a person's quality of life (14, 28). Putting the emphasis on buildings being reassuring and comprehensible is particularly beneficial to people with dementia (29). Providing a choice and variety of spaces to spend time, including options for privacy is also associated with enhanced quality of life (17). While these design elements have been shown to significantly improve the quality of life of older people, it is being able to decide what levels of privacy and community are wanted, and being able to control the environment, that are of greater significance to patients than the general appearance of the environment (13).

There is evidence to suggest that moving patients between beds in hospitals is common practice. This is largely done without consultation and against the wishes of the patient, and often during the night (13). Moves occur more frequently in patients approaching the end of life as privacy is prioritized and patients are moved to more 'appropriate' areas for dying; it is relatively common for patients to be moved several times before death (30). Patients in hospitals often develop a strong attachment to their bed area and many strongly dislike being moved. Placing dying patients on multi-occupancy wards does necessitate a potentially unwelcome move at the very end of life; hospital wards with single rooms virtually remove the need for this.

Recommendations for improved hospital environments

It is apparent from research carried out on the impact of environment on patient well-being that hospital environments are not always optimal for older people reaching the end of life (13, 14). Recommendations for improving hospital environments clearly need to take careful consideration of available research evidence and comparisons with other care settings can also be helpful in developing an optimal environment. An important aim of the modern hospice movement in the UK is to provide an environment which facilitates the provision of good palliative care, whilst fulfilling the diverse individual needs of patients and their families. The hospice movement has been lauded for its recognition of the importance of environment for patients reaching the end of life. Whilst it is acknowledged that environmental and design challenges still exist in many hospices, hospitals can learn valuable lessons from the dedicated recognition of environmental features in the hospice setting. Such features include architectural considerations, creating an interior designed to put patients and families at ease, spaces which engender a sense of calm, light, space, peace, and supportive order, and landscaped gardens providing places of refuge and sanctuary (26).

Other care settings in which environmental and design features are highly prioritized include children's hospitals. Clearly these are settings which serve a distinct population with specific needs and requirements; however, the level of consideration given to environmental features of children's care settings is striking in comparison to that of adult care settings. The design of children's care environments commonly incorporates consultation with children and parents in order that young patients can be involved in influencing their environment. For example, the Evelina Children's Hospital in London opened in 2005 and involved young patients and their families in shaping the environment and architecture of the hospital from the earliest stages of design (31). In stark contrast to this approach to design, hospital inpatients, service user groups, and carers are rarely consulted regarding the design of new adult hospitals.

Whilst resource restrictions may prevent designers and architects from meeting the preferences and requirements of all patients, some consultation with the people who are going to be using the facility is crucial for creating an optimum environment within this setting.

As older patients can reside in hospital settings for long periods of time, a potentially useful way of taking environmental design forward is attempting to create 'home' in hospital. To emulate a more 'homelike' environment, single rooms would be most appropriate for this population. However, while single rooms eliminate the need to move patients around so often, particularly at the end of life, consideration needs to be given to patients who welcome the company and support of others.

In order to maintain a symbolic connection to their home, patients should be actively encouraged to bring personal items into the hospital. This helps to create a homely appearance and appropriate storage, shelving and picture hooks should be in place to house these personal objects. Additionally, while correct equipment in line with regulations is necessary, this should be concealed where possible. To maintain some level of autonomy, patients should be offered control over their immediate environment, for example being able to open and close curtains or windows and regulate heating and cooling. Improvements in sound insulation, sound absorption, and nurse call systems can be helpful in eliminating unwanted noise and make the environment more comfortable.

Provision of a choice of communal indoor areas as well as outdoor spaces provides opportunities for socializing and mutual support for both patients and relatives. Hospitals need to improve overnight facilities for relatives and this can be achieved by providing more space in single rooms, positioning furniture appropriately, and providing enough chairs to accommodate visitors. Bereavement suites can offer private space to break bad news to relatives. Gardens and outdoor spaces should be well cared for and accessible without the assistance of staff. For patients who are unable to go outside, the bed can be positioned suitably in relation to the windows, which should have low sills to maximize views of interesting outdoor spaces. Most importantly, consultation with patients, their families, and staff should be undertaken from the earliest stages of design when new hospitals are being planned.

Whilst these recommendations are intended as practical guidelines, it is recognized that inevitable resource restrictions mean it may not always be possible to enact all of these recommendations in practice. In order to achieve these recommendations, serious consideration needs to be given to the small but expanding evidence base for the significant impact of environment on patient well-being. Important lessons can also be learnt from the priority ascribed to environmental aspects of different care settings such as hospices and children's hospitals. Post-occupancy evaluations and encouraging better practice and fuller understanding of the briefing process at the beginning of a project are critical to the success of therapeutic environments. Historically both aspects have been seriously neglected, and improved hospital environments can only be achieved if this is recognized and acted upon (32). Service user groups, carer organizations, and bereavement groups should also be consulted for input when considering improvements to hospital environments for people reaching the end of life. The concept of involving service users in health care research is now an accepted and necessary component of any new research study. The same consideration of the views and opinions of the people for whom hospital environments are designed for would benefit not only the patients, but also the architects and the design teams charged with delivering improved care environments. Improving hospital environments for dying patients is a clear priority when considering ways in which end of life care can be improved. More research is needed to facilitate recognition and change at the highest level.

References

1. World Health Organization (2004). *The Solid Facts: Palliative Care.* Copenhagen: WHO Regional Office for Europe.

2. Department of Health (2008). *End of Life Care Strategy for England.* London: Department of Health.

3. Gomes B, Higginson IJ (2008). Where people die (1974—2030): past trends, future projections and implications for care. *Palliative Medicine,* 22(1): 22–31.

4. World Health Organization (2004). *Better Palliative Care for Older People.* Copenhagen: WHO Regional Office for Europe.

5. Dunnell K (2008). *Ageing and mortality in the UK: National Statistician's Annual Article on the Population.* London: Office for National Statistics.

6. Higginson IJ, Sen-Gupta GJA (2000). Place of care in advanced cancer: a qualitative systematic literature review of patient preferences. *Journal of Palliative Medicine,* 3(3): 287–300.

7. Gott M, Seymour J, Bellamy G, Clark D, Ahmedzai S (2004). Older people's views about home as a place of care at the end of life. *Palliative Medicine,* 18: 460–7.

8. Marie Curie Cancer Care (2004) *Valuing Choice–Dying at home.* London: Marie Curie Cancer Care.

9. Heath H, Phair L (2000). Living environments and older people. *Nursing Older People,* 12(8): 21–5.

10. Lishman G (2009). *Age Concern responds to Health Secretary Alan Johnson's announcement on mixed sex wards (28.01.09).* Available at: http://www.ageconcern.org.uk/AgeConcern/mixed-wards-response-280109. asp. (Accessed 3 December 2009.)

11. Ellis G, Langhorne P (2005). Geriatric wards in acute hospitals. *Age & Ageing,* 34(4): 417–8.

12. Lawton MP, Nahemow L (1973). Press-competence model of person-environment interaction. In MA Matteson, ES McConnell (eds) *Gerontological Nursing: concepts and practice.* Philadelphia, PA: WB Saunders Co.

13. Lawson B, Phiri M (2003). *The architectural healthcare environment and its effects on patient health outcomes: a report on an NHS estates funded research project.* London: NHS Estates.

14. Parker C, Barnes S, McKee K, Morgan K, Torrington J, Tregenza P (2004). Quality of life and building design in residential and nursing homes for older people. *Ageing & Society,* 24: 941–62.

15. Netten A (1993). *A Positive Environment? Physical and Social Influences on People with Senile Dementia in Residential Care.* Aldershot: Ashgate.

16. Morgan DG, Stewart NJ (1998). Multiple occupancy versus private rooms on dementia care units. *Environment and Behavior,* 30(4): 487–503.

17. Barnes S (2006). Space, choice and control, and quality of life in care settings for older people. *Environment & Behaviour,* 38(5): 589–604.

18. Heyland D K, Dodeck P, Rocker G, Groll D, Gafni A, Pichora D, et al. (2006). What matters most in end of life care: perceptions of seriously ill patients and their family members. *Canadian Medical Association Journal,* 174: 1–9.

19. Lawson B, Wells-Thorpe J (2002). The effect of the hospital environment on the patient experience and health outcomes. *Journal of Healthcare Design and Development.* March: 27–32.

20. Hawker S, Kerr C, Payne S, Seamark D, Davis C, Roberts H, et al. (2006). End of life care in community hospitals: the perceptions of bereaved family members. *Palliative Medicine,* 20: 541–7.

21. Barnes S (2006). Space, choice and quality of life in care settings for older people. *Environment and Behaviour,* 38: 589–604.

22. Rigby J, Payne S, Froggatt K (2010). What evidence is there about the specific environmental needs of older people who are near the end of life and are cared for in hospices or similar institutions? A literature review. *Palliative Medicine,* **24**(3): 268–85.

23. Franklin LL, Ternestedt BM, Nordenfelt L (2006). Views on dignity of elderly nursing home residents. *Nursing Ethics,* **13**: 130–46.

24. Ulrich RS (1984). View through a window may influence recovery from surgery. *Science,* **224**(4647): 420–1.

25. Brawley EC (1997). *Designing for Alzheimer's Disease: Strategies for creating better care environments.* New York: John Wiley and Sons Inc.

26. Warpole K (2009). *Modern hospice design: the architecture of palliative care.* Oxford: Routledge.

27. Manser M (1989). The architecture of institutions for demented persons. In J Wertheimer, P Baumann, M Gaillard, P Schwed (eds), *Innovative Trends in Psychogeriatrics,* pp. 22–7. Basle: Karger.

28. Passini R, Pigot H, Rainville C, Tetreault MH (2000). Wayfinding in a nursing home for advanced dementia of the Alzheimer's type. *Environment and Behavior,* **32**(5): 684–710.

29. Marshall M (1992). Designing for disorientation. *Access by Design,* **58**: 15–17.

30. Vagnair A, Forster R (2003). A room for dying in: Patient's need or nurses' fantasy? *European Journal of Palliative Care,* **10**: 168–9.

31. Guys & St Thomas's (2009). Evelina Children's Hospital opens for business. Available at: http://www.guysandstthomas.com/news/newsarchive/archive0305/evelinaopens.aspx. (Accessed 4 December 2009.)

32. Nightingale F (1946). *Notes on Nursing.* Philadelphia, PA: JB Lippincott.

Section 5

Some thoughts on priorities for research, education, and service development

Chapter 21

End of life care for older people with dementia: priorities for research and service development

Murna Downs

People fear both living and dying with advanced dementia. They fear both for very good reasons. They fear *living with advanced dementia* because they do not expect to experience a good life with dementia (1) and there is overwhelming evidence to suggest that this is an accurate appraisal (2). Indeed living well with advanced dementia is something of an oxymoron. Advanced dementia is commonly portrayed as a 'living death' for the person and a 'living bereavement' for the carer. Technical fixes, including inappropriate use of feeding tubes, are common, in the absence of evidence of their doing good and concern that they do harm (2–5). *Dying with dementia* is no more attractive, being associated with aggressive medical intervention rather than a more palliative approach emphasizing dignity and comfort (6).

These concerns about living and dying with advanced dementia are borne out by recent evidence which, in England, led to a Public Account Committee Report in 2008 on dementia (7). This was swiftly followed in 2009 by the Department of Health's National Dementia Strategy entitled *Living well with dementia* (8). The strategy outlined a 5-year plan to *transform* the quality of care provided to people with dementia and their families. Recognition of the unacceptability of the neglect of people with dementia and their families is not restricted to England; the European Commission, along with a growing number of Member States (e.g. Netherlands, Norway) have developed strategies on dementia, as have Australia and as is Canada.

With this context in mind, quality end of life care is a key priority for people with advanced dementia. Yet in addressing this key priority we are faced with an apparent contradiction. As we challenge the erroneous link between advanced dementia and both the death of the person and the death of hope for quality of life, we must place equal emphasis on ensuring improved care of people with advanced dementia who are dying.

People with advanced dementia can live for several years (9, 10) reliant on others for their entire daily needs (11). The National Council for Palliative Care describes end of life care as help that is provided to those with advanced, progressive, incurable illnesses to live as well as possible until they die (12).

What constitutes quality end of life care for people with advanced dementia?

There is consensus that quality end of life care for people with advanced dementia comprises the following components:

Person-centred care

Person-centred care includes both care for *the person* and care for *the whole person* (13).

Care for the person

We are in a highly unusual circumstance where people with advanced dementia are at risk of no longer being seen as a person and, if they are, as no longer being seen to be the same person they were before (14–17). This makes a key task of end of life care for people with dementia being the reinstatement of the person as a human being, with the same rights and entitlements to well-being as all human beings (16, 18). The controversial call for people with dementia to consider terminating their life in order to prevent the burden of their care falling on their families and the health care system (see, e.g. 19) is a chilling reminder of the compelling need to reinstate the human worth and entitlement of life with advanced dementia.

A significant percentage of people with advanced dementia live in care homes. Research conducted in these settings leaves us with some concern as to the quality of attention paid to the person (20, 21) and the inappropriate use of antipsychotic medication in these settings (22). There is, however, a growing evidence base, using the gold standard of randomized trials, which demonstrate effective approaches to ensuring we maintain a focus on the person as a unique human being with emotional and social as well as physical needs (23–25). Fossey et al. demonstrated a significant reduction in neuroleptic medication when such a person-centred approach was adopted (24). What is now needed is to embed this evidence in practice; for which action and translational research may well be the most effective route (26).

Care for the whole person

Care for the whole person refers to equal weight being given to emotional, medical, physical, psychological, and spiritual needs (27). The tendency for care for people with advanced dementia to focus on treating a medical need (e.g. difficulty with swallowing) with a technical fix (e.g. feeding tube) without due regard to the resulting loss of human contact or sensory pleasure or physical discomfort is a growing concern (3, 28). Care for the whole person requires that we challenge the (curative) practice of medicine to keep a person alive at all costs with the approach of palliative care which is guided by ensuring comfort and dignity for the person.

Support for the family

This requires that family are afforded their rightful place as partners in care of their relative, as well as recognized as having support and information needs of their own. Yet our literature is littered with the neglect of family perspectives and experience and expertise (29) which Nolan et al.'s relationship-centred care strives to address (30). Care for people with advanced dementia will place the family in the role of decision-maker and much can be done to minimize the stress associated with this role. Addressing interfamily conflict can be done with facilitated family meetings (31). There is also a need to address communication between families and professionals as well as between professionals themselves (32).

Support for care staff

Care staff who work closely with the person with advanced dementia need adequate preparation (training and education) and emotional support. Yet we know the emotional side of this work is neglected and viewed as not a legitimate part of the job, leading to burnout and, at the time of the resident's death, the phenomenon of 'disenfranchised grief' (33). It is now recognized that care home staff are poorly prepared for their role (34) and, recently, Clare argues for the need to train staff in awareness of the needs of people with advanced dementia (35).

Decision-making and advanced planning

The Department of Health's *National Dementia Strategy* (2009) places significant emphasis on improving the end of life care for people with dementia (8). Its main suggestion for achieving this is to involve people with dementia and their carers in planning end of life care, recognizing the principles outlined in the Department of Health's *End of life care strategy* (36). As such, it is really focused on terminal care. Advanced care planning has a role to play in ensuring quality terminal care, but it by no means guarantees it. The recent 2009 report from the Nuffield Council on Bioethics describes the limitations of advanced care planning (18).

Terminal care

Care provided in the last weeks and days of life is generally regarded as terminal care. Quality terminal care includes the provision of psychological, social, and spiritual support to people with dementia and their families throughout the last phase and into bereavement. It will include excellent medical (e.g. pain management) and physical (e.g. skin and mouth care) care. It will also require a recognition that predicting or even identifying the terminal phase in advanced dementia is notoriously difficult.

What needs to be in place to ensure quality end of life care?

- Recognizing dementia as a terminal illness which if you do not die with it, you will die from it (6, 37)
- Having an explicit policy regarding end of life care for people with dementia (6)
- Having clinical and practice guidelines in the care of people with advanced dementia (6)
- Training and education in appropriate end of life care directed at the general public, people with early dementia, families, care staff, and professionals (6)
- Systematic research on palliative care for people with advanced dementia including the development of appropriate outcome measures (4, 38)
- Action research on changing the culture of care for people with advanced dementia (39, 40)
- Ensuring the inclusion of people with dementia in research on end of life care, which may require education for research ethics panels.

References

1. Moniz-Cook ED, Manthorpe J, Carr I, Gibson G, Vernooij M (2006). Facing the future. A qualitative study of older people referred to a memory clinic prior to assessment and diagnosis, *Dementia*, 5(3): 375–95.
2. National Audit Office (2007). *Improving Services and support for people with dementia*. London: TSO.
3. Heath I (2009). Memento mori. *InnovAiT*, 2(8): 503–4.
4. Sampson EL, Ritchie CW, Lai R Raven PW, Blanchard MR (2005). A systematic review of the scientific evidence for the efficacy of a palliative care approach in advanced dementia. *International Psychogeriatrics*, 17(1): 31–40.
5. Gillick MR (2004). Rethinking the role of tube feeding in patients with advanced dementia. *New England Journal of Medicine*, 342(3): 206–10.
6. Sachs GA, Shega JW, Cox-Hayley D (2004). Barriers to excellent end-of-life care for patients with dementia. *Journal of General Internal Medicine*, 19(10): 1057–63.

7. House of Commons Public Accounts Committee Report (2008). *Improving services and support for people with dementia*. London: House of Commons Committee of Public Accounts.

8. Department of Health (2009). *Living Well with Dementia: A national dementia strategy*. London: The Stationery Office.

9. Lynn J, Adamson DM (2003). *Living well at the end of life. Adapting health care to serious chronic illness in old age*. Washington, DC: Rand Health.

10. Lunney JR, Lynn J, Foley DS, Lipson S, Guralnik JM (2003). Patterns of functional decline at the end of life. *Journal of the American Medical Association*, **289**: 2387–92.

11. Burns A, Winblad B (eds) (2006). *Severe dementia*. Chichester: John Wiley and Sons.

12. National Council for Palliative Care and Alzheimer's Society (2006). *Exploring palliative care for people with dementia*. London: National Council for Palliative Care.

13. Downs M (2010). Person-centred care as supportive care. In JC Hughes, M Lloyd-Williams, GA Sachs (eds) *Supportive care for the person with dementia*. Oxford: Oxford University Press.

14. Hughes JC, Robinson L, Volicer L (2005). Specialist palliative care in dementia. *British Medical Journal*, **330**: 57–8.

15. Jennings B (2004). Alzheimer's disease and the quality of life. In KJ Doka (ed) *Living with grief: Alzheimer's disease*, pp. 247–58. Washington, DC: Hospice Foundation of America.

16. Kitwood T (1997). *Dementia reconsidered: The person comes first*. Buckingham: Open University Press.

17. Sabat S (2001). *The experience of Alzheimer's disease: Life through a tangled veil*. Oxford: Blackwell.

18. Nuffield Council on Bioethics (2009). *Dementia: Ethical issues*. London: Nuffield Council on Bioethics.

19. Beckford M (2008). Baroness Warnock: Dementia sufferers may have a 'duty to die'. *The Telegraph*, 18 September. Available at: http://www.telegraph.co.uk/news/uknews/2983652/Baroness-Warnock-Dementia-sufferers-may-have-a-duty-to-die.html.

20. Ballard C, Fossey J, Chithramohan R, Howard R, Burns A, Thompson P, et al. (2001). Quality of care in private sector and NHS facilities for people with dementia: cross sectional survey *British Medical Journal*, **323**: 426–7.

21. Cohen-Mansfield J, Creedon M, Malone T, Parpura-Gill A, Dakheel M, Heasly C (2006). Dressing of cognitively impaired nursing home residents: Description and analysis. *The Gerontologist*, **46**(1): 89–96.

22. All-Party Parliamentary Group on Dementia (2008). *Always a last resort: Inquiry into the prescription of antipsychotic drugs to people with dementia living in care homes*. London: Alzheimer's Society.

23. Chenoweth L, King MT, Jeon Y-H, Brodaty H, Stein-Parbury J, Norman R, et al. (2009). Caring for aged dementia care resident study (CADRES) of person-centred care, dementia care mapping and usual care in dementia: a cluster-randomised trial. *Lancet Neurology*, **8**(4): 317–25.

24. Fossey J, Ballard C, Juszczak E, James I, Alder N, Jacoby R, et al. (2006). Effect of enhanced psychosocial care on antipsychotic use in nursing home residents with severe dementia: cluster randomised trial *British Medical Journal*, **332**: 756–61.

25. Sloane P, Hoeffer B, Mitchell C, McKenzie DA, Barrick AL, Rader J, et al. (2004). Effect of person-centred showering and the bath towel on bathing associated aggression, agitation, and discomfort in nursing home residents with dementia: A randomized, controlled trial. *Journal of the American Geriatrics Society*, **52**(11): 1795–804.

26. Burgio LD (2010). Disentangling the translational sciences: A Social Science perspective, *Research and Theory for Nursing Practice: An International Journal*, **24**(1): 56–63.

27. Hughes JC, Lloyd-Williams M and Sachs GA (eds) (2010) *Supportive care for the person with dementia*. Oxford: Oxford University Press.

28. Sampson EL, Candy B, Jones L (2009). Enteral tube feeding for older people with advanced dementia. *Cochrane Database Systematic Review*, **2**: CD007209.

29. Davies S, Nolan M (2004). 'Making it better': Self-perceived roles of family caregivers of older people living in care homes: A qualitative study. *International Journal of Nursing Studies*, **43**(3): 281–91.

30. Nolan MR, Davies S, Brown J, Keady J, Nolan J (2004). Beyond 'person-centred' care: a new vision for gerontological nursing. *International Journal of Older People Nursing*, **13**(3a): 45–53.

31. Zarit SH, Zarit JM (2007). *Mental disorders in older adults*, 2nd edn. New York: Guilford.

32. Levenson R (2004). Lessons from the end of life. *British Medical Journal*, **329**(7476): 1244.

33. Moss MS Moss SZ Rubinstein RL, Black HK. (2003). The metaphor of 'family' in staff communication about dying and death. *Journal of Gerontology, Psychological Science Social Science*, **58**(5): S290–6.

34. All Party Parliamentary Group on Dementia (2009). *Prepared to care: Challenging the dementia skills gap*. London: APPG.

35. Clare L (2010). Awareness in people with severe dementia: review and integration. *Ageing and Mental Health*, **14**(1): 20–32.

36. Department of Health (2009). *End of life care strategy*. London: The Stationery Office.

37. Volicer L (2007) Goals of care in advanced dementia: quality of life, dignity and comfort. *Journal of Nutrition, Health and Ageing*, **11**(6): 481.

38. Birch D, Draper J (2008). A critical literature review exploring the challenges of delivering effective palliative care to older people with dementia. *Journal of Clinical Nursing*, **17**(9): 1144–63.

39. Chang E, Daly J, Johnson A, Harrison K, Easterbrook S, Bidewell J, Stewart H, et al. (2009). Challenges for professional care of advanced dementia, *International Journal of Nursing Practice*, **15**(1): 41–7.

40. Monteleoni C, Clark E (2004). Using rapid-cycle quality improvement methodology to reduce feeding tubes in patients with advanced dementia: before and after study. *British Medical Journal*, **329**(7464): 491–4.

Chapter 22

Evidence, evidence, and evidence: future priorities for research and service development in improving palliative care for older people

Irene J. Higginson

Hospices and the global palliative care movement were undoubtedly one of the great successes of the 20th century. But is that enough for the 21st century? Senior politicians, policy-makers, and others have questioned the level of evidence for some of the practices within hospices and medicine for older people (1). And indeed hospice, palliative care, and gerontology staff all want to improve care as much as possible, and to do this evidence is needed.

Evidence in palliative and end of life care comes forward in three main forms. There is evidence of need, of importance (to those affected by cancer and to society), and evidence of an effective solution (2). Sadly, there has been too little investment in palliative care research and also in research among older people. Typically most trials of drug and other therapies exclude people over the age of 75 or even 65 years, or people with many comorbidities, because such people are difficult to research. And there is very little spending on research in palliative care. Analysis by the NCRI Analysis of the National Cancer Research Portfolio 2002–2006 shows that less than 0.2% (i.e. less than 20 pence in every £100) of research spent by charities and government on cancer is on palliative and end of life care in the UK (3). A far smaller proportion of that is spent on specifically on the oldest people—so we are probably talking about only a few pence in every £100. In other diseases the amount spent on research is probably much less than this. Despite this very low investment it is impressive that a good amount of research has been undertaken in palliative and end of life care, and has produced results that have improved practice and care.

Unfortunately the low level of investment has led to research of the cheaper kind, which is largely concerned with the first two forms of evidence, rather than developing or discovering better services or treatments, and evaluating these using robust methods. Without doubt there is ample evidence of need for effective supportive and palliative care among patients, including older people. This is evidenced by studies over many years that have demonstrated concern and problems in communication, information, psychological support, symptom control, care of the dying, bereavement support, care for patients and families, the need to involve users, palliative care, spiritual support, social support, and the need to orientate services around the issues faced by patients and families at a time when patients and families themselves are feeling vulnerable and often are less able to be proactive or demanding. There is also evidence that people value palliative care and regard it as a high priority (2).

But it is for the third type of evidence where the major gaps in research exist. There is a particularly acute gap in research which follows a programmatic pattern in which one study leads to and builds on the previous work, or where smaller exploratory or needs-based studies lead to trials testing interventions. This gap is shown in the evidence review for the National Institute of Health and Clinical Excellence (NICE, UK) in supportive and palliative cancer care (2, 4–6) and in the US National Institutes of Health Systematic Review End of Life Care (7, 8). More recently a review undertaken by for the Service Development and Organisation (SDO) in the UK on end of life care reached similar conclusions. Specifically for older people, better practice guidance on the palliative care for older people has been produced for the World Health Organization (WHO) (9, 10). There are some great examples of innovative practice and care, but not enough on the evaluation of these practices.

Gaps in defining the interventions

In all systematic reviews and evidence appraisals two main difficulties are encountered in understanding the services. First, in many instances the intervention was not clearly described and defined. This limitation may result from a lack of publishing space within journals. However, lack of information about interventions makes drawing conclusions about their relevance in different circumstances and settings more difficult. It also makes it difficult for others to independently and accurately reproduce this in another setting.

The second problem is that when information about the interventions is available the interventions often vary greatly from setting to setting, making it difficult to draw conclusions about the overall effectiveness of a group of interventions. This is demonstrated clearly in the area of specialist palliative care, where teams work in different ways with different policies, different staffing mixes and different training backgrounds. Thus, it is difficult to draw conclusions about the best model of working (2, 6).

Populations, patients, and carers or families

Conducting research with patients who are highly distressed, have severe symptoms or are dying is very difficult. Many studies make extremely bold and rigorous attempts to recruit from representative samples of patients and families and to collect data in an ethical, sensitive, and meaningful way. However, it is important to make sure that studies select patients who are older, some of whom may have cognitive impairment. These groups are often missed but require methods such as face-to-face interviewing, or observation, all methods which are more difficult and costly to conduct (11, 12).

Opportunities and next steps

An important opportunity exists in palliative care for older people. There is a new demographic pressure leading to a growing future need for palliative care (13), and a new population, which will be older, and with more comorbidities, and complex social situations than in the past. Therefore, treatments need to be tested among older people, and new models of care may need to be developed. These models of care could be developed using modern research methods guidance, such as the Medical Research Council (MRC) (14) guidance on the development and evaluation of complex interventions. Studies which integrate quantitative and qualitative methods, or use them sequentially, are likely to be able to capture the more important outcomes for patients and understand what these mean in clinical practice (15).

A major challenge in the field of palliative core care for older people is to use outcome measures that are sensitive and appropriate to the intangible nature of critical issues such as symptom control, psychological well-being, quality of life, quality of death, quality of care, and yet short enough to be used in practice (16, 17). Great progress has been made in developing robust and sensitive outcome measurement and these measures are now available and are being further refined, including through European collaboratives, such as the PRISMA collaborative, spanning Europe (18). Progress is now needed into ways to better measure the costs and cost-effectiveness of treatments and models of care (19).

Dame Cicely Saunders is universally seen as the founder of the modern hospice movement, but she wasn't content with that, she wanted research and from that more education. Created by Cicely Saunders International (a new charity focused on creating a centre for research) and King's College London, the Cicely Saunders Institute opened in May 2010. This will also form a centre for palliative care research and development, demonstrating to all that research is needed. This group is also a WHO Collaborating Centre for Palliative Care and Older People, to help ensure research reaches policy makers. Other centres are being established on palliative and end of life care, including the European Centre for Palliative Care in Trondheim, Norway, and groups of excellence, in Houston, Texas, New York, and across Canada, Australia, and Europe. These centres, along with other strong groups will all aid the development of future high quality research and training in research in palliative care.

From the gaps in knowledge priorities emerge. These are:

Direction and nature of research

1. Future research should focus on determining effective solutions rather than on re-determining need, because there is a wealth of evidence regarding need and importance, and a relative dearth of evidence regarding effective solutions.
2. New services and many existing services should be developed or continued to be developed within an evaluation framework, which is rigorous and properly funded.
3. Research funders should invest in research programmes in both supportive and palliative care. These should be sufficiently substantial, sustained, and robust to ensure studies involve and measure aspects important to users, determine effectiveness and experience, and achieve appropriate power.
4. Studies should use appropriate validated outcomes measures and be multiprofessional, if appropriate.

Interventions and population

5. Detailed descriptions of interventions and service configurations should be made available when evaluations are published.
6. Wherever possible studies should use a research base to develop interventions, building on existing research and indicating where interventions deviate from those already established.
7. Future research should compare different service configurations and interventions.
8. Clear descriptions of the populations, patients, and carers included seen by individual services and comparison of how these compare with the general population need to be made. Specifically these should include older people, including those from different cultures.

Areas of particular need

9. Research in settings where older people are especially concentrated, such as nursing homes, at home, as well as in hospitals and hospices.
10. Research into the cost-effectiveness of new models of care which allow for patients with longer trajectories of illness and with comorbidities, rather than single diseases.

11. Research into the cost-effectiveness of new models of support for caregivers.

12. Research into the cost-effectiveness of treatment and care for the symptoms that particularly affect older people and currently have been relatively neglected, such as breathlessness (common in cancer, chronic obstructive pulmonary disease, and heart failure), fatigue, weakness, and cachexia (common in dementia, heart failure, and cancer).

References

1. Higginson IJ (2010). Palliative care in the tennies: What can we expect? (Editorial). *Journal of Palliative Medicine*, **13**(4): 355–6.

2. Gysels M, Higginson IJ (2004). *Improving supportive and palliative care for adults with cancer: Research Evidence*. London: National Institute of Clinical Excellence.

3. National Cancer Research Institute (2008). *Analysis of the National Cancer Research Porfolio*. London: NCRI.

4. Higginson IJ, Finlay I, Goodwin DM, Cook AM, Hood K, Edwards AGK, et al. (2002). Do hospital-based palliative teams improve care for patients or families at the end of life? *Journal of Pain & Symptom Management*, **23**: 96–106.

5. Higginson IJ, Finlay IG, Goodwin DM, Hood K, Edwards AGK, Cook A, et al. (2003). Is there evidence that palliative care teams alter end-of-life experiences of patients and their caregivers? *Journal of Pain & Symptom Management*, **25**: 150–68.

6. Higginson IJ (2004). It would be NICE to have more evidence? *Palliative Medicine*, **18**: 85–6.

7. Dy SM, Shugarman LR, Lorenz KA, Mularski RA, Lynn J (2008). A systematic review of satisfaction with care at the end of life. *Journal of the American Geriatrics Society*, **56**(1): 124–9.

8. Lorenz KA, Lynn J, Dy SM, Shugarman LR, Wilkinson A, Mularski RA, et al. (2008). Evidence for improving palliative care at the end of life: a systematic review. *Annals of Internal Medicine*, **148**(2): 147–59.

9. Davies E, Higginson IJ (2004). *Better palliative care for older people*. Denmark: World Health Organization.

10. Hall S, Petkova H, Tsouros A, Costantini M, Higginson IJ (2010). *Palliative Care for Older People: Better Practice*. Copenhagen: WHO Regional Office for Europe.

11. Bennett MI, Davies EA, Higginson IJ (2010). Delivering research in end-of-life care: problems, pitfalls and future priorities. *Palliative Medicine*, **24**: 456–61.

12. Costantini M, Beccaro M (2009). Health services research on end-of-life care. *Current Opinion in Supportive and Palliative Care*, **3**(3): 190–4.

13. Gomes B, Higginson IJ (2008). Where people die (1974–2030): past trends, future projections and implications for care. *Palliative Medicine*, **22**(1): 33–41.

14. Craig P, Dieppe P, Macintyre S, Michie S, Nazareth I, Petticrew M (2008). Developing and evaluating complex interventions: the new Medical Research Council guidance. *British Medical Journal*, **337**: a1655.

15. Lewin S, Glenton C, Oxman AD (2009). Use of qualitative methods alongside randomised controlled trials of complex healthcare interventions: methodological study. *British Medical Journal*, **339**: b3496.

16. Higginson IJ, Gao W (2008). Caregiver assessment of patients with advanced cancer: concordance with patients, effect of burden and positivity. *Health and Quality of Life Outcomes*, **6**: 42.

17. Higginson IJ, Gao W, Jackson D, Murray J, Harding R (2010). Short-form Zarit Caregiver Burden Interviews were valid in advanced conditions. *Journal of Clinical Epidemiology*, **63**(5): 535–42.

18. Harding R, Higginson IJ (2010). PRISMA: A pan-European co-ordinating action to advance the science in end-of-life cancer care. *European Journal of Cancer*, **46**(9): 1493–50.

19. Gomes B, Harding R, Foley KM, Higginson IJ (2009). Optimal approaches to the health economics of palliative care: report of an international think tank. *Journal of Pain & Symptom Management*, **38**(1): 4–10.

Chapter 23

Priorities for research and service development in primary care to improve end of life for older people

Scott A. Murray

Primary care has a greater potential than any other service or setting to make a positive difference in the end of life care for older people. There are four main reasons. Firstly, primary care can deal with older people with all progressive life-threatening illnesses, not just a specific diagnostic or specialist grouping. Secondly, primary care can start end of life care for older people as soon as this would be beneficial and not just in the last days or weeks of life. Thirdly, all dimensions of need—physical, psychological, social, and spiritual—can be addressed by professions who have holistic care as a mindset. Finally, primary care can help more older people be cared for and die at home and in care homes, if that is their wish. The provision of palliative care in the community by generalists such as general practitioners and district nurses is now sometimes referred to internationally as Primary Palliative Care. The Primary Palliative Care Research Group at Edinburgh University has led work using various innovative concepts and methods to develop these four potential areas for development of palliative care in the community, which are now summarized in turn.

Primary care can develop end of life care for all people who are dying of a progressive illness

Figure 23.1 illustrates the typical trajectories of physical decline at the end of life. Each general practitioner with an average of 2000 registered patients has approximately 20 deaths per year. Only two are from acute causes, and on average five are from cancer, six occur due to organ failure (such as heart failure or chronic obstructive pulmonary disease), and seven now occur in older persons after a period of physical or cognitive frailty. General practitioners are encouraged by some governments to identify patients in their last year of life and thus most practices in the UK have 'supportive and palliative care registers' to identify such people. General practitioners are now realizing that cancer patients tend to die after a relevantly short period of illness whereas organ failure takes months or years and that people on the frailty trajectory often take many years (1–3). This identification of older persons as the main group in need of a palliative care approach means that older people are increasingly considered and assessed for care planning including end of life issues. There is thus a structure in place, assisted by the Gold Standards Framework documentation (http://www.goldstandardsframework.nhs.uk/), and also a policy directive, at least in the UK, for primary care to identify, assess, and plan care for older persons.

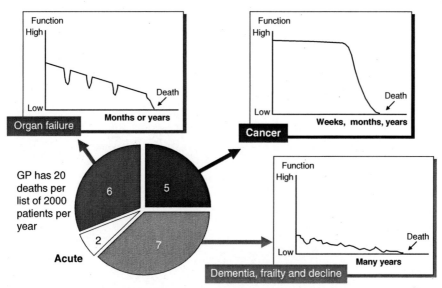

Fig. 23.1 Typical trajectories of physical decline at the end of life: acute, intermittent, and gradual decline (2).

Primary care can start end of life care as soon as it would be useful

Figure 23.2 illustrates appropriate care near the end of life with a diagram that was initially used concerning cancer care. With cancer there was a period when a cure was attempted, but when a cure could no longer be planned, palliative care then intervened. The new and better concept, however, is that supportive and palliative care should start at diagnosis of a life-threatening illness and gradually increase while disease-modifying care may decrease. This model and understanding can be applied to all people with a progressive illness including organ failure and frailty (4, 5). As debility increases from specific illnesses or general frailty, people can be considered for a palliative approach. Provision of palliative care should be triggered not by diagnosis, or even prognosis, but according to need. Another specific trigger for consideration for a holistic palliative approach might be admission to a care home, as this is generally done to increase supportive care. Yet another criteria could be the need of a certain amount of hours of care in the community. Further research is needed to identify when a palliative approach is appreciated by patients and when it is associated with favourable outcomes for patients, and what outcomes are best measured.

Primary care can improve end of life care for the elderly by addressing and meeting their multidimensional needs

Although death has been 'medicalized' over the last few years, death is clearly a four-dimensional activity. Work clarifying how these four different dimensions may change at the end of life has been done with cancer and organ failure patients and further work is necessary with the elderly so that proactive and planned care can be offered when it is most likely to be necessary, and focus on the dimension of care that is needed. See Figure 23.3 for typical physical, social, psychological, and spiritual end of life trajectories in people with lung cancer (6). Especially as there are some practical interventions that meet the needs of people with spiritual distress, such as dignity therapy,

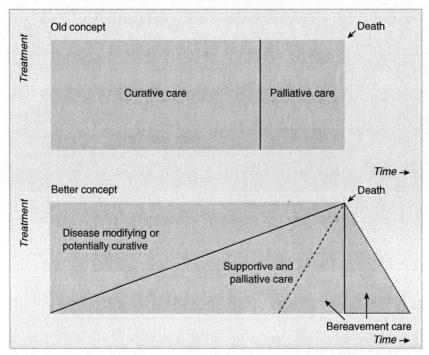

Fig. 23.2 Appropriate care near the end of life: from disease modifying to active palliation. Reproduced from Murray SA, Kendall M, Boyd K, Sheikh A (2005). Illness trajectories and palliative care. *British Medical Journal*, **330**: 1007–11. Copyright © 2005 BMJ Publishing Ltd.

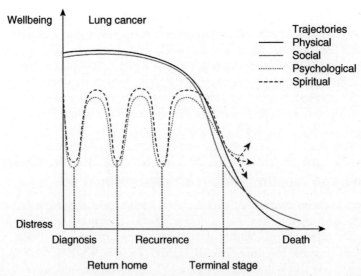

Fig. 23.3 Typical physical, social, psychological and spiritual end of life trajectories in people with lung cancer.

REFERENCES | 259

such exploratory research is necessary in older people. Spiritual needs can be defined as issues relating to meaning and purpose, and may not be expressed using religious language. Simply spending time listening can help people who are suffering psychologically or spiritually (7).

Developing primary care services at the end of life can help more people die at home or in homes, if they wish

Only about 19% of people die at home in the UK, and this figure rises to around 35% if we include care homes. Research suggests that over 60% of people would like to die at home if this were a realistic possibility for them. Work in some general practices where the Gold Standards Framework is routine suggests that around 40% of people can die at home if they are identified and their needs are assessed and planned for earlier rather than later. An action research in a study in all care homes in Midlothian, Scotland in 2008 showed that introducing advance care planning routinely in nursing homes reduced admissions to hospital in the last year of life by 50% (8). Research with specialist palliative care nurses in hospices and with general practitioners in the community has found, however, that advance care planning has many barriers to overcome, including firstly identifying people and assessing them before planning can start. Thus research is needed to identify how best people can be identified and for a palliative approach at the end of life whether they are dying from frailty or from complex comorbidities.

Conclusions

The average age of people who die from cancer or organ failure is 74 years and thus the vast majority of people in developing countries now die old after a period of physical, social, and often psychological decline. Primary care is ideally placed to reach and serve the whole population and to provide care where people wish. Primary care can, moreover, provide supportive care from diagnosis of a life-threatening illness (including dementia) and to people with all conditions and also their carers. Primary care clinicians have the potential to provide this given adequate training and support from specialist geriatric and palliative care services. Further research is urgently required to identify how this can be best delivered.

Acknowledgements

We thank the Scottish Government and Macmillan Cancer Support for funding much of the work leading to these insights.

References

1. Lunney JR, Lynn J, Foley DS, Lipson S, Guralnik JM (2003). Patterns of functional decline at the end of life. *Journal of the American Medical Association*, **289**: 2387–92.
2. Murray SA, Kendall M, Boyd K, Sheikh A (2005). Illness trajectories and palliative care. *British Medical Journal*, **330**: 1007–11.
3. Lynn J (2008). Reliable comfort and meaningfulness. Making a difference campaign. *British Medical Journal*, **336**: 958–9.
4. World Health Organization (2004). *Palliative care: the solid facts*. Geneva: WHO.
5. Murray SA (2008). Meeting the challenge of palliation beyond cancer. *European Journal of Palliative Care*, **15**: 213.
6. Murray SA, Kendall M, Grant E, Boyd K, Barclay S, Sheikh A (2007). Patterns of social psychological and spiritual decline towards the end of life in lung cancer and heart failure. *Journal of Pain and Symptom Management*, **34**: 393–402

7. Grant E, Murray SA, Kendall M, Boyd K, Tilley S, Ryan D (2004). Spiritual issues and needs: perspectives from patients with advanced cancer and non-malignant disease. A qualitative study. *Palliative & Supportive Care*, **2**: 371–8

8. Hockley J, Watson J, Oxenham D, Murray SA. The integrated implementation of two end of life care tools in nursing care homes in the UK: an in-depth evaluation. *Palliative Medicine*, 2010;24:828.

Chapter 24

Priorities for specialist palliative care: an Australian perspective

Margaret O'Connor

One hundred and thirty-eight thousand Australians die each year and the majority of these are of people aged 70 years and over. Thus, in recent years, an important focus for palliative care service delivery is care of older people facing the end of life. This chapter discusses the shift in specialist palliative care service provision that has occurred over the last 10 years or so, as the population ages and palliative care has become a more integrated part of mainstream health care systems.

An important shift in palliative care in Australia has been the significant investment in skilling the primary health care workforce, in the recognition that not all dying people and their families require specialist palliative care and it would be impossible for services to meet the expectation of providing care for all dying people. This means that specialist services have predominantly become consultative services to generalist providers and this work is more frequently involving consultation into residential aged care homes.

How history influences present models

Traditional hospice care has been part of Australia's health care system since early colonial times with the Irish Sisters of Charity establishing the first Hospice in Sydney in 1898 (1, 2). Large bed-based hospices grew around the country, mostly built in settings separate from other health facilities and care of the dying remaining unacknowledged and hidden. A hospice was seen as a haven for the dying that protected them from the pressures of the acute hospital system (3). With an often protracted length of stay, the hospices were distinctive from nursing homes, only because the population in aged care homes at the time was not necessarily frail, vulnerable, or dying. Until the 1990s, there was little recognition that the work of the hospice and the nursing home had anything in common.

Even with 'modern' palliative care becoming an integral part of health care systems during the last 15 years or so, palliative care and aged care continued to work separately from each other. However, with the increase in comorbidities of aged care home residents, there was a growing awareness that the core work of both aged and palliative care services was to look after people 'who are finishing' (4). Separateness resulted in an inequitable system whereby a younger person dying of cancer at home could receive the range of specialist palliative care services required, but an older person dying of perhaps an undiagnosed condition in residential aged care, had little access to specialist palliative care services. There developed a resultant entrenched attitude of disregard for the death of an older person, as 'decrepit' (5). Besides this care inequity, organizational disparities have endured, like models of care, levels of funding, and staff skill mixes, and are highlighted as barriers for the easy transfer of palliative care knowledge into residential aged care environments (6–8).

Melding the expertise of palliative care and aged care

With growing government awareness of the real and anticipated costs of aged care, both current and in the future, a range of sweeping changes were introduced by the Aged Care Act (1997), including the deregulation of staffing (9). The changes precipitated by the Act, did not necessarily reflect the changing demographics of much older, more dependent people making up the residential aged care population and being resident for shorter periods before death (10). The concept of 'ageing in place' was introduced, meaning that as much as possible, care needs were to be provided where the person resides, instead of them needing to move. O'Connor and Pearson (11) argued that if 'ageing in place' was to be a complete concept for residential aged care settings, then in recognition of the numbers of deaths that occur, 'dying in place' logically followed.

Accreditation of all residential aged care homes became a requirement in 2001 and included the provision of palliative care; however, it was unclear as to how aged care services were faring, given the constraints on staffing and funding (9, 12).

Current models of care

Perhaps arising from the focus on older people created by the International Year of the Older Person in 1999, in the early 2000s, the Australian Government's National Palliative Care Programme funded a large national project to develop evidence-based guidelines: *Guidelines for a Palliative Approach in Residential Aged Care* (13) (see Chapter 19, this volume) Working on the definition of a 'palliative approach' the guidelines sought to provide a framework for:

- Enhancing the care of residents and their families by offering them a palliative approach when appropriate, and
- Increasing the knowledge and range of skills of staff in providing the palliative approach in caring for residents and their families (13).

The philosophy of a palliative approach takes a positive attitude towards death and dying requiring open discussions about death and dying, between the aged care team, residents, and their families. Care is holistic, providing active comfort to reduce symptoms and distress and includes identifying the resident's wishes regarding their end-of-life care (13). The guidelines have been widely distributed to approximately 4000 services, with companion guidelines almost completed on a palliative approach for aged care in the community setting.

The role of specialist community palliative care services has increased as aged care services seek to use the guidelines and meet accreditation requirements. Formal evaluation of the impact of the guidelines is yet to occur, but there has been some criticism about their lack of use (10). Anecdotally, specialist community palliative care services have found their work expanding into residential aged care homes in their local area. These services are called upon to provide consultation on individual residents, manage symptoms especially pain, liaise with general practitioners, and deliver educational programmes, with little additional funding to support these increased activities.

Formalized local service linkages based on geography may well be the way to provide local support to the melding of palliative care and aged care expertise. Such partnerships between specialist palliative care and aged care services, and perhaps based on the guidelines, need to address a consistent programme of professional support and include adequate remuneration. These linkages may be a key to both ensuring that the dying older person's needs are met as well as alleviating the need to move them to hospital (5). Recognition of the breadth of this work through appropriate funding would assist in embedding the role of specialist palliative care in care of the dying person in residential aged care homes.

References

1. Redpath, R (1998). Palliative care in Australia. In Ramadge J (ed) *Australian nursing practice and palliative care: its origins, evolution and future,* vol. 9, pp. 1–17. Canberra: Royal College of Nursing Australia.

2. O'Connor, M (2002). *The veils of death: Understanding dying in residential aged care. A discourse analysis of policy.* Doctor of Nursing Thesis. Melbourne: La Trobe University.

3. McNamara, B (2001). *Fragile lives: death, dying and care.* Crows Nest: Allen & Unwin.

4. Knepfner G (1989). *Nursing for Life.* Sydney: Pan Books.

5. O'Connor, M (2009). Decrepit death as a discourse of death in older age: implications for policy. *International Journal of Older People Nursing,* **4**: 263–71.

6. Palliative Care Australia (1999). *Discussion Paper: Palliative Care in Aged Care Facilities.* Canberra: Palliative Care Australia.

7. Whittaker E, Kernohan G, Hasson F, Howard V, McLaughlin D (2007). Palliative care in nursing homes: exploring care assistants' knowledge. *International Journal of Older People Nursing,* **2**: 36–44.

8. Froggatt K (2001). Palliative care and nursing homes: where next? *Palliative Medicine,* **15**: 42–8.

9. Angus J, Nay R (2003). The paradox of the Aged Care Act 1997: the marginalisation of nursing discourse. *Nursing Inquiry,* **10**: 130–8.

10. Andrews-Hall S, Howe A, Robinson A (2007). The dynamics of residential aged care in Australia: 8 year trends in admissions, separations and dependency. *Australian Health Review,* **31**: 611–22.

11. O'Connor M, Pearson A. (2004). Ageing in place–dying in place–competing discourses for care of the dying in aged care policy. *Australian Journal of Advanced Nursing,* **22**: 31–7.

12. Allen S, Francis K, Chapman Y, O'Connor M (2007). Multipurpose services and palliative care: emerging funding challenges and possible solutions. *Asia-Pacific Journal of Health Management,* **2**: 51–5.

13. Australian Government, Department of Health & Ageing (2006). *Guidelines for a Palliative Approach in Residential Aged Care.* Canberra: National Palliative Care Program.

Chapter 25

Inter-disciplinary perspectives

Sabine Pleschberger

Being an interdisciplinary endeavour, end of life care for older people is comprised of a number of health professions and academic disciplines involved in research and practice in the field. Apart from individual knowledge and competencies, how these professions and disciplines work together plays a crucial role for the quality of care provided. This is equally true for the quality of research. Therefore this chapter refrains from a specific disciplinary perspective to identify the future development of a research agenda for end of life care for older people. Rather, the focus will be on the relevance of some overarching themes, such as user involvement, gender issues, organizational issues, research methodology and ethics, all of which transgress disciplinary boundaries. These issues require an interdisciplinary approach which goes beyond an additive model of multidisciplinary perspectives but implies close interaction and reflection of the researchers involved throughout the whole research processes.

Connecting disciplines, fields, and professions

With palliative care on the one hand and old age care on the other hand we have two well established international disciplines both with an impressive body of knowledge based on clinical experience and academic research.

Nevertheless, both disciplines have a history of neglecting end of life care for older people. Palliative care was developed in light of terminal diseases like cancer and has so far neglected to pay attention to the specific needs and living conditions of older people (1). In 2002 the World Health Organization's definition of palliative care was broadened to explicitly refer to other disease groups and specific demographic groups, including children and older people (2). They gave specific consideration to older people in a policy paper published in 2004 (3). In geriatrics and gerontology, end of life issues have received little attention due to the dominance of discourses promoting health and productive ageing up to the late 1990s (4, 5). However, changing demographics, for example the emergence of the 'oldest old' age cohort, as well as new approaches to dementia care, have led to raised awareness of end of life issues in these disciplines in recent years (6, 7). Shared concerns and shared challenges have been highlighted, yet research that systematically connects knowledge and evidence of palliative care and old age care is just in its infancy (8). In order to improve end of life care for older people a policy of promoting collaboration in research and practice between palliative care specialists, geriatricians and further academic disciplines will be vital.

User involvement in end of life care for older people

User involvement has become a rather unchallenged norm in health and social care in recent years. The importance of valuing individual experience at all levels of service delivery and research is beyond question; however, getting this right is a complex endeavour. This is even more the case in the field of end of life care for older people: who are the 'users' within this context, what are the issues they should be involved in, and how can effective involvement be achieved (9)? Small and Sargaent provide us with essential conceptual work to reflect upon the concept of user involvement and define its potential, challenges, and limits in this area in their contribution for this book (see Chapter 8, this volume).

Finding ways to involve older people and their families in end of life care issues is, obviously, an interdisciplinary initiative which combines social work and palliative care as well as drawing upon discourses of participation in gerontology (10–12). Approaches such as peer education groups to implement advance care planning, or community development which aims to build capacity in all nature of end of life matters at a local level, are promising in this regard (13, 14).

All models make clear, however, that user involvement is usually time consuming and costly (11), which is why effective user involvement requires increased resources in research and practice.

Old age care as gendered territory

There is striking evidence of gender differences at the end of life: to begin with, there is a lower chance that women will die at home when compared with men in all ages (15). Due to their higher life expectancy, women are more often affected by diseases of old age, such as dementia. Both factors contribute to the development of care homes as 'female' places over the last years. Finally, it is women who predominantly take on caring roles, be they formal or informal (16). Therefore, those dealing with end of life care for older people inevitably enter gendered territory and should thoroughly consider gender issues at all levels of action.

Research itself also needs to consider the influence of gender at all stages of the research process and consideration of issues for older people at the end of life should be better integrated within the renowned body of gender theory. If research neglects the issue of gender the existing discrimination of women is likely to be perpetuated (17).

Integrated care and organizational issues

A considerable number of older people—and this number will be growing in coming decades—are spending their last days of life in an institution like a hospital or care home (18). Therefore, a research agenda towards improving end of life care has to consider models of introducing good end of life care to these institutions. Developing skills and training individual staff is important, although organizational development also plays a vital role in this respect (19, 20).

Transitions in place at the end of life are often problematic for dying people; hence a policy of 'ageing in place' should incorporate the aim of 'dying in place'. In order to achieve that, services of care need to be arranged and organized differently. In this respect, research on integrated health and social care for older persons is highly relevant, though it mostly leaves out the challenges of dying (21). Strengthening the tradition of research on integrated models of care by a focus on end of life is an important goal here and, overall, research in end of life care has to move beyond the individual and strengthen its focus on organizations and communities.

Decision-making in end of life care

Due to the rapid developments in medicine and technology and the broad range of interventions in critical care, the death of a person is nowadays connected to another person's decision to either hasten or postpone death. Especially in old age, where recognizing dying is typically no simple undertaking, ethical decision-making is at the forefront of good end of life care (22, 23).

Nevertheless, decision-making in end of life care is a far from easy process with a range of perspectives to be considered, including the legal, ethical, and clinical, as well as those of patients and their families. In light of this, a number of more or less complex instruments and procedures have been developed to help facilitate decision-making, such as living wills, advance directives, and advance care planning. How these meet the needs of older people, their influences on the relationships of carers and patients, and other ways of attaining 'good decisions' is yet to be explored.[1]

Research methodology and ethics

Older women and men who usually have complex needs when approaching the end of life should be at the core of any agenda on developing end of life care for older people. The employment of qualitative methods—commonly involving interviews and focus groups or, less commonly, observation—is a central means of accessing older people's perspectives about end of life care issues. Although approaches like these are usually considered more sensitive than others they still raise a number of methodological as well as ethical questions which have to be better reflected and discussed in light of end of life issues for older people (24).

While useful in reminding researchers of the particular sensitivity needed to protect participants from harm, the concept of vulnerability might support ageism through systematically excluding older people from end of life research in general (25). Instead, research itself should incorporate ethical sensitivity in all phases of the process. Much has already been done in reflecting upon research in the field of palliative care and there is now a need to link the discipline more closely with feminist research and transdisciplinary research, as well as geriatrics and gerontology (26–28).

Conclusion

In short, in order to face the challenge of improving end of life care for older people it will be vital to bring together expertise from various disciplines and fields in research as well as in practice. This refers first and foremost to palliative care and old age care—gerontology and geriatrics—but has to go beyond this as well. All of the issues outlined above obviously cut across disciplinary boundaries which imply that research has to include various perspectives at all levels. This might be realized through interdisciplinary approaches and might even enter transdisciplinary ground. How this kind of research can be established, organized, and financed should therefore be of major concern internationally when considering methods to improve end of life care for older women and men.

References

1. WHO (1990). *Cancer pain relief and palliative care*. Report of a WHO Expert Committee. Geneva: World Health Organization.
2. WHO (2002). *National Cancer Control Programmes. Policies and managerial Guidelines*. Geneva: World Health Organization.
3. Davies E, Higginson I (2004). *Better Palliative Care for Older People?* Copenhagen: WHO Regional Office for Europe.

---

[1] Indeed there is substantial research on these issues in the USA, although it has to be considered that different legal frameworks might impede the interpretation of results (29, 30).

4. Heller A, Pleschberger S (2008). Palliative Versorgung im Alter. In A Kuhlmey, D Schaeffer (eds) *Alter, Gesundheit und Krankheit,* pp. 382–400. Bern: Verlag Hans Huber.

5. Butler RN (1985). Health, productivity and ageing: an overview. In RN Butler, HP Gleason (eds) *Productive Ageing,* pp. 114–25. New York: Springer.

6. Small N, Froggatt K, Downs M (2007). *Living and Dying with Dementia. Dialogues about Palliative Care.* Oxford: Oxford University Press.

7. Kojer M, Heimerl K (2009). Palliative Care ist ein Zugang für hochbetagte Menschen—ein erweiterter Blick auf die WHO—Definition von Palliative care. *Zeitschrift für Palliativmedizin,* **10**: 154–61.

8. Seymour JE, Clark D, Philp I (2001). Palliative care and geriatric medicine: shared concerns, shared challenges. *Palliative Medicine,* **15**: 269–70.

9. Stevens T (2008). Involving or using? User involvement in palliative care. In S Payne, J Seymour, C Ingleton (eds) *Palliative Care Nursing. Principles and Evidence for Practice,* pp. 55–70. Maidenhead: Open University Press.

10. Beresford P, Ashead L, Croft S (2007). *Palliative Care, Social Work and Service Users. Making Life Possible.* London: Jessica Kingsley Publishers.

11. Walker A (1993). Towards a European agenda in home care for older people: convergencies and controversies. In A Evers, GH van der Zanden (eds) *Better Care for Dependent People Living at Home,* pp. 301–33. Bunnik: LSOB.

12. Small N (2005). User voices in palliative care. In C Faull, Y Carter, L Daniels (eds) *Handbook of Palliative Care,* pp. 61–74. Oxford: Blackwell.

13. Sanders C, Seymour JE, Clarke A, Gott M, Welton M (2006). Development of a peer education programme for advance end-of-life care planning: an action research project with older adults. *International Journal of Palliative Nursing,* **12**(5): 216–23.

14. Kellehear A (2005). *Compassionate Cities: Public Health and End-Of-Life Care.* London: Routledge.

15. Gomes B, Higginson IJ (2006). Factors influencing death at home in terminally ill patients with cancer: systematic review. *British Medical Journal (Clinical research ed.),* **332**(7540): 515–21

16. Payne S, Hudson P, Grande G, Oliviere D, Tishelman C, Pleschberger S, et al. (2010). White Paper on improving support for family carers in palliative care: part 1. *European Journal of Palliative Care,* **17**(5): 238–45.

17. Backes G, Lasch V, Reimann K (eds) (2006). *Gender, Health and Ageing. European perspectives on Life Course, Health Issues and Social Challenges.* Heidelberg: VS Verlag für Sozialwissenschaften.

18. Froggatt K, Payne S (2006). A survey of end-of-life care in care homes: issues of definition and practice. *Health and Social Care in the Community,* **14**(4): 341–8.

19. Abbey J, Froggatt K, Parker D, Abbey B (2006). Palliative care in long-term care: a system in change. *International Journal of Older People Nursing,* **1**: 56–63.

20. Heller A, Dinges S, Heimerl K, Reitinger E, Wegleitner K (2003). Palliative Kultur in der stationären Altenhilfe. *Zeitschrift für Gerontologie und Geriatrie,* **36**: 360–5.

21. Leichsenring K, Alaszewski AM (eds) (2004). *Providing Integrated Health and Social Care for Older Persons. A European Overview of Issues at Stake. Public Policy and Social Welfare, Vol. 28.* Aldershot: Ashgate.

22. Hockley J, Froggatt K (2006). The development of palliative care knowledge in care homes for older people: the place of action research. *Palliative Medicine,* **20**(8): 835–43.

23. Pleschberger S, Wenzel, C, Hornek, A (2009). The process of recognising dying–Anything but a simple diagnosis. *European Journal of Palliative Care,* 11th Congress of the European Association of Palliative Care, Vienna, 7–10 May 2009, Abstracts: 93.

24. Seymour JE, Payne S, Reid D, Sargeant A, Skilbeck J, Smith P (2005). Ethical and methodological issues in palliative care studies: the experiences of a research group. *Journal of Research in Nursing,* **10**(2): 169–88.

25. Addington-Hall J (2007). Introduction. In J Addington-Hall, E Bruera, J Higginson, S Payne (eds) *Research Methods in Palliative Care*, pp. 1–8. Oxford: Oxford University Press.

26. Grande G, Ingleton C (2008). Research in palliative care. In S Payne, J Seymour, C Ingleton (eds) *Palliative Care Nursing. Principles and Evidence for Practice*, pp. 625–42. Maidenhead and New York: Open University Press.

27. Nowotny H, Scott P, Gibbons M. (2001). *Re-Thinking Science—Knowledge and the Public in an Age of Uncertainty*. Cambridge: Polity Press.

28. Reitinger E (2009). *Transdisziplinäre Praxis*. Forschen im Sozial- und Gesundheitswesen. Heidelberg: Carl Auer Verlag.

29. Quill TE, McCann R (2003). Decision making for the cognitively impaired. In SR Morrison, DE Meier (eds) *Geriatric Palliative Care*, pp. 332–41. New York: Oxfords University Press.

30. Sampson EL, Richie CW, Lai R, Raven PW, Blanchard MR (2005). A systematic review of the scientific evidence for the efficacy of a palliative care approach in advanced dementia. *International Psychogeriatrics*, **17**(1): 31–40.

Chapter 26

Workforce capacity issues: a New Zealand perspective

Jackie Robinson and Christine Ingleton

In common with other developed countries, the New Zealand health policy framework envisages an innovative, creative, and sustainable workforce that can meet the increasingly complex needs of service users and achieve optimal standards in quality of life based on integrated teamwork (1). These laudable aspirations are taking place against a backdrop of challenges, which include: changes in population demographics; changes to workforce composition with problems recruiting and retaining heath care workers; and difficulties delivering appropriate, cost-effective, and flexible education and training to ensure health professionals are equipped with the skills to provide high-quality care. All these challenges have implications for those involved in the commissioning, planning, and delivery of palliative care for older people. These are discussed in turn in the rest of this chapter.

Changes in population demographics

Demographic change asserts a major influence on the demand for health care services. An ageing population will result in an increasing need for palliative care in the coming years. Statistics New Zealand has predicted that from 2001 to 2021 the population aged over 65 years will increase from 461,000 to 792,000. Moreover, in this period it has been forecast that those aged over 85 years will increase from 48,639 to 105,400 (2). It has been predicted that by 2021 the proportion of non-European people aged over 65 years will increase by 242%. According to the 2006 census the four largest ethnic groups are New Zealand European (67.6%), Maori (14.6%), Asian (9.2%), and Pacific people (6.9%). Maori and Pacific people are affected more by chronic health conditions such as diabetes, cardiac disease, and cancer. The proportion of older people from these ethnic groups is increasing (3). This is a group that will require care at the end of life which reflects the uniqueness of their culture, value, and beliefs. This may not easily be delivered in the dominant 'Western' health care environment of New Zealand. More discussion is needed on understanding the needs of older Maori people whose experiences are structured not only through membership of an indigenous cultural group, but profoundly by the legacy of colonialism.

Workforce composition

In New Zealand, there is a lack of robust data regarding the composition of the health care workforce. Before 2005 there were no routine national workforce data collection systems in place. In 2001 it was estimated that there were 107,000 people working in the health and disability sector in New Zealand (1). This includes registered health practitioners, support workers (including administration staff), and complimentary health workers. Nursing makes up a large proportion of this workforce, at 40% of the registered workforce, of which 90% are female. The Medical Council has indicated that nearly 11,000 doctors currently hold current practicing certificates and over 40% of the medical workforce are women. The fact that woman make up a great majority of the health care workforce will therefore require employers to be flexible about work hours to accommodate care giving and family commitments. Moreover, the average age of health care workers in New Zealand is increasing, with the average age for doctors and nurses being 45 years (4). The impact of this has been highlighted by the Ministry of Health who have predicted that if health and disability services were to retain their current share of the working age population, demand for labour will outstrip supply by 2011 (1). Considering that this scenario is predicted to evolve into a severe global shortage, understanding the factors that influence job satisfaction should be viewed as a pressing priority.

Worryingly, we know less about the composition of the 'unregistered workforce' as information is not routinely collected. However, it is estimated to be as many as 50,000 people, almost half the total health and disability workforce in New Zealand. It is unclear how many are involved in direct patient care although it is known that most are working in the residential care setting, caring for the most vulnerable and frail. This workforce is mainly made up of woman who are relatively low paid and work part-time, often with no guaranteed hours (1).

Delivering education and training

Key to appropriate palliative care management is ensuring an adequately trained workforce. Within New Zealand, the need to improve 'generalist' palliative care management is well recognized (5). Generalist palliative care providers are those who provide palliative care as an integral part of standard clinical practice (6). They include the majority of the 100,000 people working in the health and disability sector. These providers work across multiple clinical settings including hospital, community, and residential care settings. By contrast, specialist palliative care providers are those who have undergone specific training in palliative care. They work in hospice services and hospital palliative care teams and their role is direct care of those patients with complex palliative care needs and provision of education and support to the generalist provider (6).

We know from a recent gap analysis of specialist palliative care providers in New Zealand that there are only approximately 380 full-time equivalents working in specialist palliative care services (7). It is this relatively small group of people that are charged with the responsibility for educating and supporting the 100,000 people providing generalist palliative care at a time when health budgets are under even more pressure to deliver more for less. Furthermore, palliative care is going to be challenged by the management of highly complex health and social care needs. Formerly acute diseases become chronic diseases in old age. This is likely to be combined with people experiencing greater numbers of comorbidities, especially older people. This will mean that a different type of workforce will be required in specialist palliative care. For example, demands for specialist professionals to become advisors, educators, and consultants (on pain and symptom control) to generalists who actually deliver care in their usual health care environments will make workforce planning and delivery of education and training complex and challenging. Ensuring a workforce is equipped with the skills and knowledge to deliver palliative care requires a coordinated approach to workforce development acknowledging that each group has unique learning needs relative to the population of patients they care for.

Future priorities

The changing demographics are daunting when considering future workforce planning and provision of education and training. The evolving model of palliative care has moved away from primarily end of life care for those with cancer when all options for further treatment have been exhausted, to a more inclusive model of care delivery available to those who need it regardless of diagnosis or care setting. This care is delivered by all clinicians regardless of discipline or specialty and is expected to run concurrently alongside life-prolonging treatment. This broadening of service delivery has placed a significant demand on the palliative care workforce and its traditional model of care delivery. As such, developing capability, strengthening capacity, and facilitating collaboration between health professionals and service providers is a priority to ensure we meet the increasing demands for high-quality palliative care in a climate where increasing funding is unlikely, certainly in the short term.

Those working in specialist palliative care services in New Zealand now have an opportunity to challenge 'the norm' and identify opportunities to develop new and innovative ways of working, particularly in advanced nursing practice roles such as the nurse specialist and the nurse practitioner. Nurses in these roles have the potential to influence service development and contribute to national policy in palliative care whilst remaining immersed in the clinical environment. To ensure these roles are used to their full potential, organizational change is required to support these nurses to contribute fully to the development of an integrated palliative care model across the continuum of care.

Reaching out to the 'unregistered workforce' who are a significant group in terms of size and who work predominantly in the residential care setting is a particular priority. This care setting has been notoriously difficult to influence in terms of general residential care improvements. A number of factors may contribute to this difficulty including: the largely independent and fragmentary nature of residential care provision, the slow development of networks for providers, and the high turnover of staff that these particular organizations are often faced with (8). In addition, working in residential aged care settings has not traditionally been seen as particularly high status among health professionals and other workers, and this has also impacted on the continuity of any training initiatives which have been attempted (9).

Conclusions

There are key challenges facing the health workforce in New Zealand in ensuring appropriate palliative care provision for an ageing population. In order to address these it is important that palliative care is increasingly articulated as a core skill of all health care professionals and that specialist palliative care providers are trained and funded to teach and support these frontline providers of care for those with chronic life-limiting conditions. This moves palliative care provision (whether generalist or specialist) back into the mainstream and requires a focus particularly on advanced nursing practice roles to bridge old and new models, cancer and non-malignant provision, acute and chronic care, care for the young and old, and provision for indigenous people and those from varying ethnic backgrounds. In this way the vision of appropriate palliative care available for all who require it, regardless of age, ethnicity, diagnosis, or care setting may be realized.

References

1. Ministry of Health (2006). *Health Workforce Development: An Overview*. Wellington: Ministry of Health.
2. New Zealand Institute of Economic Research (2004). *Ageing New Zealand and Health and Disability Services: Demand Projections and Workforce Implications, 2001–2021*. Discussion document. Wellington: Ministry of Health.
3. Public Health Intelligence Group (2003). *Decades of Disparity. Ethnic Mortality Trends in New Zealand 1980–1999 (2003)*. Public Health Intelligence Occasional Bulletin No. 16. Wellington: Ministry of Health.
4. Health Workforce Advisory Committee (2003). *The NZ Health Workforce: A stocktake of issues and capacity 2001*. Wellington: Health Workforce Advisory Committee.

5. Ministry of Health (2001). *The NZ Palliative Care Strategy*. Wellington: Ministry of Health.

6. Ministry of Health (2007). New Zealand Palliative Care: A working definition. Wellington: Palliative Care Sub-committee, NZ Cancer Treatment Working Party.

7. Ministry of Health (2009). *Gap Analysis of Specialist Palliative Care in New Zealand*. Wellington: Ministry of Health.

8. Ingleton C, Froggatt K (2009). Commentary on Hewison A, Badger F, Clifford C and Thomas K. Delivering 'Gold Standards' in end of life care in care homes: a question of teamwork? *Journal of Clinical Nursing*, **18**: 1812–15.

9. Nolan M, Davies S, Brown J, Wilkinson A, Warnes T, McKee K, et al. (2008). The role of education and training in achieving change in care homes: a literature review. *Journal of Research in Nursing*, **13**: 411–33.

Conclusion

Merryn Gott and Christine Ingleton

The intention of this book was to open up the issue of ageing and end of life care to critical reflection and debate. Experts from a range of disciplines have identified a need to know more—more about the current end of life experiences of older people and their families, more about what currently works well (and what doesn't), and more theoretical understanding to ensure action is informed by critical thinking and reasoned debate. This book must therefore be seen only as the first step in a lengthy process, not as an end in itself.

What we have been reminded of is the sheer scale of the challenge. The proportion of older people globally will double by 2050; there will be particular growth in the numbers of those aged over 85. The demographics, in themselves, are therefore daunting when considering future palliative care provision. However, in addition, authors have highlighted that current provision needs rethinking; a disjuncture has been identified between the priorities of decision-makers and those of older people themselves. To further complicate the situation, the nature of the palliative care population is changing, both in terms of the diseases people will be dying from and the settings in which they will be living during the last years of their lives. At the same time, there will be fewer younger family members available to provide care and this responsibility will increasingly fall to older carers. An increasing proportion of older people are also likely to live alone.

There will be other difficult questions to consider. How to deploy health technologies to improve quality, rather than just quantity, of life? How to tackle the insidious ageism that has the potential to taint older people's end of life experiences and decision-making? How to improve care in all settings and ensure that dying in a 'home-like' environment, if that is what is desired, can be achieved in institutions? How to ensure better support and educate family carers to provide the care they may want, or may have no option but to provide? How to ensure all 'professionals' working with older people perceive palliative care as a fundamental component of their role and not an add-on, to be done if there's time and if there are no 'specialists' on hand? And all this at a time when health budgets globally are under ever more pressure to deliver more for less.

Some would frame this as a catastrophe in waiting. However, in a discussion of 'health promoting palliative care', Kellehear, Rumbold (and others) appear to offer hope. The potential to reframe the negatives into positives—to recognize the potential of communities to provide care, and acknowledging the key role that older people can play in this regard. 'Involvement' must certainly be prioritized, whether that's in terms of enabling individual older people to make decisions about their care if they so choose, initiating debates with the wider public about appropriate palliative care provision, or providing communities with the resources, and potentially affording them some responsibility, to care for older people at the end of life. For health professionals, the message must be an increased emphasis on palliative care as 'core business'; this is not just about 'being educated' by specialists, but being encouraged to see palliative care as relevant to anyone working with older people.

The need for theoretical, as well as practical, developments in this area has also been high-lighted. Whilst service planning may be seen as an atheoretical activity, in reality, what is done (and not done) to whom, is obviously informed by a set of ideas, and ideals, rooted in a particular sociocultural and historical context. It is also a profoundly political activity and it is important to recognize that older people, as a group, typically have little political leverage. It has been hypothesized that this may change, that future cohorts of older people may improve the nature of palliative and end of life care provision themselves, through individual and collective action. However, critical gerontologists remind us that 'old age' is unlikely to ever be an attractive identity, particularly given the continued growth of anti-ageing medicine and ever increasing availability of, and pressure to use, age-resisting technologies.

If there is one message that unifies the discussions throughout this book, it is the need for greater integration. Integration between gerontology and palliative care, integration between services for older people and those who are dying, integration between family carers and 'profes-sionals', integration between 'decision-makers' and communities, integration between theory and practice, and integration between 'specialist' and 'generalist' palliative care providers. The need to improve palliative and end of life care for older people is a global priority. In order that good intentions translate into action, debate and discussion between as many different interested parties will be critical. Within this context, we are all interested parties.

Index